Neuroradiology Imaging

CASE REVIEW SERIES

Series Editor

David M. Yousem, MD, MBA

Associate Dean for Professional Development

Johns Hopkins School of Medicine

Director of Neuroradiology, Vice Chairman of Program Development

Johns Hopkins Medical Institution

Baltimore, Maryland

Other Volumes in the CASE REVIEW Series

Brain Imaging

Breast Imaging

Cardiac Imaging

Duke Review of MRI Principles

Emergency Radiology

Gastrointestinal Imaging

General and Vascular Ultrasound

Genitourinary Imaging

Head and Neck Imaging

Musculoskeletal Imaging

Nuclear Medicine

Obstetric and Gynecologic Ultrasound

Pediatric Imaging

Spine Imaging

Thoracic Imaging

Neuroradiology Imaging

CASE REVIEW SERIES

Salvatore V. Labruzzo, DO

Major, US Army Medical Corps
Staff Neuroradiologist, MRI Section Chief
William Beaumont Army Medical Center
El Paso, Texas;
Russell H. Morgan Department of Radiology and
Radiological Science
Neuroradiology Division
Johns Hopkins Medical Institution
Baltimore, Maryland

Laurie A. Loevner, MD

Professor of Radiology, Otorhinolaryngology: Head
and Neck Surgery, and Neurosurgery
Department of Radiology
University of Pennsylvania Medical Center
Hospital of the University of Pennsylvania
Philadelphia, Pennsylvania

Efrat Saraf-Lavi, MD

Associate Professor of Radiology
Neuroradiology Section
Medical Director of Applebaum MRI Center
University of Miami, Miller School of Medicine
Miami, Florida

David M. Yousem, MD, MBA

Associate Dean for Professional Development
Johns Hopkins School of Medicine
Director of Neuroradiology, Vice Chairman of
Program Development
Johns Hopkins Medical Institution
Baltimore, Maryland

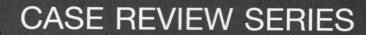

ELSEVIER

ELSEVIER

1600 John F. Kennedy Blvd.
Ste 1800
Philadelphia, PA 19103-2899

NEURORADIOLOGY IMAGING: CASE REVIEW SERIES   ISBN: 978-0-323-41726-6

Library of Congress Cataloging-in-Publication Data

Names: Labruzzo, Salvatore V., author. | Loevner, Laurie A., author. | Saraf-Lavi, Efrat, author. | Yousem, David M., author. | Absorption in part of (expression): Yousem, David M. Head and neck imaging. Fourth edition. | Absorption in part of (expression): Loevner, Laurie A. Brain imaging. 2nd ed. | Absorption in part of (expression): Saraf-Lavi, Efrat. Spine imaging. Third edition.
Title: Neuroradiology imaging / Salvatore V. Labruzzo, Laurie A. Loevner, Efrat Saraf-Lavi, David M. Yousem.
Other titles: Case review series.
Description: Philadelphia, PA : Elsevier, [2017] | Series: Case review series | "Content for this title came from Head and Neck Imaging, 4e, Brain Imaging, 2e, and Spine Imaging, 3e." | Includes bibliographical references and index.
Identifiers: LCCN 2016013341 | ISBN 9780323417266 (pbk. : alk. paper)
Subjects: | MESH: Nervous System Diseases–diagnosis | Head–radiography | Neck–radiography | Brain–radiography | Spinal Diseases–radiography | Neuroradiography | Examination Questions | Case Reports
Classification: LCC RC386.6.R3 | NLM WL 18.2 | DDC 616.8/047572–dc23 LC record available at http://lccn.loc.gov/2016013341

Executive Content Strategist: Robin Carter
Content Development Specialist: Jillian Crull
Publishing Services Manager: Catherine Jackson
Project Manager: Rhoda Howell
Design Direction: Amy Buxton

Printed in China

Last digit is the print number: 9   8   7   6   5   4   3   2   1

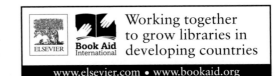

To my sons, Mason and Gavin. Have strong minds and strong hearts. Share both with each other always. I love you.

Dad

I have been very gratified by the popularity and positive feedback that the authors of the Case Review series have received on the publication of the editions of their volumes. Reviews in journals and online sites as well as word-of-mouth comments have been uniformly favorable. The authors have done an outstanding job in filling the niche of an affordable, easy-to-access, case-based learning tool that supplements the material in *The Requisites* series. I have been told by residents, fellows, and practicing radiologists that the Case Review series books are the ideal means for studying for oral board examinations and subspecialty certification tests.

Although some students learn best in a noninteractive study book mode, others need the anxiety or excitement of being quizzed. The selected format for the Case Review series (which consists of showing a few images needed to construct a differential diagnosis and then asking a few clinical and imaging questions) was designed to simulate the board examination experience. The only difference is that the Case Review books provide the correct answer and immediate feedback. The limit and range of the reader's knowledge are tested through scaled cases ranging from relatively easy to very hard. The Case Review series also offers feedback on the answers, a brief discussion of each case, a link back to the pertinent *The Requisites* volume, and up-to-date references from the literature.

We are ready for the new boards! The Case Reviews are now available in an e-book format on ExpertConsult.com that allows for greater portability and functionality via electronic access. Personally, I am very excited about the future. Join us.

David M. Yousem, MD, MBA

What a brilliant idea! Sal Labruzzo has taken the best of the Brain, Spine, and Head and Neck editions and created a one-stop shop Neuroradiology edition that allows a general overview of the field in a case-based format. The cases have been placed into one voice, that of Dr. Labruzzo, and they have been hand-picked for demonstrating the pathology the best. For nearly one fourth of the cases, Dr. Labruzzo has created physics questions and follow-up questions that are ideal for a preparation for the general radiology and neuroradiology subspecialty board examinations. Brilliant, I say!

Take Dr. Labruzzo's great idea and combine it with the expertise of the original authors from the University of Pennsylvania (Laurie Loevner), the University of Miami (Efrat Saraf-Lavi), and Johns Hopkins University (me, myself, and Irene?) and you have an excellent addition to the Case Review series. All of the authors endorsed the idea of taking the best of the best and making it better, and Dr. Labruzzo has achieved that. For those who want more in-depth knowledge, the individual Brain, Spine, and Head and Neck editions are still available and will provide even greater challenges … and expertise.

Thank you to all my coauthors for combining to make this outstanding work.

David M. Yousem, MD, MBA

I am honored that Dr. David Yousem invited me to write this first edition of *Neuroradiology Imaging: Case Review Series*. I wrote this book with the generous help of Jillian Crull, Content Development Specialist, and support of Robin Carter, Executive Content Strategist, at Elsevier.

Before writing this edition, I examined the newest of Dr. Laurie A. Loevner's *Brain Imaging*, Dr. David M. Yousem's *Head and Neck Imaging*, and Dr. Efrat Saraf-Lavi's *Spine Imaging: Case Review Series*. Each of these talented authors' prior efforts laid the foundation for this book and from these books I cherry-picked the best and most relevant cases to neuroradiology practice. As some disease processes manifest differently in the various areas covered in these sources, I also combined cases and therefore eliminated redundancies. This brings all of neuroradiology review into one go-to source.

In keeping with the format of the diagnostic radiology CORE exam, maintenance of certification examinations (MOC), and neuroradiology subspecialty examination (CAQ), questions are proposed in single-best-answer multiple-choice format. Additionally, new questions regarding physics and patient management have been added.

The images provided for each case have been updated from prior editions of the Case Review series, and selected images are reprinted on the answer and discussion pages with more thorough explanations. By minimizing your need to flip back and forth to the question page, this book allows for more efficient studying.

The discussion section for each case has been segmented for easier review and much of the text has been updated to include the most contemporary classification systems and nomenclature related to anatomy and disease.

The cases and images in this book were submitted from the authors' institutions, and the modalities include standard CT and MRI, MR and CT angiography, MR spectroscopy, PWI, DWI, and SWI. Select images from digital subtraction angiography and select relevant radiographs are also included in some cases. The cases are also cross referenced to the fourth edition of *Neuroradiology: The Requisites* by Drs. David Yousem and Rohini Nadgir, which provides an easy resource for those of you who are lucky enough to have that excellent text.

Authoring and editing this book has been a pleasurable experience. I have a desire to teach and this book allows me to reach those of you who have a desire to learn. I hope that you enjoy and learn as much from reading this book as I did co-authoring it.

I thank my wife, Sally, for her patience and unwavering support in my career and during this recent endeavor. I thank the Neuroradiology Division at Johns Hopkins Medical Institutions, especially Dr. David Yousem for his mentorship and support.

Sincerely,
Salvatore V. Labruzzo, DO

CONTENTS

Opening Round

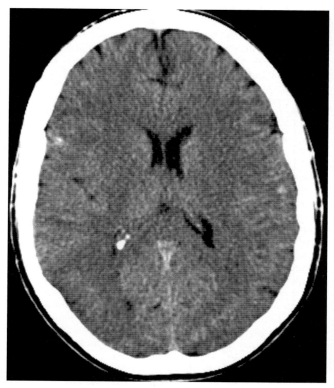

Figure 1-1 Patient A.

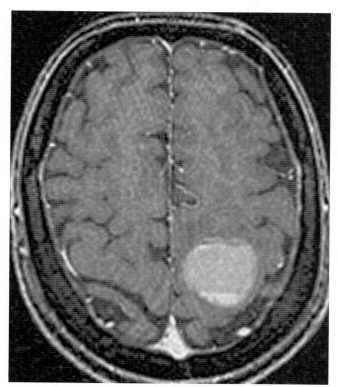

Figure 1-2 Patient B.

HISTORY: Withheld.

1. What is the most likely single diagnosis for both of these cases?
   A. Acute arterial infarcts
   B. Venous infarcts
   C. Hemorrhagic metastasis
   D. Hereditary hemorrhagic telangiectasia

2. A lesion with high attenuation on computed tomography (CT) and T2 signal hypointensity on magnetic resonance imaging (MRI) is *least* likely which of the following?
   A. Acute hemorrhage
   B. A hypercellular tumor
   C. A proteinaceous lesion
   D. Calcified
   E. Acute infarct

3. How often is metastatic disease to the brain a solitary metastasis?
   A. Less than 25%
   B. 25% to 50%
   C. 51% to 75%
   D. More than 75%

4. What type of parenchymal metastases may be associated with little or no edema such that they are missed on T2-weighted imaging and are readily identified only on gadolinium-enhanced images?
   A. White matter
   B. Brainstem
   C. Cortical
   D. Dural

CASE 1

Hemorrhagic Metastases: Melanoma

1. **C.** Hemorrhagic metastasis. In Figure 1-1 there are multifocal hyperdense lesions because of hemorrhage. In Figure 1-2 there is a mass with fluid level. Acute arterial infarcts rarely bleed, venous infarct–related hematomas tend not to be as small as in Figure 1-1, and hereditary hemorrhagic telangiectasia (HHT) is much less common than hemorrhagic metastasis and rarely would result in a single large hemorrhage.

2. **E.** Acute infarct. These tend to have normal to low attenuation on CT and normal to hyperintense signal on T2-weighted MRI.

3. **B.** 25% to 50%.

4. **C.** Cortical. White matter and brainstem lesions tend to have more edema than cortical lesions. Dural lesions are by definition not parenchymal and do not typically cause parenchymal edema.

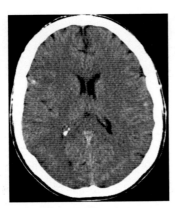

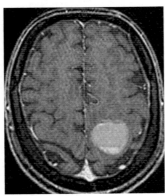

Comment

Metastatic disease is among the most common causes of intracranial masses in adults. Metastases are often multiple; however, in 30% to 50% of cases, they occur as an isolated lesion on imaging. Enhanced MRI is clearly more sensitive than CT in detecting cerebral metastases. Metastases are typically circumscribed masses that demonstrate variable enhancement patterns (solid, peripheral, or heterogeneous). Metastases are often associated with a disproportionate amount of surrounding edema, manifested on T2-weighted images as increased signal intensity in the adjacent white matter.

Metastases typically occur at the gray-white matter interface because tumor cells lodge in the small-caliber vessels in this location. Metastatic deposits can also involve the cortex. With cortical metastases in particular, edema may be absent such that metastatic lesions could be missed on T2-weighted imaging. Therefore, it is essential to give intravenous contrast to patients with suspected brain metastases. Studies examining the role of double- and triple-dose gadolinium have shown that although higher doses of contrast reveal more lesions than does a single dose, this often occurs in patients whose standard-dose study already shows more than one metastasis. Therefore, management in these patients is not affected, and multidose gadolinium is neither indicated nor recommended. In patients with no or a single metastasis on single-dose gadolinium, higher doses of contrast material yield additional metastases in less than 10% of cases.

Hypointensity (T2-weighted shortening) may be seen with blood products; as a result of the paramagnetic effects of melanin; and when lesions have calcification, hypercellularity, or proteinaceous material.

Vascular tumors, such as renal and thyroid carcinoma, and melanoma have a propensity to bleed, but because breast and lung carcinomas are much more common, a hemorrhagic metastasis is more likely to be related to one of these cancers. In the case of a single cerebral hemorrhagic mass, primary brain tumors, such as glioblastoma, should be considered.

Cases in Point

In both cases seen here, the patients have hemorrhagic metastatic melanoma. Patient A has multiple small metastases at the gray-white junction (Figure 1-1), and Patient B has a solitary large hemorrhagic metastasis with a fluid-hemorrhage level (Figure 1-2).

References

Anzalone N, Scotti R, Riva R. Neuroradiologic differential diagnosis of cerebral intraparenchymal hemorrhage. *Neurol Sci.* 2004;24:S3-S5.

Gaul HP, Wallace CJ, Crawley AP. Reverse enhancement of hemorrhagic brain lesions on postcontrast MR: detection with digital image subtraction. *AJNR Am J Neuroradiol.* 1996;17:1675-1680.

Cross-Reference

Neuroradiology: THE REQUISITES, 4th ed, pp 72-74.

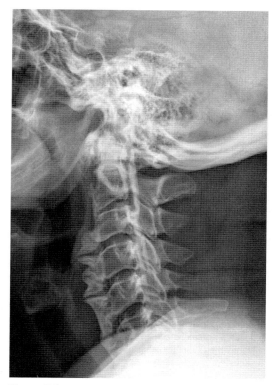

Figure 2-1

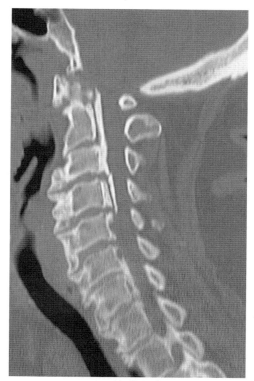

Figure 2-2

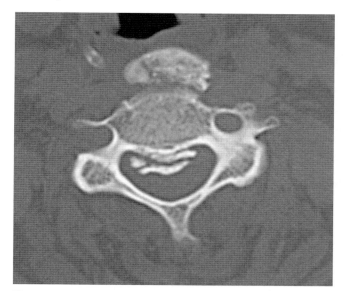

Figure 2-3

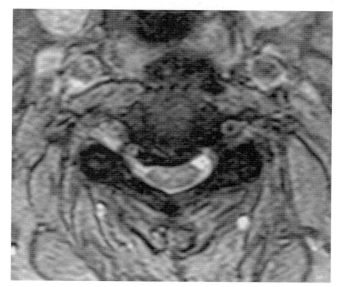

Figure 2-4

HISTORY: A 55-year-old man presents with myelopathy.

1. What is the single best diagnosis?
   A. Multilevel disc herniations
   B. Ossification of ligamentum flavum
   C. Ossification of the posterior longitudinal ligament
   D. Calcified meningioma

2. Which vertebral levels are most severely involved with this entity?
   A. C2-C4
   B. C4-C6
   C. C7-T2
   D. T3-T5

3. Which one of the four types of OPLL, according to the classification based on computed tomography (CT) appearance, may be difficult to differentiate from an osteophyte?
   A. Type I
   B. Type II
   C. Type III
   D. Type IV

4. What is the preferred and most effective treatment for this entity?
   A. Observation
   B. Canal expansive laminoplasty
   C. Anterior discectomy and fusion
   D. External beam radiotherapy

CASE 2

Ossification of Posterior Longitudinal Ligament

1. **C.** Ossification of the posterior longitudinal ligament (OPLL). This is the typical appearance for OPLL, not herniations, meningiomas, or ligamentum flavum ossification.

2. **B.** C4-C6. These are the most commonly involved levels.

3. **D.** Type IV. This is located posterior to the disc space. Type I is continuous, type II is segmental at the vertebral body level, and type III is mixed I and II.

4. **B.** Canal expansive laminoplasty. This is the preferred treatment. The other proposed answers are not acceptable treatment options.

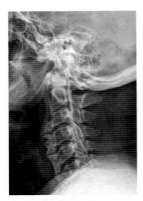

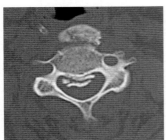

Comment

Demographics and Clinical Findings

OPLL generally produces severe central canal stenosis and significant myelopathy. Patients typically present in the sixth decade with upper and lower extremity weakness, dysesthesias, and neck pain.

Pathophysiology

OPLL begins with calcification and progresses to frank ossification, first in the upper cervical spine and later in the lower cervical and upper thoracic spine. OPLL can be associated with ligamentum flavum calcification or ossification and, when combined, these processes can result in circumferential compression of the cord. Association of OPLL with diffuse idiopathic skeletal hyperostosis, as seen in Figures 2-1 and 2-2, has also been reported.

Imaging

CT scan and plain films are probably preferable to magnetic resonance imaging (MRI) to identify subtle calcification or ossification. Four types of OPLL have been proposed on the basis of the CT appearance: (1) continuous, which extends confluently over several vertebral bodies (27% of cases); (2) segmental, which is one or several separate lesions behind the vertebral bodies (39%); (3) mixed continuous and segmental (29%) (see Figure 2-2); and (4) circumscribed, mainly located posterior to a disc space (5%). The shape of OPLL on axial images varies and may be mushroom-like, cubic, round, or tandem (Figure 2-3). MRI is valuable for identifying cord compression (Figure 2-4). The ossified ligament may have fatty marrow and increased signal on T1-weighted images and on T2-weighted fast spin echocardiographic images. An important finding on CT or MRI is that the calcification or ossification usually occurs along the length of the ligament and can be seen at the level of the pedicles; this helps differentiate OPLL from osteophytes and calcified herniated discs, which should be present at the level of the disc space only.

Management

Numerous studies have shown clinical benefits when multilevel disease is treated with a canal-expansive laminoplasty procedure. This procedure usually includes levels C3 through C7. There is little to no role for anterior discectomy. In cases of severe spinal cord impingement, myelopathy may be progressive and severely debilitating. Although some patients are observed, the effects of OPLL are not self-limiting.

References

Koyanagi I, Iwasaki Y, Hida K, et al. Magnetic resonance imaging findings in ossification of the posterior longitudinal ligament of the cervical spine. *J Neurosurg.* 1998;88(2):247-254.

Nagata K, Sato K. Diagnostic imaging of cervical ossification of the posterior longitudinal ligament. In: Yonenobu K, Nakamura K, Toyama Y, eds. *OPLL: Ossification of the Posterior Longitudinal Ligament.* Tokyo, Japan: Springer Japan; 2006.

Cross-Reference

Neuroradiology: THE REQUISITES, 4th ed, pp 545, 548-549.

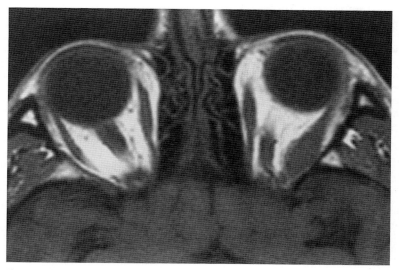

Figure 3-1

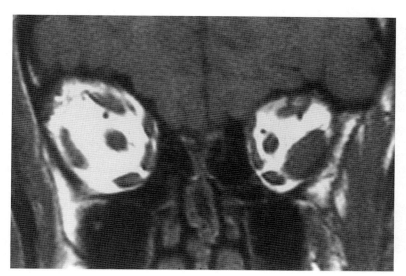

Figure 3-2

HISTORY: Pain.

1. Which of the following *should not* be considered in the differential diagnosis for extraocular muscle enlargement?
   A. Thyroid ophthalmopathy
   B. Orbital pseudotumor
   C. Meningioma
   D. Metastasis

2. What is the most common cause of nontraumatic proptosis?
   A. Orbital pseudotumor
   B. Metastasis
   C. Thyroid ophthalmopathy
   D. Lymphoma

3. Which symptom is not typical for orbital pseudotumor?
   A. Pain
   B. Decreased ocular motility
   C. Proptosis
   D. Disequilibrium

4. What structure runs between the superior rectus muscle and the optic nerve?
   A. Lacrimal artery
   B. Superior ophthalmic vein
   C. Central retinal artery
   D. Lacrimal nerve

CASE 3

Orbital Pseudotumor

1. **C.** Meningioma. Intraorbital meningiomas tend to occur along the optic nerve–sheath complex, not directly involving the extraocular muscles. Answer options A and B commonly result in enlargement of the extraocular muscles, and metastasis (answer option D) can occur anywhere in the orbit.

2. **C.** Thyroid ophthalmopathy is the most common cause of proptosis, excluding trauma.

3. **D.** Disequilibrium. The classic triad of orbital pseudotumor is pain, decreased ocular motility, and proptosis.

4. **B.** Superior ophthalmic vein. The lacrimal artery and nerve are in the superolateral orbit. The central retinal artery is in the optic nerve–sheath complex.

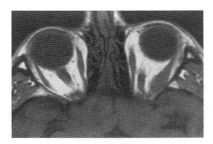

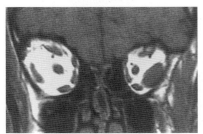

Comment

Presentation

Orbital pseudotumor, also known as idiopathic orbital inflammatory syndrome, is a nonspecific inflammation of unknown cause that involves the contents of the orbit. Clinical presentations include proptosis, pain, and decreased ocular motility. This disorder is usually unilateral (Figures 3-1 and 3-2) but is bilateral in less than 10% of patients.

Differential Diagnosis

Orbital pseudotumor should be considered a diagnosis of exclusion, with evaluation directed at eliminating other causes of orbital disease. Underlying systemic disorders should be considered, including sarcoid, lymphoma, connective tissue disease, Wegener granulomatosis, and autoimmune disorders.

Clinical and Imaging Features

In the early stages of orbital pseudotumor, histologic features are characterized by inflammation and edema, with an abundance of lymphocytes, plasma cells, and giant cells. In the late stages of disease, fibrosis may be abundant. Orbital pseudotumor has a spectrum of manifestations, including myositis (see Figures 3-1 and 3-2), dacryoadenitis (lacrimal gland involvement), periscleritis (uveal and scleral thickening), or retrobulbar soft tissue abnormality. In myositis, pseudotumor can involve one or more muscles, and unlike thyroid ophthalmopathy, it often involves the tendinous insertion of the muscle as well as the muscle bellies. When idiopathic inflammation primarily involves the cavernous sinus and the orbital apex, it is referred to as Tolosa-Hunt syndrome. Ophthalmoplegia is secondary to involvement of cranial nerves III through VI in the cavernous sinus.

Because orbital pseudotumor radiologically can appear similar to a variety of disease processes, the patient's history is important (pseudotumor is classically associated with pain and acute onset).

Treatment

Importantly, there is usually a dramatic response to steroids that may be useful in confirming the diagnosis of pseudotumor. A small percentage of patients do not respond to steroids and can require radiation or chemotherapy.

Reference

Jacobs D, Galetta S. Diagnosis and management of orbital pseudotumor. *Curr Opin Ophthalmol.* 2002;13:347-351.

Cross-Reference

Neuroradiology: THE REQUISITES, 4th ed, pp 335-336.

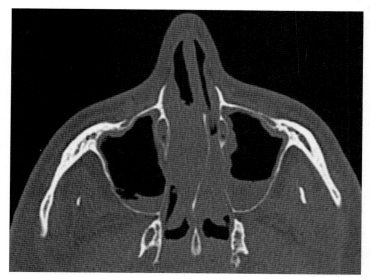

Figure 4-1

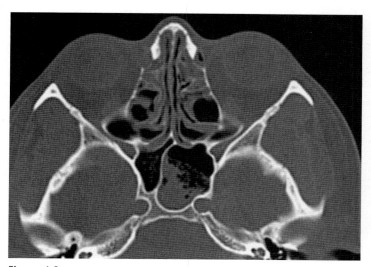

Figure 4-2

HISTORY: A young adult complains of nasal congestion and a runny nose.

1. Which of the following is the most likely diagnosis for the imaging findings presented?
   A. Sinonasal polyposis
   B. Mucocele
   C. Acute sinusitis
   D. Sinonasal adenocarcinoma

2. Which of the following is *true* about sinusitis?
   A. Acute sinusitis in a patient who is receiving a bone marrow transplant is associated with increased mortality.
   B. Acute sinusitis in a patient who is receiving a bone marrow transplant is associated with transplant rejection.
   C. Chronic sinusitis in a patient who is receiving a bone marrow transplant is associated with decreased mortality.
   D. Screening for sinusitis in a patient receiving a bone marrow transplant has little value.

3. The routes of paranasal sinus drainage include which of the following?
   A. Frontal sinuses to nasolacrimal duct
   B. Maxillary sinus to inferior meatus
   C. Posterior ethmoid to spheno-ethmoidal recess
   D. Anterior ethmoid to agger nasi

4. Which finding is *not* indicative of chronic sinusitis?
   A. Air-fluid levels
   B. Mucosal thickening
   C. Osteitis
   D. Polyps
   E. Mucous retention cysts

CASE 4

Acute Sinusitis

1. **C.** Acute sinusitis. The fluid levels are a common finding in acute sinusitis.

2. **A.** Acute sinusitis in a patient who is receiving a bone marrow transplant is associated with increased mortality. The other answer options are false.

3. **C.** Posterior ethmoid to spheno-ethmoidal recess. The frontal, anterior ethmoid, and maxillary sinuses drain into the middle meatus.

4. **A.** Air-fluid levels. This is not common to chronic sinusitis. The other answer options are common to chronic sinusitis.

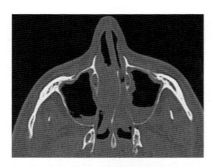

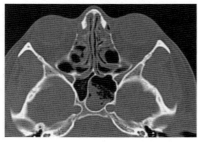

Comment

Imaging Findings

The imaging findings that imply acute sinusitis include new mucosal thickening, air-fluid levels (Figure 4-1), and air bubbles in sinus secretions (Figure 4-2) even in the absence of an air-fluid level. The misconception that mucosal edema/thickening occurs only in chronic sinusitis is rampant, but one of the authors, who underwent serial imaging of himself during the course of 14 days of antibiotics and intranasal steroid therapy, demonstrated that mucosal thickening appears and resolves over that period of time along with symptoms.

Sites of Obstruction

When reviewing cases of chronic and acute sinusitis, clinicians should note the potential obstructive sites that may be the underlying cause of the sinusitis. Radiologists should report on areas of mucosal thickening and narrowings of the maxillary sinus ostia, hiatus semilunaris, infundibulum, and middle meatus in cases of maxillary and ethmoid sinusitis. For frontal sinusitis, the frontal (ethmoidal) recess and middle meatus should be scrutinized. For posterior ethmoid and sphenoid sinusitis, the spheno-ethmoidal recess should be assessed for obstruction.

Pathogens

Viral and bacterial microorganisms are the usual culprits in an immunocompetent individual with acute sinusitis. Rhinoviruses, influenza virus, parainfluenza virus, and respiratory syncytial virus are the leading viral pathogens. *Streptococcus pneumoniae, Haemophilus influenzae, Moraxella catarrhalis, Streptococcus pyogenes,* and *Staphylococcus aureus* constitute the usual bacteria.

Reference

Wittkopf ML, Beddow PA, Russell PT, Duncavage JA, Becker SS. Revisiting the interpretation of positive sinus CT findings: a radiological and symptom-based review. *Otolaryngol Head Neck Surg.* 2009; 140(3):306-311.

Cross-Reference

Neuroradiology: THE REQUISITES, 4th ed, pp 417-424.

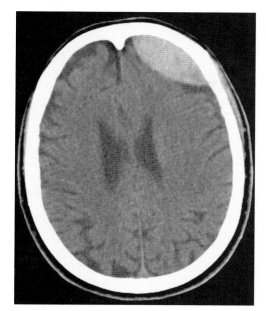

Figure 5-1

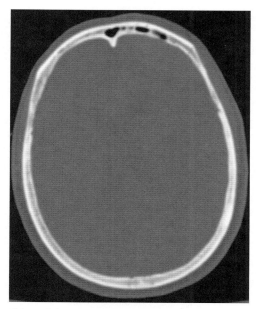

Figure 5-2

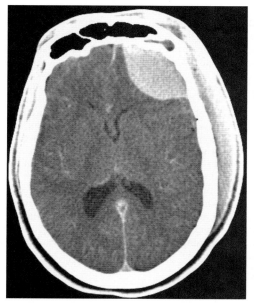

Figure 5-3

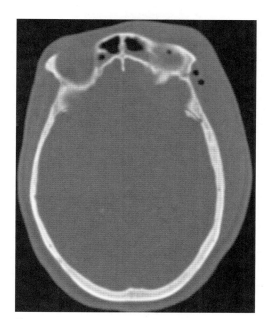

Figure 5-4

HISTORY: Fall.

1. What is the most common cause for this abnormality?
   A. Arteriovenous fistula
   B. Trauma
   C. Supratherapeutic anticoagulation
   D. Hemorrhagic tumor

2. What type of extra-axial hematoma is most usually associated with a skull fracture?
   A. Subarachnoid hematoma
   B. Subdural hematoma
   C. Epidural hematoma
   D. Subgaleal hematoma

3. This collection is located between which tissue layers?
   A. Pia and arachnoid
   B. Arachnoid and inner dural reflections
   C. Calvarium and outer periosteum
   D. Dura and inner calvarium

4. What is the most common source of an epidural hematoma?
   A. Venous sinus injury
   B. Middle meningeal artery injury
   C. Tears of the bridging veins
   D. Intracranial hypotension

CASE 5

Acute Epidural Hematoma and Associated Linear Fracture of the Frontal Bone

1. **B.** Trauma. Overall, the most common cause of any intracranial hemorrhage is trauma.

2. **C.** Epidural hematoma. This is because of laceration of meningeal arteries or veins.

3. **D.** Dura and inner calvarium. Answer options A, B, and C represent different potential spaces other than the epidural space.

4. **B.** Middle meningeal artery (MMA) injury. Although venous sinus injury may result in epidural hematoma, MMA injury is more common. Tears of bridging veins and intracranial hypotension result in subdural blood.

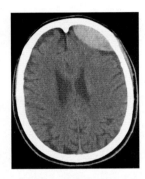

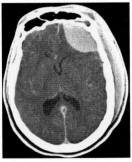

Comment

There are two anatomic types of confined extra-axial collections or hematomas, namely, subdural and epidural. On computed tomographic imaging, acute epidural hematomas are hyperdense extra-axial masses that can usually be distinguished from acute subdural hematomas based on their shape and location relative to the calvarial sutures. Epidural hematomas are usually confined by the cranial sutures because the dura is adherent to the periosteum of the inner calvarium. This results in the biconvex or lenticular shape (Figures 5-1 and 5-3) of these collections, which occur between the dura and the periosteum. In comparison, subdural hematomas cross sutural boundaries because they occur deep to the dura, occupying the space between the dura and pia arachnoid along the surface of the brain. As a result, subdural collections or hematomas tend to be crescentic, similar to a sliver of the moon.

In the vast majority of cases (80% to 90%), epidural hematomas are secondary to a direct laceration of the meningeal arteries (most commonly the middle meningeal artery) by an overlying skull fracture (Figures 5-2 and 5-4). In a small percentage of cases (<20%), epidural hematomas occur as a result of tearing of meningeal arteries in the absence of a fracture. This is most commonly seen in children and may be related to transient depression of the incompletely ossified soft calvarium, resulting in laceration of a meningeal artery. Most arterial epidural hematomas occur in the temporal region, although they may be seen in the frontal or temporoparietal regions.

Epidural hematomas caused by venous rather than arterial injury are much less common. Venous epidural hematomas are usually the result of tearing of a dural venous sinus related to an underlying calvarial fracture. They are most common in the posterior fossa as a result of injury to the transverse or sigmoid sinuses, and they are most often seen in the pediatric population. Unlike arterial epidural hematomas and subdural hematomas, venous epidural hematomas can extend across the tentorium cerebelli and involve both the supratentorial and infratentorial compartments. These can also occur in a paramedian location over the cerebral convexities or in the middle cranial fossa as the result of a tear in the superior sagittal or sphenoparietal sinus, respectively.

Other traumatic sequelae that occasionally are seen in the setting of epidural hematomas include pseudoaneurysms of the meningeal artery (most commonly the middle meningeal artery) and arteriovenous fistulas if a fracture lacerates both the middle meningeal artery and vein, resulting in their communication.

Reference

Hamilton M, Wallace C. Nonoperative management of acute epidural hematoma diagnosed by CT: the neuroradiologist's role. *AJNR Am J Neuroradiol.* 1993;13:853-859.

Cross-Reference

Neuroradiology: THE REQUISITES, 4th ed, pp 153-154.

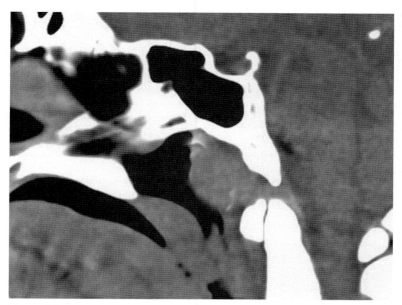

Figure 6-1

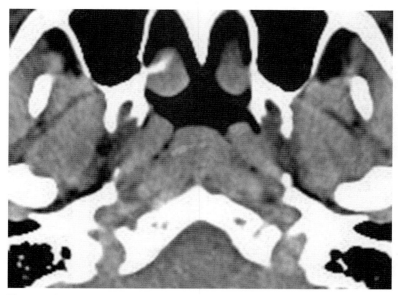

Figure 6-2

HISTORY: A 52-year-old woman presents with ear congestion.

1. What is the most common cause for this imaging finding?
   A. Upper respiratory tract infection
   B. Lymphoma
   C. Tornwaldt cyst
   D. Nasopharyngeal carcinoma

2. What type of lymphoma has a predilection for the nasopharynx?
   A. Hodgkin lymphoma
   B. Burkitt lymphoma
   C. Undifferentiated carcinoma
   D. Non-Hodgkin lymphoma

3. What is the best imaging finding that suggests lymphoid hyperplasia rather than tumor?
   A. High signal on T2-weighted image
   B. Striated enhancement pattern
   C. Crenated nodularity
   D. Cyst formation

4. What is the most common cause of obstructive sleep apnea in children?
   A. Tonsillar enlargement
   B. Uvular hypertrophy
   C. Adenoidal hypertrophy
   D. Lingual thyroid glands

CASE 6

Adenoidal Hypertrophy

1. **A.** Upper respiratory tract infection. This condition is the most common cause of adenoidal and other tonsillar hypertrophy.

2. **D.** Non-Hodgkin lymphoma. This type of lymphoma has a particular predilection to the tonsillar tissues.

3. **B.** Striated enhancement pattern. This pattern provides reassurance that the condition is simply adenoidal hypertrophy of a benign nature.

4. **C.** Adenoidal hypertrophy. This also leads to other conditions such as otitis media.

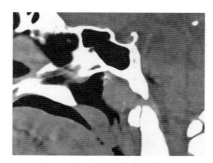

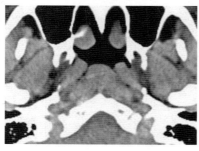

Comment

Associations with Lymphoid Hyperplasia

Lymphoid hyperplasia can affect the nasopharyngeal adenoidal tissue, the palatine tonsils, and the lingual tonsil tissue (Figures 6-1 and 6-2). It may be associated with lymph node enlargement as well. Most cases are reactive to adjacent inflammation, such as an upper respiratory or sinonasal tract infection; however, chronic illnesses such as human immunodeficiency virus (HIV), collagen vascular diseases, and immunosuppressive conditions (such as that after organ transplantation) may also lead to such enlargements. Patients with atopic or seasonal allergies may have more lymphoid tissue present. Epstein-Barr virus (EBV) is the virus most closely associated with adenoidal hypertrophy, which is problematic because EBV also is associated with nasopharyngeal carcinoma. However, virtually all viruses can cause enlargement of the adenoid pad in children and even in adults whose adenoids had previously atrophied.

Effect of Lymphoid Hyperplasia

Adenoidal hypertrophy can lead to snoring, chronic mouth breathing, obstructive sleep apnea, and otitis media. Secondary right-sided heart failure and pulmonary hypertension may coexist.

Age and Nasopharyngeal Adenoidal Prominence

Adenoidal tissue enlarges in the first decade of life, but by the end of the second decade, it should regress. When tissue in the nasopharynx is enlarged in an adult, particularly if obstructing the eustachian tube, the clinician should consider the possibility of carcinoma and lymphoma. A linear striated enhancement pattern provides reassurance that the condition is simply adenoidal hypertrophy of a benign nature.

Reference

Rout MR, Mohanty D, Vijaylaxmi Y, Bobba K, Metta C. Adenoid hypertrophy in adults: a case series. *Indian J Otolaryngol Head Neck Surg.* 2013;65(3):269-274.

Cross-Reference

Neuroradiology: THE REQUISITES, 4th ed, pp 440, 492.

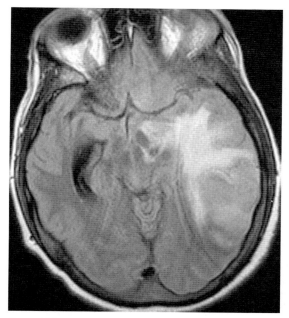

Figure 7-1

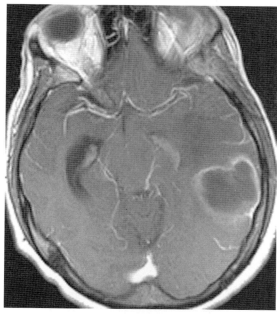

Figure 7-2

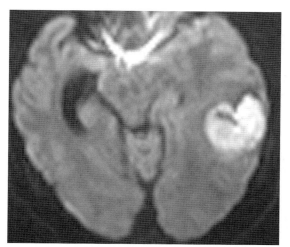

Figure 7-3

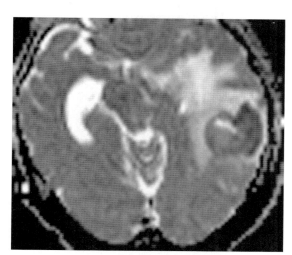

Figure 7-4

HISTORY: Withheld.

1. What is the most likely diagnosis?
   A. Venous infarct
   B. Encephalitis
   C. Abscess
   D. Hematoma

2. Regarding necrotic metastases, what is the most common cell type to result in this appearance?
   A. Melanoma
   B. Adenocarcinoma
   C. Squamous cell carcinoma
   D. Thyroid carcinoma

3. What is the most excepted cause for low apparent diffusion coefficient (ADC) within abscesses?
   A. Increased viscosity as a result of high cellularity
   B. Elevated protein content
   C. Blood products usually within the abscess
   D. Infarcted tissue

4. What are the most common cerebral locations for pyogenic brain abscesses?
   A. Anterior cerebral artery distribution
   B. Posterior cerebral artery territory
   C. Middle cerebral artery distribution
   D. Superior cerebellar artery

CASE 7

Pyogenic Brain Abscess

1. **C.** Abscess. The well-defined restricted diffusion, degree of vasogenic edema, and the peripheral enhancement make abscess the most likely diagnosis.

2. **B.** Adenocarcinoma.

3. **A.** Increased viscosity as a result of high cellularity. Although this is the most accepted explanation, other theories may exist. The other answer options have not been accepted or have been disproven.

4. **C.** Middle cerebral artery distribution. The frontal and parietal lobes are the most common locations.

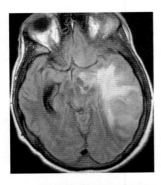

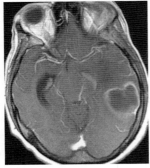

Comment

The development of a pyogenic brain abscess (Figures 7-1 through 7-4) may be divided into four stages: early cerebritis (1 to 3 days), late cerebritis (4 to 9 days), early capsule formation (10 to 13 days), and late capsule formation (14 days and after). The length of time required to form a mature abscess varies from approximately 2 weeks to months. In the mature abscess there is a collagen capsule that is slightly thinner on the ventricular side than on the cortical margin; this may be related to differences in perfusion. The presence of a dimple or small evagination pointing toward the ventricular margin from a ring-enhancing lesion should raise suspicion for an abscess. This is also important because intraventricular rupture and ependymitis can occur and are associated with a very poor prognosis. In the presence of a mature abscess, there is relatively little surrounding cerebritis and edema compared with the early stages of abscess formation. A circumferential rim that is isointense to slightly hyperintense to white matter on unenhanced T1-weighted images and hypointense on T2-weighted images may be present around a brain abscess. This appearance may be related to the presence of collagen, free radicals within macrophages, or small areas of hemorrhage. Diffusion-weighted imaging may be very helpful because the high signal intensity of the pus-filled necrotic center might show restricted diffusion (low ADC), differentiating an abscess from a necrotic neoplasm, as in this case (see Figures 7-3 and 7-4). Restricted diffusion is likely the result of the elevated viscosity within the abscess.

Management

The management of a mature brain abscess is surgical drainage and antibiotic therapy. Cerebritis and early abscesses can be managed with antibiotics and should be followed closely with magnetic resonance imaging (MRI) and clinically for signs of improvement or deterioration. Successful management monitored with serial MRI examinations will show a decrease in the surrounding edema, mass effect, and associated enhancement. It is important to remember that radiologic findings lag behind clinical improvement, and enhancement can persist for months. Resolution of an abscess can result in an area of gliosis with small calcifications.

References

Nowak DA, Rodiek SO, Topka H. Pyogenic brain abscess following haematogenous seeding of a thalamic haemorrhage. *Neuroradiology.* 2003;45:157-159.

Stadnik TW, Damaerel P, Luypaert RR, et al. Imaging tutorial: differential diagnosis of bright lesions on diffusion-weighted MR images. *Radiographics.* 2003;23:e7.

Tung GA, Rogg JM. Diffusion-weighted imaging of cerebritis. *AJNR Am J Neuroradiol.* 2003;24:1110-1113.

Cross-Reference

Neuroradiology: THE REQUISITES, 4th ed, pp 179-182.

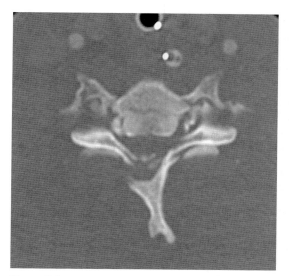

Figure 8-1

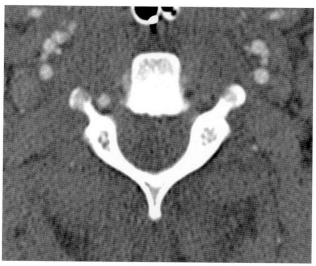

Figure 8-2

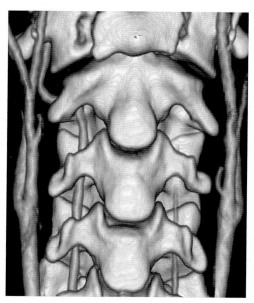

Figure 8-3

HISTORY: A 24-year-old man was found unconscious after diving from a boat.

1. What should be included in the differential diagnosis?
   A. Left vertebral artery pseudoaneurysm
   B. Left vertebral artery dissection
   C. Left vertebral artery aneurysm
   D. Left carotid artery occlusion

2. What is the most common mechanism associated with traumatic vertebral artery occlusion?
   A. Distractive flexion injury
   B. Unilateral facet dislocation
   C. Compression fracture
   D. Hyperextension injury

3. In the evaluation of a non–contrast enhanced computed tomography (CT) scan of the cervical spine for trauma, fracture of which of the following vertebral structures would most likely explain injury to the vertebral artery, indicating CT angiography for further evaluation?
   A. Spinous process
   B. Transverse foramen
   C. Transverse process
   D. Lamina

4. Which of the following statements regarding traumatic vascular injuries to the neck is true?
   A. In penetrating neck trauma, vertebral artery injury is more common than carotid injury.
   B. Vertebral artery injury is more common than carotid injury in cervical blunt trauma.
   C. Most injuries to the vertebral artery occur near its origin (V1 segment).
   D. Extremity weakness is the most common complaint in patients with symptomatic vertebral artery injury.

17

CASE 8

Traumatic Vertebral Artery Occlusion

1. **B.** Left vertebral artery dissection. There is absent contrast opacification of the distal V2 segment of the left vertebral artery.

2. **A.** Distractive flexion injury. Vertebral artery dissection occurs in 28% to 75% of these injuries, more commonly than the other answer options, even at the low end. Hyperextension injury was once thought to be more commonly associated, but more recent research shows otherwise.

3. **B.** Transverse foramen. Because the vertebral artery courses within these bony canals, injury to the vessel can occur associated with fractures.

4. **B.** Vertebral artery injury is more common than carotid injury in cervical blunt trauma. As opposed to penetrating trauma, vertebral artery injury is more common than carotid injury in patients with blunt cervical trauma.

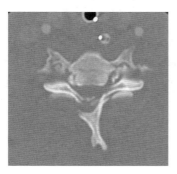

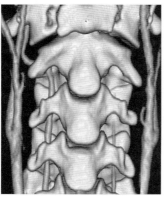

Comment

Relevant Anatomy

The vertebral artery is anatomically divided into four segments: segment V1, from its origin at the subclavian artery to the level of the transverse foramen at C6 or C7; segment V2, the transforaminal course from C6 to C1 (Figure 8-3); segment V3, from C1 to the dura; and segment V4, from the dura to its termination in the basilar artery. The transforaminal segment is the most commonly injured secondary to stretching of the artery or from displaced fractures of the foramen (Figure 8-1).

Pathophysiology

Vascular injuries to the neck may be the result of blunt or penetrating trauma. With the advent of helical CT and the increased use of magnetic resonance angiography (MRA), traumatic vertebral artery injury has been proven to be more common than previously reported: it is seen in 25% of cases of acute major cervical trauma. Distraction flexion injury has been identified as the most common spinal mechanism of injury. Vascular lesions to the vertebral arteries include occlusion, pseudoaneurysm, dissection, transection, intimal flap, and arteriovenous fistula formation. The most common lesion in blunt neck trauma for both the carotid and the vertebral arteries is vascular occlusion (Figures 8-2 and 8-3), likely the result of intimal injury and subsequent thrombosis of the vessel.

Imaging

CT angiography plays a central role in the evaluation of acute trauma patients. The wide availability and fast acquisition of CT makes CT angiography the initial test of choice. The intravascular contrast agent allows evaluation of vascular structures with equivalent accuracy compared with catheter angiography in blunt neck trauma. Magnetic resonance imaging has also proven useful in evaluation for vertebral artery injury, mainly in cases of vascular occlusion.

Management

Most vertebral artery injuries are clinically silent, and spontaneous recanalization of vascular occlusion has been documented. Infrequently, vertebrobasilar ischemia may occur, particularly in cases of inadequate collateral circulation. Given the poor prognosis of brainstem ischemia, early recognition and prompt management with anticoagulation, embolization, or surgical ligation is usually implemented to prevent secondary injury.

References

Chokshi F, Munera F, Rivas L, et al. 64-MDCT angiography of blunt vascular injuries to the neck. *AJR Am J Roentgenol.* 2011;196(3): W309-W315.

Taneichi H, Suda K, Kajino T, et al. Traumatically induced vertebral artery occlusion associated with cervical spine injuries: prospective study using magnetic resonance angiography. *Spine (Phila Pa 1976).* 2005;30(17):1955-1962.

Torina P, Flanders A, Carrino J, et al. Incidence of vertebral artery thrombosis in cervical spine trauma: correlation with severity of spinal cord injury. *AJNR Am J Neuroradiol.* 2005;26(10): 2645-2651.

Cross-Reference

Neuroradiology: THE REQUISITES, 4th ed, p 33.

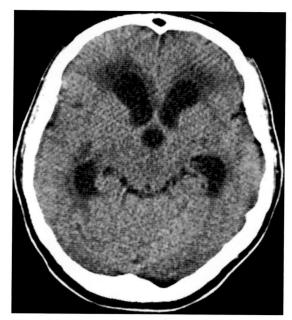

Figure 9-1

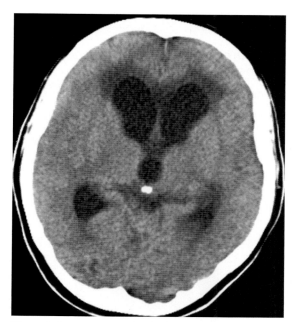

Figure 9-2

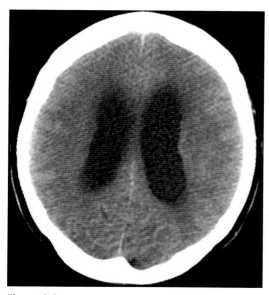

Figure 9-3

HISTORY: Altered mental status, fever, photophobia.

1. What is the primary imaging finding?
   A. Cerebral edema
   B. Hydrocephalus
   C. Tectal glioma
   D. Brain atrophy

2. What secondary imaging findings in this case indicate that this condition is likely acute?
   A. Ventricular dilation
   B. Transependymal cerebrospinal fluid (CSF) flow
   C. Sulcal effacement
   D. Subarachnoid hemorrhage

3. What type of hydrocephalus is present?
   A. Noncommunicating
   B. Hereditary
   C. Communicating
   D. Obstructive

4. The medical intern would like to assess for subarachnoid hemorrhage in this patient. What is the most prudent information to discuss with the intern?
   A. Subarachnoid hemorrhage is not visible on the computed tomography (CT) scan and therefore it is unnecessary to perform other examinations.
   B. Lumbar puncture (LP) is contraindicated because of the risk of brain herniation.
   C. Magnetic resonance imaging (MRI) can be performed prior to LP to exclude impending herniation.
   D. There is subarachnoid hemorrhage present on imaging, and a CT angiogram is necessary to identify an occult aneurysm. Perform emergent LP to confirm.

CASE 9

Acute Hydrocephalus Secondary to Meningitis

1. **B.** Hydrocephalus. The ventricles are markedly dilated.

2. **B.** Transependymal CSF flow. There is periventricular confluent hypoattenuation.

3. **C.** Communicating. Noncommunicating and obstructive hydrocephalus are synonymous. This patient has a clinical presentation for meningitis often resulting in communicating hydrocephalus.

4. **B.** LP is contraindicated because of the risk of brain herniation. This patient needs a transcalvarial shunt/drain placed.

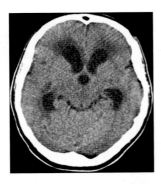

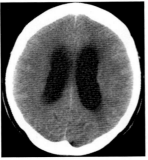

Comment

Obstructive hydrocephalus can be categorized as communicating or noncommunicating. Noncommunicating hydrocephalus is usually related to obstruction of CSF flow at some level within the ventricular system and is commonly related to neoplasms; however, infection, hemorrhage, cysts, or congenital lesions (synechiae, webs, arachnoid cysts) may be responsible. Communicating hydrocephalus typically results from obstruction of the arachnoid villi, foramen magnum, or tentorial incisura. Common causes of communicating hydrocephalus include inflammation of the meninges (meningitis, as in this case; the patient has bacterial meningitis); ventriculitis, subarachnoid hemorrhage, and carcinomatous meningitis. Obstruction of the arachnoid villi in these situations is usually related to high protein concentrations, hemorrhage, or hypercellularity of the CSF. In bacterial meningitis, purulent exudate in the subarachnoid spaces over the cerebral convexities and in the basilar cisterns, where CSF flow is more sluggish, results in impairment of CSF absorption by the arachnoid villi.

On imaging, dilation of the anterior third ventricle (Figures 9-1 and 9-2) in particular is most indicative of hydrocephalus and should not be present in normal subjects or in patients with atrophy. Elevation and thinning of the corpus callosum, best appreciated on sagittal MRI, is present in more than 75% of cases of hydrocephalus. Acute hydrocephalus may manifest with hypodensity around the ventricles on CT scans or hyperintensity on magnetic resonance T2-weighted images in the periventricular white matter because of transependymal flow of CSF (Figures 9-1 through 9-3). Compensated long-standing hydrocephalus usually does not present with this finding. Treatment of noncommunicating and communicating hydrocephalus is different. Noncommunicating hydrocephalus often requires surgery (e.g., resection of a neoplasm), whereas communicating hydrocephalus is usually treated with shunting.

LP is contraindicated in cases such as this one because the patient will be at risk for herniation. MRI will not reliably determine if the patient will herniate or not during or after LP. No subarachnoid blood is identified on these images; further hunting for it is not necessary in this setting, and the patient should be treated appropriately as discussed earlier.

References

Daoud AS, Omari H, Al-Shayyab M, Abuekteish F. Indication and benefits of computed tomography in childhood bacterial meningitis. *J Trop Pediatr.* 1998;44:167-168.

Gammal TE, Allen MB, Brooks BS, Mark EK. MR evaluation of hydrocephalus. *AJR Am J Roentgenol.* 1987;149:807-813.

Cross-Reference

Neuroradiology: THE REQUISITES, 4th ed, pp 230-262.

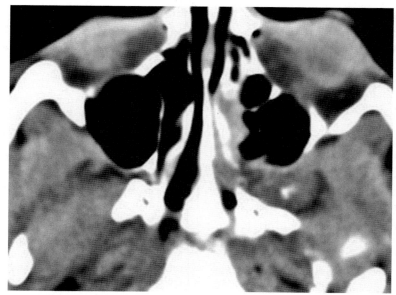

Figure 10-1

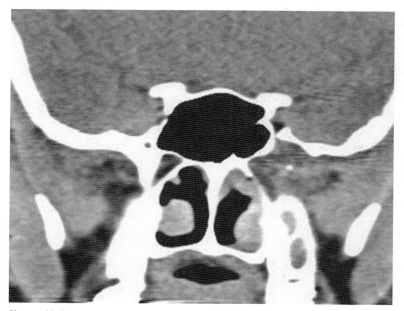

Figure 10-2

HISTORY: 25-year-old woman with left-sided sinus pain.

1. Which of the following is the best diagnosis for the imaging findings presented?
   A. Schwannoma
   B. Meningioma
   C. Epidermoid
   D. Squamous cell carcinoma
   E. Chondrosarcoma

2. Which cranial nerve is intrinsic to the pterygopalatine fossa (PPF)?
   A. V_1
   B. V_2
   C. V_3
   D. VII

3. Which benign vascular tumor has a predilection for the PPF?
   A. Meningioma
   B. Hemangioma
   C. Juvenile nasopharyngeal angiofibroma
   D. Venous vascular malformation

4. For what malignancy is perineural spread most common?
   A. Squamous cell carcinoma
   B. Nasopharyngeal carcinoma
   C. Adenoid cystic carcinoma
   D. Melanoma

CASE 10

Trigeminal Schwannoma

1. **A.** Schwannoma. Meningioma would be unusual outside the central nervous system. Epidermoid would be cystic. Squamous cell carcinoma would have mucosal extension. Chondrosarcoma does not occur at this site. Schwannoma can occur in the PPF.

2. **B.** V_2. The second division (V_2) of the cranial nerve V (trigeminal nerve) is the maxillary nerve, and it is associated with the PPF (with a ganglion there). The mandibular nerve (V_3) is associated with foramen ovale, and the ophthalmic nerve (V_1) goes through the superior orbital fissure and branches into lacrimal, frontal, and nasociliary nerves.

3. **C.** Juvenile nasopharyngeal angiofibroma. This benign tumor commonly infiltrates the PPF from its origin at the sphenopalatine foramen.

4. **C.** Adenoid cystic carcinoma. Squamous cell carcinoma and melanoma do not demonstrate perineural spread as commonly as adenoid cystic carcinoma, which has a 50% to 60% rate of perineural spread. Nasopharyngeal carcinoma grows here by direct spread, not by perineural extension.

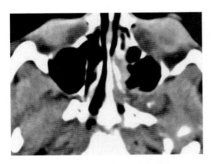

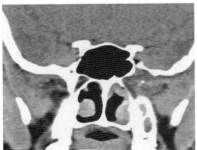

Comment

Anatomy of the Pterygopalatine Fossa

The main structures of the PPF are branches of the maxillary nerve, pterygopalatine ganglion, internal maxillary artery branches, and nerve of the pterygoid canal (Vidian nerve). It sits just behind the maxillary sinus but leads from the palate to the intracranial compartment. The Vidian nerve receives innervation from parts of the superficial petrosal branch of cranial nerve VII, and it receives parasympathetic innervation from the deep petrosal sympathetic plexus.

Exits from the Pterygopalatine Fossa

Exits from the pterygopalatine fossa include the greater and lesser palatine canals inferiorly, the Vidian canal and foramen rotundum posteriorly, the sphenopalatine foramen and palatovaginal canal medially, the inferior orbital fissure anterolaterally, and the pterygomaxillary fissure laterally. Spread to and from these regions by tumors that have a propensity for perineural spread (adenoid cystic carcinoma in particular) may fill the PPF. Skin lesions such as basal cell carcinoma or aggressive melanomas, mucosal squamous cell carcinomas of the pharynx and oral cavity, and nasopharyngeal carcinoma may also invade the PPF via the nerves.

Tumors of the Pterygopalatine Fossa

The most common primary tumors of the PPF are schwannomas (Figures 10-1 and 10-2). Juvenile nasopharyngeal angiofibromas frequently inhabit the same space. Secondary spread is usually either from perineural spread of tumors or directly from sinonasal, facial, or nasopharyngeal primary cancers.

Reference

Williams LS. Advanced concepts in the imaging of perineural spread of tumor to the trigeminal nerve. *Top Magn Reson Imaging.* 1999;10(6):376-383.

Cross-Reference

Neuroradiology: THE REQUISITES, 4th ed, pp 44-46.

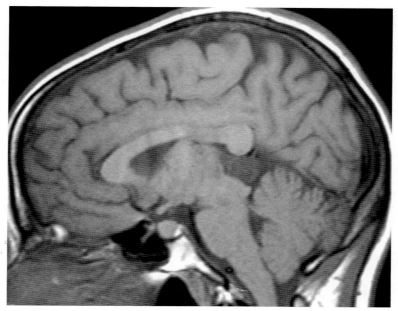

Figure 11-1

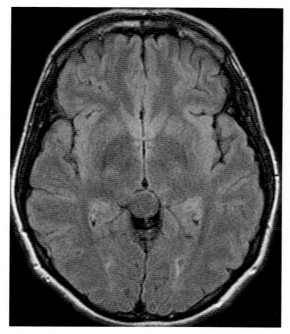

Figure 11-2

HISTORY: Withheld.

1. Within what structure is the abnormality demonstrated?
   A. Tectal plate
   B. Splenium of the corpus callosum
   C. Vermis
   D. Pineal gland

2. Mass effect on what structure causes Parinaud syndrome?
   A. Tectal plate
   B. Pineal gland
   C. Dorsal pons
   D. Corpus callosum

3. Which of the following is a sign or symptom of Parinaud syndrome?
   A. Lateral gaze disturbance
   B. Vertigo
   C. Hydrocephalus
   D. Nystagmus

4. What would be the most appropriate next step in management?
   A. Perform contrast-enhanced magnetic resonance imaging (CEMRI).
   B. Make a neurosurgical referral for biopsy.
   C. Perform magnetic resonance spectroscopy.
   D. Perform contrast-enhanced computed tomography (CT).

CASE 11

Pineal Cyst

1. **D.** Pineal gland.

2. **A.** Tectal plate. Also known as dorsal midbrain syndrome.

3. **D.** Nystagmus. Parinaud syndrome is characterized by vertical gaze palsy, pupillary light-near dissociation, and convergence-retraction nystagmus.

4. **A.** Perform CEMRI. A pineal cyst typically presents with thin rim enhancement. Nodular enhancement is more indicative of a pineal neoplasm such as pineocytoma. CT is less sensitive, no accepted use for spectroscopy has been determined, and biopsy would not be recommended without further noninvasive characterization.

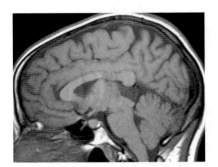

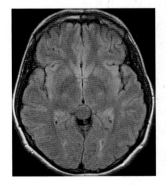

Comment

The pineal gland develops during the second month of gestation as a diverticulum in the diencephalic roof of the third ventricle. Pineal cysts are common incidental findings on MRI of the head obtained for unrelated indications and are seen in 1% to 4% of patients. In autopsy series, cystic lesions of the pineal gland have been found in 20% to 40% of specimens. Masses of the pineal gland can cause mass effect on the tectum and the aqueduct, resulting in paralysis of upward gaze (Parinaud syndrome) and hydrocephalus or headache, respectively. However, even large pineal cysts rarely are symptomatic. Pineal cysts are variable in size, and 50% of cysts identified on MRI are larger than 1 cm. Studies have shown that overall, the majority of cysts do not change in size; however, small changes in size (increases and decreases) have been noted. Enlargement of these cysts may be caused by increased cyst fluid or intracystic hemorrhage. Rare cases of pineal apoplexy have been reported in which there may be sudden death as a result of intracystic hemorrhage and acute hydrocephalus.

Pineal cysts are less common in young children and are usually seen in middle-aged adults, suggesting that these cysts might develop in late childhood or adolescence and later involute. Pineal cysts are homogeneous on MRI (Figures 11-1 and 11-2). They are typically well demarcated and round or oval and have a thin or imperceptible wall. On proton density–weighted and fluid-attenuated inversion recovery imaging (as in this case), the cyst contents are often hyperintense relative to cerebrospinal fluid. Nodular enhancement of the wall should not be present with cysts. Asymptomatic, larger cysts can cause tectal deformity.

Reference

Barboriak DP, Lee L, Provenzale JM. Serial MR imaging of pineal cysts: implications for natural history and follow-up. *Am J Roentgenol.* 176:2001;737-743.

Cross-Reference

Neuroradiology: THE REQUISITES, 4th ed, p 80.

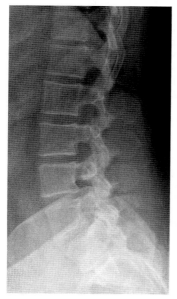

Figure 12-1

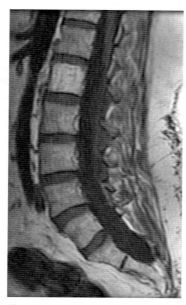

Figure 12-2

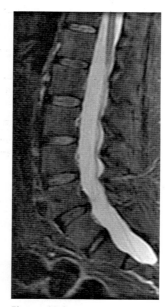

Figure 12-3

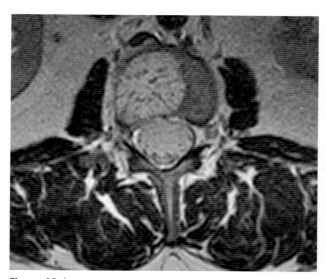

Figure 12-4

HISTORY: A 63-year-old man presents with a 2-year history of lower back pain.

1. What is the single best diagnosis?
   A. Giant cell tumor
   B. Fat island
   C. Metastatic disease
   D. Hemangioma

2. The hyperintensity observed on the T1-weighted image is due to which of the following components of the lesion?
   A. Vessels
   B. Fat
   C. Cartilage
   D. Marrow edema

3. Which of the following statements regarding vertebral hemangioma management is *false?*
   A. Embolization is advocated before surgery for compressive lesions.
   B. Resection and partial corpectomy is an accepted treatment of noncompressive lesions.
   C. No treatment is needed for asymptomatic vertebral hemangiomas.
   D. Painful lesions with minimal or no compression can be treated with embolization alone.

4. What statement is true regarding the technique utilized in Figure 12-3?
   A. This is a standard sagittal T2 spin echo (SE) sequence.
   B. This is considered opposed phase imaging.
   C. A frequency-selective saturation radio frequency (RF) pulse with the same resonance frequency of adipose has been applied, followed by a homogeneity spoiling gradient.
   D. A 90-degree inversion pulse is applied at the null point of adipose.

CASE 12

Benign Vertebral Hemangioma

1. **D.** Hemangioma. Although this lesion contains fat, the "polka-dot" appearance on Figure 12-4 and the vertical trabeculation on Figure 12-2 make hemangioma the most likely diagnosis.

2. **B.** Fat. Fat is bright on both standard T1 and T2 sequences.

3. **B.** Resection and partial corpectomy for noncompressive lesions. This is not advocated. The other answer options are true statements.

4. **D.** A 90-degree inversion pulse is applied during short tau inversion recovery (STIR) imaging. Fat signal is suppressed, although not by standard fat saturation as described in answer option C. This is not opposed phase imaging such as a Dixon technique.

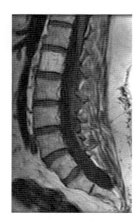

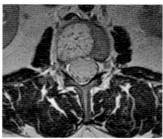

Comment

Background and Clinical Findings

Vertebral hemangiomas are benign vascular lesions of the vertebral column that occur in 10% of the general population, on the basis of autopsy studies in adults. Incidence increases with age, and there is a slight female predominance. They are usually incidental, asymptomatic, and solitary and become symptomatic in 1% of affected individuals. Symptoms include back pain and radicular pain. Symptoms are thought to develop by the following mechanisms: (1) vascular expansion of the vertebra leading to direct compression of nerve roots or the thecal sac or both, (2) subperiosteal extension resulting in an extradural mass causing sac or cord compression, and (3) compression fractures secondary to replacement of bone by the hemangioma. Rarely, a vertebral hemangioma may cause bleeding with epidural hematoma or vascular steal with spinal cord ischemia. Pregnancy may contribute to the development of aggressive and symptomatic hemangiomas, which is hypothesized to be because of an increase in blood volume and cardiac output.

Histopathology

Histologically, hemangiomas result from proliferation of normal capillary and venous structures. Approximately 20% to 30% of hemangiomas are multiple. The lesions are usually rounded with discrete margins. They vary from subcentimeter in size to replacing the entire vertebral body. Lesions are most commonly limited to the vertebral body; 10% to 15% extend into the posterior elements. Hemangiomas rarely arise primarily from the posterior elements.

Imaging

Vertebral hemangiomas exhibit a classic radiographic appearance of coarse vertical striations owing to thickening of bony trabeculae. This appearance has been described as a characteristic "honeycomb" or "corduroy cloth" pattern; the overall density of the vertebral body is decreased because of the presence of fatty marrow (Figure 12-1). Computed tomography (CT) scan shows low attenuation interspersed with thickened bony trabeculae appearing as multiple dots, representing a cross section of reinforced trabeculae with a characteristic "salt-and-pepper" or "polka-dot" appearance on axial images. Conventional magnetic resonance imaging (MRI) is less definitive. MRI-histologic correlation from autopsy specimens has shown that the signal intensity patterns observed on MRI are related to the relative proportion of fat, vessels, and interstitial edema. Areas with high signal intensity on T1-weighted images contain a larger proportion of marrow occupied by fat (Figures 12-2 and 12-3), whereas areas with high signal intensity on T2-weighted images contain a larger proportion of vessels and edema. These signal characteristics also differ from the signal characteristics of metastatic lesions, which have decreased signal intensity on T1-weighted images and increased signal intensity on T2-weighted images. As with CT scan, the thickened bony trabeculae on MRI axial images result in a "salt-and-pepper" or "polka-dot" pattern (Figure 12-4). For more difficult indeterminate cases, CT scan can be used to problem solve because it is more sensitive to the characteristic osseous remodeling of hemangiomas than MRI. If necessary, follow-up examinations can be performed to ensure stability. Angiography confirms the vascular nature of these tumors, and preoperative embolization is useful in many cases.

Management

Most patients with asymptomatic vertebral hemangiomas can be observed. Treatment options include surgery with decompression or resection and stabilization, transarterial embolization, vertebroplasty, kyphoplasty, and radiation therapy.

References

Baudrez V, Galant C, Vande Berg BC. Benign vertebral hemangioma: MR-histological correlation. *Skeletal Radiol.* 2001;30(8):442-446.

Ropper AE, Cahill KS, Hanna JW, et al. Primary vertebral tumors: a review of epidemiologic, histological, and imaging findings, Part I: benign tumors. *Neurosurgery.* 2011;69(6):1171-1180.

Cross-Reference

Neuroradiology: THE REQUISITES, 4th ed, pp 582, 585.

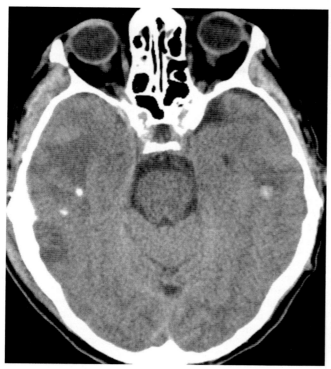

Figure 13-1

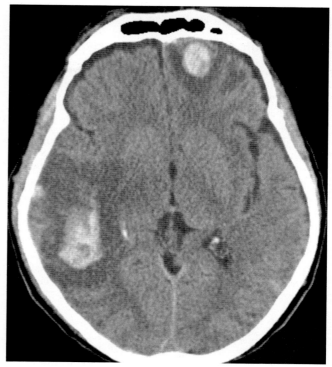

Figure 13-2

HISTORY: Trauma.

1. What is the single best diagnosis?
   A. Epidural hematoma
   B. Supratherapeutic anticoagulation
   C. Hemorrhagic contusions
   D. Diffuse axonal injury

2. The most correct statement regarding prognosis and management is which of the following?
   A. A Glasgow Coma Scale (GCS) score of 12 correlates with mild traumatic brain injury.
   B. A GCS score of E2V3M5 means the patient opens his eyes to verbal command.
   C. The best eye response score for the GCS is 4.
   D. A patient with a GCS score of 15 has no injury and can be discharged without further evaluation.

3. Blood-fluid levels are often seen in patients with traumatic brain injury (TBI) with which of the following?
   A. Lacerated bridging veins
   B. Treated atrial fibrillation
   C. More severe trauma
   D. Less severe trauma

4. Which structure has an intact blood-brain barrier?
   A. Pituitary stalk
   B. Pineal gland
   C. Choroid plexus
   D. Optic nerve

CASE 13

Hemorrhagic Contusion: Closed Head Injury

1. **C.** Hemorrhagic contusions. Multiple parenchymal hematomas in the distribution demonstrated with surrounding vasogenic edema in the setting of trauma are compatible with hemorrhagic contusions.

2. **C.** The best eye response score for the GCS is 4. The GCS is a quick prognostic exam. Mild TBI is a score of 13 or higher, and 8 or less is severe TBI. A patient's GCS score does not always correlate with the injury sustained and can change from the time of injury. See Table 13-1.

3. **B.** Treated atrial fibrillation. The mainstay of medical treatment for atrial fibrillation is anticoagulation. Blood dyscrasias or the use of anticoagulation is associated with fluid-fluid levels within hematomas. The degree of trauma is not associated with this finding.

4. **D.** Optic nerve. The optic nerves have an intact blood-brain barrier and therefore do not normally enhance with contrast as the other answer options would.

Table 13-1 GLASGOW COMA SCALE

Eye Response	Verbal Response	Motor Response
1. No eye opening	1. No verbal response	1. No motor response
2. Open to pain	2. Incomprehensible	2. Extension to pain
3. Open to verbal	sounds	3. Flexion to pain
command	3. Inappropriate words	4. Withdrawal from pain
4. Open	4. Confused	5. Localizing pain
spontaneously	5. Oriented	6. Obeys commands

Adapted from Teasdale G, Jennett B. Assessment of coma and impaired consciousness. A practical scale. *Lancet.* 1974;2:81-84.

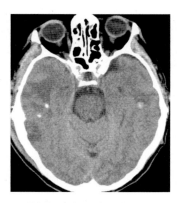

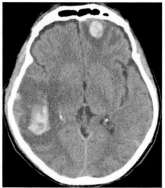

Comment

Hemorrhagic contusions are among the most common TBIs. Contusions represent petechial hemorrhages in the cortex that can extend into the adjacent white matter and are often associated with adjacent subarachnoid blood (Figures 13-1 and 13-2). They tend to occur along the superficial surfaces of the brain and are the result of acceleration forces (e.g., boxing) and deceleration forces (e.g., motor vehicle accident with head impact, such as against the steering wheel or side window) that cause the brain to rub along surfaces where there are prominent osseous ridges or dural reflections. The anterior and inferior portions of the temporal and frontal lobes, the posterolateral temporal lobes, and the occipital poles are typically contused in acceleration-deceleration injuries, as in this case (see Figures 13-1 and 13-2). The surfaces of these portions of the brain rub against the floor and anterior walls of the anterior and middle cranial fossae, sphenoid wings, temporal bones, and petrous ridges. Hemorrhagic contusions can also occur in the setting of penetrating trauma (gun and knife injuries, depressed skull fractures, or iatrogenic causes). Contusions can also occur along the convexities of the cerebral hemispheres adjacent to the midline as a result of the brain's rubbing against the rigid falx or the surface of the inner table of the calvaria.

Imaging findings depend on when the patient is imaged relative to the time of injury. In the acute setting, hemorrhages are hyperdense and are often associated with surrounding hypodensity that represents edema. Acute hemorrhagic contusions are hypointense on T2-weighted, fluid-attenuated inversion recovery, and gradient echo magnetic resonance imaging, with surrounding high signal intensity due to edema. Long-term follow-up shows resolution of the hemorrhage, encephalomalacia in the area of traumatized brain, and hemosiderin in the contusion bed.

Reference

Oertel M, Kelly DF, McArthur D, et al. Progressive hemorrhage after head trauma: predictors and consequences of the evolving injury. *J Neurosurg.* 2002;96:109-116.

Cross-Reference

Neuroradiology: THE REQUISITES, 4th ed, pp 159, 161, 165.

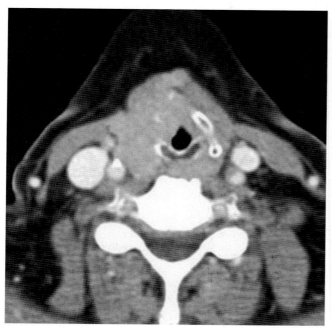

Figure 14-1

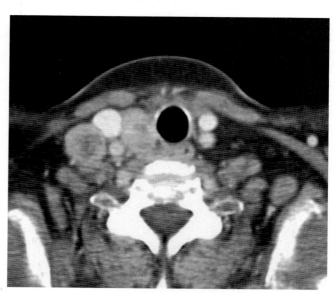

Figure 14-2

HISTORY: A middle-aged man presents with voice changes and a palpable neck mass.

1. Which of the following should *not* be included in the differential diagnosis for the imaging findings presented?
   A. Laryngeal cancer
   B. Thyroid cancer
   C. Esophageal cancer
   D. Piriform sinus cancer

2. In what percent of cases does thyroid cancer erode the larynx?
   A. 1% to 5%
   B. 6% to 10%
   C. 11% to 15%
   D. More than 15%

3. In what percent of cases does thyroid cancer erode the trachea?
   A. 1% to 5%
   B. 6% to 10%
   C. 11% to 15%
   D. More than 15%

4. In what percent of cases does thyroid cancer erode the esophagus?
   A. 1% to 5%
   B. 6% to 10%
   C. 11% to 15%
   D. More than 15%

CASE 14

Thyroid Cancer

1. **C.** Esophageal cancer. Thyroid cancer is invading the thyroid cartilage on the right and has right-sided nodal metastases. Laryngeal cancer and piriform sinus cancer can also be included in the differential diagnosis because they also may erode cartilage, but the site of esophageal cancer is too remote.

2. **B.** 6% to 10%. Thyroid cancer typically erodes the larynx in 6% to 10% of cases.

3. **B.** 6% to 10%. Thyroid cancer typically erodes the trachea in 6% to 10% of cases.

4. **A.** 1% to 5%. Thyroid cancer typically erodes the esophagus in 1% to 5% of cases. Esophageal erosion is less common than laryngotracheal invasion.

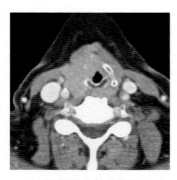

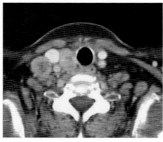

Comment

Invasion of Adjacent Structures by Thyroid Cancer

Laryngeal and tracheal invasion by thyroid cancer is uncommon because thyroid cancer is often detected while it is still indolent, often as an incidental finding. Imaging findings are most accurate for tracheal invasion when one identifies soft tissue in the cartilage (Figure 14-1), an intraluminal mass, and tumor encircling the trachea by 180 degrees or more. These findings, in combination, yield 100% sensitivity and 84% specificity. To detect esophageal invasion, the radiologist should look for abnormal T2-weighted wall signal, enhancement in the esophageal wall, or circumferential involvement by greater than 180 degrees. The incidence of aerodigestive system invasion by thyroid cancer varies by the histologic subtype. Anaplastic carcinoma, although a very rare subtype, invades the airway in as many as 20% of cases, whereas the well-differentiated papillary and follicular cancers are much less likely to do so. Strap muscle involvement is the most common type of extrathyroidal spread, followed by involvement of the trachea, larynx, recurrent laryngeal nerve, and esophagus. These structures may be infiltrated by direct spread of the thyroid cancer or via metastatic lymph nodes (Figure 14-2), particularly those in a paratracheal location. When invasion occurs, hemoptysis, stridor, difficulty breathing as a result of aspiration of blood, and viscus perforation may lead to superimposed infection and other complications.

Neck Masses

Lymph nodes and thyroid nodules are the most common palpable abnormalities in the neck in adults, whereas reactive lymph nodes are the most common palpable neck abnormalities in children.

Reference

Honings J, Stephen AE, Marres HA, Gaissert HA. The management of thyroid carcinoma invading the larynx or trachea. *Laryngoscope.* 2010;120(4):682-689.

Cross-Reference

Neuroradiology: THE REQUISITES, 4th ed, pp 519-521.

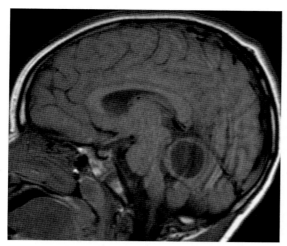

Figure 15-1

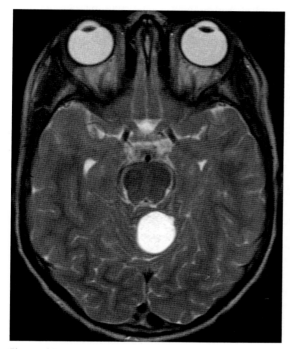

Figure 15-2

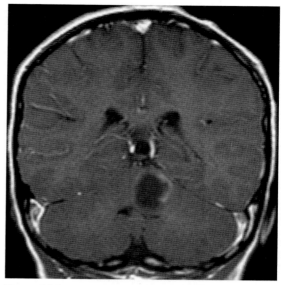

Figure 15-3

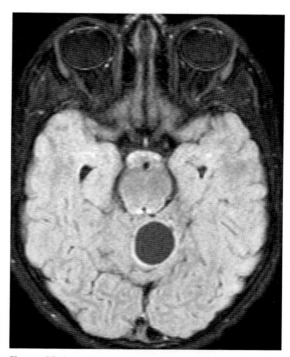

Figure 15-4

HISTORY: Altered gait.

1. What is the most likely diagnosis for a cystic mass arising within the cerebellum of a child?
   A. Hemangioblastoma
   B. Pilocytic astrocytoma
   C. Medulloblastoma
   D. Ependymoma

2. What is the typical clinical presentation of pediatric posterior fossa masses?
   A. Headache, vomiting, and ataxia
   B. Headache, nausea, and bitemporal hemianopsia
   C. Headache and unilateral blindness
   D. Ataxia and bitemporal hemianopsia

3. What is the name for the curved artifact identified in the first image (sagittal T1WI)?
   A. Pulsation
   B. Chemical shift
   C. Aliasing
   D. Gibbs (truncation)

4. What disorder is associated with pilocytic astrocytomas involving the visual pathway?
   A. Tuberous sclerosis
   B. Neurofibromatosis type 2 (NF2)
   C. Neurofibromatosis type 1 (NF1)
   D. Sturge-Weber syndrome

CASE 15

Juvenile Pilocytic Astrocytoma of the Cerebellum

1. **B.** Pilocytic astrocytoma. Although a hemangioblastoma can present as a cerebellar cystic mass, this is usually seen in adults. Medulloblastoma and ependymoma typically arise from the fourth ventricle and not from the cerebellum.

2. **A.** Headache, vomiting, and ataxia. The pediatric fossa masses typically manifest with symptoms related to mass effect and hydrocephalus, including headache, vomiting, and ataxia.

3. **D.** Gibbs (truncation). The alternating signal intensity lines parallel to the curvature of the posterior calvarium are caused by errors in K-space approximation and occur at interfaces of significantly different signal intensities such as the calvarium and brain parenchyma and the vertebra and cerebrospinal fluid.

4. **C.** Neurofibromatosis type 1 (NF1). Approximately one third of patients with pilocytic astrocytomas of optic pathways have NF1. Approximately 15% of patients with NF1 develop pilocytic astrocytomas, most commonly of the visual pathway.

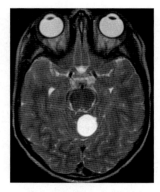

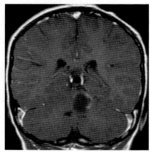

Comment

Astrocytomas are the most common intracranial tumors in children, accounting for up to 50% of such neoplasms. Approximately two thirds are located in the posterior fossa. Cerebellar astrocytomas and medulloblastomas are the most common infratentorial neoplasms in children. Approximately 80% of all cerebellar astrocytomas in children are of the pilocytic variety. Most patients with pilocytic astrocytomas have normal karyotypes; however, long arm deletions of chromosome 17 have been associated with them as well. It is important that radiologists and neuropathologists be able to distinguish pilocytic astrocytomas from the less common but more aggressive anaplastic fibrillary types because prognosis and management are distinctly different. Pilocytic astrocytomas represent one of the more benign forms of glial neoplasms and are classified as circumscribed gliomas by the World Health Organization. Histologically, tightly packed, piloid processes arising from tumor cells are typical, as are microscopic and macroscopic cysts. Eosinophilic granular bodies and Rosenthal fibers (astrocytic processes) are also present. The prognosis is usually excellent after surgical management. Conversely, patients with higher-grade infiltrative astrocytomas have a poor prognosis.

Imaging Characteristics

Pilocytic astrocytoma has a characteristic appearance. Typically, these tumors are well-circumscribed masses that usually arise within the cerebellar hemisphere (but can arise in the midline or vermis, as in this case), with a unilocular cyst and an enhancing solid mural nodule (Figure 15-3). Usually the cystic component follows the signal characteristics of cerebrospinal fluid on all magnetic resonance imaging pulse sequences (Figures 15-1, 15-2, and 15-4). The wall of the cyst does not usually enhance; however, rim enhancement of the cyst can occur and may be related to enhancement of normal adjacent cerebellar parenchyma. Calcification and hemorrhage are uncommon in juvenile pilocytic astrocytomas.

References

Morelli J, Runge V, Ai F, et al. An image-based approach to understanding the physics of MR artifacts. *Radiographics.* 2011;31:849-866.

Viano JC, Herrera EJ, Suarez JC. Cerebellar astrocytomas: a 24-year experience. *Child Nerv Syst.* 2001;17:607-610.

Cross-Reference

Neuroradiology: THE REQUISITES, 4th ed, p 57.

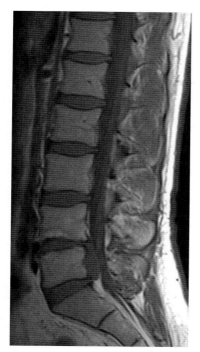

Figure 16-1

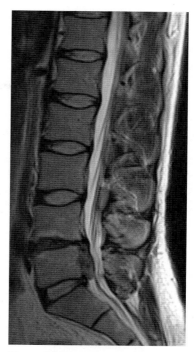

Figure 16-2

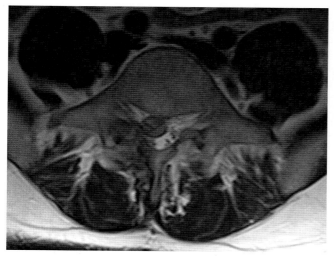

Figure 16-3

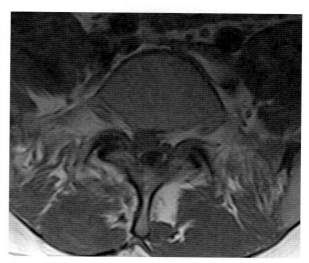

Figure 16-4

HISTORY: A 34-year-old man presents with back pain radiating to the right lower extremity that occurred after lifting his daughter.

1. Which of the following should be included in the differential diagnosis? (Choose all that apply.)
   A. Meningioma
   B. Disc protrusion
   C. Disc extrusion
   D. Discitis osteomyelitis

2. What is the frequency of disc herniation on magnetic resonance imaging (MRI) of individuals with no back pain?
   A. Less than 5%
   B. About 25%
   C. About 50%
   D. More than 75%

3. What is the frequency of bulging disc on MRI of asymptomatic individuals?
   A. Less than 5%
   B. About 25%
   C. About 50%
   D. More than 90%

4. Which of the following statements best describes an extruded disc?
   A. Disc material has a broad-based neck wider than the edges of the herniated material.
   B. Displacement of disc material involves more than 50% of the disc circumference.
   C. There is radial separation of the annular fibers.
   D. The greatest measure of the displaced disc material is greater than the base of the displaced disc material at the disc space of origin, when measured in the same plane.

CASE 16

Lumbar Disc Extrusion

1. **C.** Disc extrusion. This one happens to be inferiorly migrated. Meningiomas are typically intradural.

2. **B.** About 25%. Disc herniation is found in 27% of people with low back pain.

3. **C.** About 50%.

4. **D.** The greatest measure of the displaced disc material is greater than the base of the displaced disc material at the disc space of origin, when measured in the same plane. Choices A, B, and C define protrusion, bulge, and annular fissure, respectively.

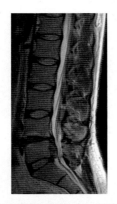

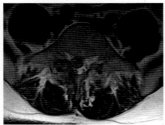

Comment

Background

Disc herniation is most common in the lumbar spine followed by the cervical spine. Lumbar disc herniation is one of the most common causes of lower back pain and often causes leg pain as well. Intervertebral disc herniation can be found in both symptomatic and asymptomatic individuals.

Histopathology

The normal intervertebral disc has an inner nucleus pulposus, which contains hydrophilic glycosaminoglycans with a lattice of collagen fibers and an outer annulus fibrosus, which contains 15 to 20 collagenous lamellae that are organized obliquely to one another. The intervertebral disc is bordered by the cartilage endplates. The disc is avascular and obtains its nutrition by diffusion from the adjacent endplates. The term *herniation* is used to describe the displacement of disc material beyond the normal confines of the disc space.

Imaging

MRI is very sensitive in delineating lumbar disc herniation and its relationship with adjacent soft tissues. On MRI, disc extrusion appears as focal, asymmetric protrusions of disc material beyond the confines of the annulus. Extruded discs are usually hypointense on T2-weighted images; however, because disc herniations are often associated with a radial annular fissure, high signal intensity in the posterior annulus is often seen.

Management

In most cases, spinal disc herniation does not require surgery. Nonsurgical methods of treatment are usually attempted first, which includes anti-inflammatory medications. Surgery is considered only as a last resort or if a patient has a significant neurologic deficit.

References

Fardon DF, Milette PC, Combined Task Forces of the North American Spine Society, American Society of Spine Radiology, and American Society of Neuroradiology. Nomenclature and classification of lumbar disc pathology. Recommendations of the combined task forces of the North American Spine Society, American Society of Spine Radiology, and American Society of Neuroradiology. *Spine (Phila Pa 1976)*. 2001;26(5):E93-E113.

Fardon DF, Williams AL, Dohring EJ, et al. Lumbar disc nomenclature: version 2.0: recommendations of the combined task forces of the North American Spine Society, the American Society of Spine Radiology and the American Society of Neuroradiology. *Spine J*. 2014;14(11):2525-2545.

Jensen MC, Brant-Zawadzki MN, Obuchowski N, et al. Magnetic resonance imaging of the lumbar spine in people without back pain. *N Engl J Med*. 1994;331(2):69-73.

Cross-Reference

Neuroradiology: THE REQUISITES, 4th ed, pp 603-604.

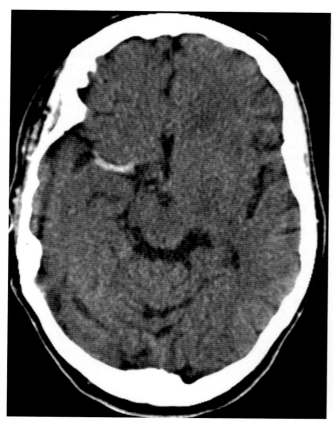

Figure 17-1

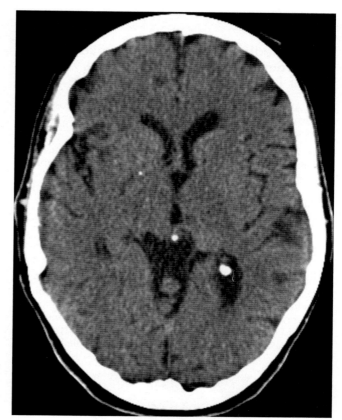

Figure 17-2

HISTORY: Altered mental status.

1. Which of the following could be included in the differential diagnosis for a hyperdense artery?
   A. Meningitis
   B. Vasculitis
   C. Subarachnoid hemorrhage
   D. Atherosclerotic plaque

2. What other presenting symptoms or signs would the patient have?
   A. Expressive aphasia
   B. Receptive aphasia
   C. Visual field cut
   D. Acute, dense left hemiplegia

3. What is meant by *penumbra* in the setting of acute stroke?
   A. The tissue with transit time prolongation and severely decreased relative cerebral blood flow and volume
   B. The tissue with unchanged perfusion values
   C. The tissue with minimal prolongation of transit time but otherwise normal perfusion values
   D. The tissue with mild to moderate elevation of transit time, moderate decrease in relative cerebral blood flow, and unchanged to mildly decreased relative cerebral blood volume

4. Which of these is another computed tomography (CT) sign of acute ischemic stroke?
   A. Hemorrhage
   B. Sulcal effacement
   C. Hyperdense cortex
   D. Encephalomalacia

CASE 17

Acute Middle Cerebral Artery Stroke: "Hyperdense" Middle Cerebral Artery and Insular Ribbon Sign

1. **D.** Atherosclerotic plaque. This may be a false positive for a true dense vessel. Check for asymmetry and use different window and level settings.

2. **D.** Acute, dense left hemiplegia. The involvement of the right internal capsule results in acute left hemiplegia. Aphasia is more commonly associated with left sided infarcts. Visual field cuts usually are due to occipital lobe infarcts (posterior cerebral artery [PCA]).

3. **D.** The tissue with mild to moderate elevation of transit time, moderate decrease in relative cerebral blood flow, and unchanged to mildly decreased relative cerebral blood volume. Penumbra, or tissue at risk, is the tissue with these perfusion values.

4. **B.** Sulcal effacement. Classic signs of acute infarct on CT include dense vessel sign, loss of insular ribbon, obscuration of gray-white interfaces, and sulcal effacement. Hemorrhage should not occur in acute ischemic stroke. Hyperdense cortex is a late finding if it occurs, as is encephalomalacia.

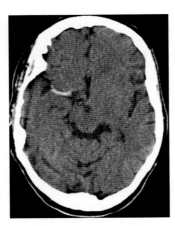

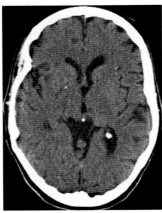

Comment

Computed Tomography

An unenhanced head CT scan remains the first-line imaging study for the emergent evaluation of acute stroke because it is readily available, rapidly performed, and sensitive in identifying acute intracranial hemorrhage.

Specific imaging findings in the assessment of acute infarct include focal parenchymal hypoattenuation (in the insular ribbon or basal ganglia for middle cerebral artery [MCA] infarcts; see Figure 17-2), cerebral mass effect manifested as sulcal effacement, and the "hyperdense" MCA sign (Figure 17-1). Initial unenhanced CT scans show hypoattenuation in up to 80% of patients with acute MCA infarcts, some degree of brain swelling in one third of cases, and hyperattenuation of the MCA in 10% to 45% of patients.

Treatment

In early infarcts, thrombolytic therapy may be used either intravenously or intra-arterially with angiographic guidance. Before interventions with thrombolytics, detection of acute hemorrhage or infarction is important because these conditions are relative contraindications to such therapy.

Prognostic Information

Ischemic changes on CT scans can predict outcome, response to thrombolytic therapy, and regions likely to become infarcted. In the European Cooperative Acute Stroke Study, there was an increased risk of fatal parenchymal hemorrhage in patients with hypoattenuating areas greater than one third the MCA territory or mass effect. Hence, these findings are considered by some to be contraindications to thrombolytic treatment. The National Institute of Neurological Disorders and Stroke (NINDS) study showed a benefit from thrombolytic agents administered intravenously within 3 hours of stroke onset, and there was a trend toward improved outcome despite initial CT-observed regions of hypoattenuation. The European Cooperative Acute Stroke study suggested that the subgroup of patients with acute stroke and without demonstrable ischemia on CT scans is also unlikely to benefit from intravenous thrombolysis.

Magnetic Resonance Imaging

Magnetic resonance imaging (MRI) is more sensitive than CT in detecting acute infarcts. MRI has also shown extension of infarctions on follow-up examinations. It is identification of this penumbra (brain tissue at risk for irreversible ischemia) that is at the heart of further development of CT and MRI techniques. It is important to protect this tissue from ischemia by applying appropriate interventions. To deliver protective agents, perfusion to this tissue is necessary.

Reference

Lev MH, Farkas J, Gemmete JJ, et al. Acute stroke: improved nonenhanced CT detection—benefits of soft-copy interpretation by using variable window width and center level settings. *Radiology.* 1999;213:150-155.

Cross-Reference

Neuroradiology: THE REQUISITES, 4th ed, pp 32-33, 224.

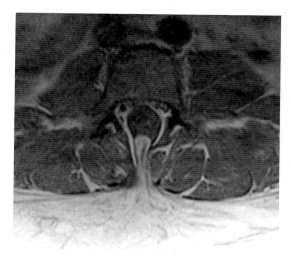

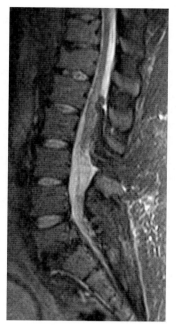

Figure 18-1

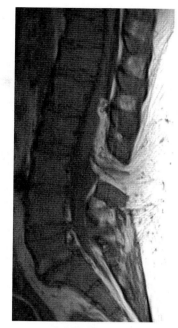

Figure 18-2

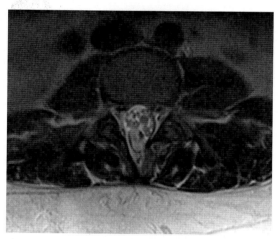

Figure 18-3

Figure 18-4

HISTORY: A 37-year-old pregnant woman is found to have a lipoma in the lower back on evaluation before epidural anesthesia.

1. What is the single best diagnosis?
   A. Dermoid
   B. Lumbar teratoma
   C. Intradural lipoma
   D. Lipomyelomeningocele

2. Is lipomyelomeningocele classified as an open or a closed spinal dysraphism?
   A. Open
   B. Closed
   C. Open in some cases and closed in others
   D. Not classified as a dysraphism

3. Which of the following statements regarding lipomyelomeningocele is true?
   A. Lipomyelomeningoceles typically manifest later in adult life.
   B. Lipomyelomeningoceles can be distinguished from intradural lipoma.
   C. Computed tomography (CT) is the preferred imaging modality.
   D. Males are affected slightly more often than females.

4. Select the most correct statement regarding magnetic resonance imaging (MRI) artifacts.
   A. Chemical shift artifact commonly occurs in the phase encoding direction.
   B. Pulsation artifact commonly occurs in the frequency encoding direction.
   C. Chemical shift artifacts occur because of differences in the Larmor frequency between fat and water being misregistered as differences in spatial position.
   D. Chemical shift artifacts are exacerbated when using fat saturation techniques.

CASE 18

Lipomyelomeningocele

1. **D.** Lipomyelomeningocele. The other choices contain fat as well but the open spinal canal, lipoma, and protrusion of the thecal sac make lipomyelomeningocele the best answer.

2. **B.** Closed. Lipomyelomeningoceles are always closed dysraphisms.

3. **B.** Lipomyelomeningoceles can be distinguished from intradural lipoma. These occur early in childhood, are differentiated by intradural lipoma by their extradural component and open dysraphism, and occur more often in females (1.5:1). MRI is the preferred imaging modality for evaluation.

4. **C.** Chemical shift artifacts occur because of differences in the Larmor frequency between fat and water being misregistered as differences in spatial position. They occur in the frequency encoding direction and can be reduced with fat saturation techniques. Pulsation artifacts occur in the phase encoding direction.

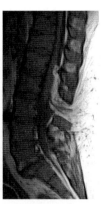

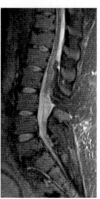

Comment

Background

Lipomyelomeningocele is a congenital lesion that is associated with spina bifida. These lesions become evident within the first few months to the first years of life, but sometimes they are discovered in older children or adults.

Classification

A simple classification scheme for spinal dysraphisms by Rossi and colleagues (2004) categorizes them as open, in which there is exposure of abnormal nervous tissues through a skin defect (myelomeningocele, myelocele), and closed, in which there is continuous skin coverage. Closed dysraphisms may be associated with a low back subcutaneous mass (lipomyelocele, lipomyelomeningocele, meningocele, or myelocystocele) or may occur without a mass (simple dysraphisms, such as tight filum terminale, filar and intradural lipomas, persistent terminal ventricle, and dermal sinus, or complex dysraphisms, such as diastematomyelia and caudal agenesis).

Imaging

MRI is the preferred imaging method for characterizing these complex malformations. Lipomyelomeningocele is distinguished from intradural lipoma by the presence of a widely bifid spinal canal and protrusion of lipoma and dural sac through the defect (Figure 18-1). The term *lipomyeloschisis* encompasses both lesions and refers to a spectrum of conditions characterized by variable protrusion of a lipoma into the associated dorsal dysraphic defect.

For the purpose of surgical management, lipomyelomeningoceles have been classified as lesions that insert caudally into the conus and lesions that attach to the dorsal surface of the conus. In the former, the lipoma may replace the filum terminale, or a separate filum may lie anteriorly. The nerve roots usually lie ventral to the lipoma. In this case, the lipoma attaches to the dorsal surface of the cord (Figures 18-1 through 18-3) with resulting cord tethering and a low position of the conus (Figure 18-4).

Management

Surgical treatment is indicated to prevent further neurologic decline. The goals of surgery are to release the attachment of the fat to the spinal cord (tethering) and reduce the bulk of the fatty tumor.

References

Rossi A, Biancheri R, Cama A, et al. Imaging in spine and spinal cord malformations. *Eur J Radiol.* 2004;50(2):177-200.

Sutton LN. Lipomyelomeningocele. *Neurosurg Clin N Am.* 1995;6(2):325-338.

Cross-Reference

Neuroradiology: THE REQUISITES, 4th ed, pp 299, 302.

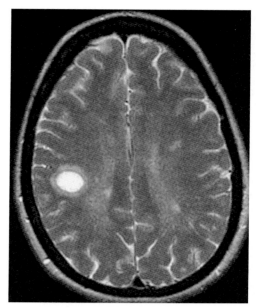

Figure 19-1 Patient A.

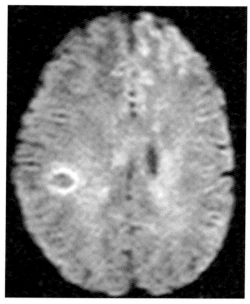

Figure 19-2 Patient A.

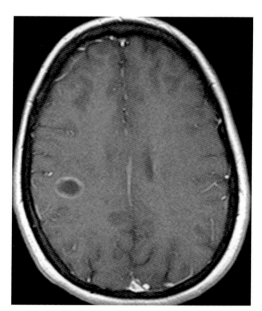

Figure 19-3 Patient A.

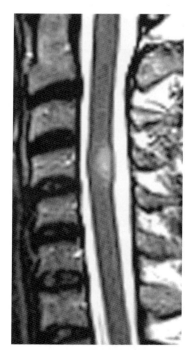

Figure 19-4 Patient B.

HISTORY: Withheld.

1. What percentage of patients with this disease have isolated spinal cord involvement?
   A. Less than 5%
   B. 5% to 15%
   C. 16% to 25%
   D. More than 25%

2. When the spinal cord is involved, where are most lesions found?
   A. Cervical region
   B. Thoracic region
   C. Conus medullaris
   D. Cauda equina

3. Which of the following findings would favor a diagnosis of a demyelinating over a neoplastic process?
   A. Spinal cord enlargement
   B. Avid solid enhancement
   C. Diffuse T2 hyperintensity in the spinal cord
   D. Scattered elongated hyperintense white matter lesions perpendicular to the longitudinal axis of the lateral ventricles

4. What serum antibody marker can help differentiate neuromyelitis optica (NMO) from multiple sclerosis (MS)?
   A. AQP4-Ab
   B. NMO-IgM
   C. Oligoclonal bands
   D. IgG4

CASE 19

Multiple Sclerosis

1. **B.** 5% to 15%. In approximately 8% to 12%. In patients presenting with myelopathy and a magnetic resonance imaging (MRI) study that reveals a cord lesion, multiple sclerosis should be considered. Evaluation should include complete spinal cord and brain MRI.

2. **A.** Cervical region. 60% to 75%.

3. **D.** Scattered elongated hyperintense white matter lesions perpendicular to the longitudinal axis of the lateral ventricles. This is the typical pattern for multiple sclerosis, although it is not diagnostic. Lesions shaped like this and radiating from the ventricles are referred to as *Dawson fingers*.

4. **A.** AQP4-Ab. This serologic marker, if positive, can help differentiate NMO from MS, allowing the treating provider to better manage the patient and prognosticate. Recombinant diagnostic assays can detect AQP4-Ab in 80% or more of patients with NMO. This antibody is also known as NMO-IgG. An IgM, answer option B, has not been identified. Oligoclonal bands are often detected in the cerebrospinal fluid, not serum, in patients with MS and NMO. IgG4 is an unassociated autoimmune marker.

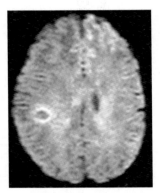

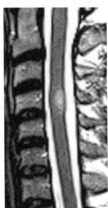

Comment

Background

MS is a demyelinating disease affecting the brain and spinal cord. It is the most common neurologic disorder in young white adults, predominately affecting women, and usually begins in the second or third decade of life. Approximately 55% to 75% of patients have spinal cord lesions at some point during the course of the disease. More than 58% of patients with cord plaques have multiple plaques. Brain lesions are not present in 20% of patients with spinal cord lesions. Of spinal cord lesions, 14% enhance.

Pathophysiology

MS is an inflammatory, demyelinating disease of the central nervous system. In pathologic specimens, the demyelinating lesions of MS, called *plaques,* appear as indurated areas—hence the term *sclerosis.* Multiple sclerosis affects the oligodendrocytes. In the acute stage, plaques have an inflammatory reaction with edema, cellular infiltration, and a spectrum of demyelination. The cause of MS is unknown, but it is likely that multiple factors act in concert to trigger or perpetuate the disease.

Imaging

On T2-weighted images, typical MS plaques (plaques fewer than two spinal segments in length and less than half the cross-sectional area of the cord) generally have a posterior or posterolateral cord location, where they involve the posterior or lateral columns. The posterior location of the enhancing nodule in Patient B (Figure 19-4) should raise suspicion that it is an MS plaque. Tumoral and nontumoral cyst formation is lacking in this case. Ring enhancement, particularly the incomplete ring sign, is a frequently observed pattern on MRI of the brain (Figure 19-3). Enhancing lesions in the brain and spine often show restricted diffusion (Figure 19-2) and some lesions, enhancing or not, may appear cystic on T2-weighted imaging (Figure 19-1). Spinal cord ring enhancement can be seen in MS, and the ring is often incomplete. The differential diagnoses for spinal cord ring enhancement should include MS in addition to neoplasm, abscess, and granulomatous disease.

Management

Ring enhancement, particularly an incomplete ring pattern, should prompt further work-up for demyelinating diseases, including MRI of the brain and cerebrospinal fluid analysis. Further evidence supporting the diagnosis of MS might preclude a need for spinal cord biopsy in patients in whom other diagnoses are suspected. Treatment consists of immunomodulatory therapy and management of symptoms. To help differentiate MS from neuromyelitis optica, a serum IgG against aquaporin 4 (AQP4-Ab) has been identified to be positive in 80% or more of patients with NMO, and the sensitivity of the exam increases as the disease progresses.

References

Bot JC, Barkhof F, Polman CH, et al. Spinal cord abnormalities in recently diagnosed MS patients: added value of spinal MRI examination. *Neurology.* 2004;62(2):226-233.

Klawiter EC, Benzinger T, Roy A, et al. Spinal cord ring enhancement in multiple sclerosis. *Arch Neurol.* 2010;67(11):1395-1398.

Loevner LA, Grossman RI, McGowan JC, et al. Characterization of multiple sclerosis plaques with T1-weighted MR and quantitative magnetization transfer. *AJNR Am J Neuroradiol.* 1995;16:1473-1479.

Cross-Reference

Neuroradiology: THE REQUISITES, 4th ed, pp 206-212.

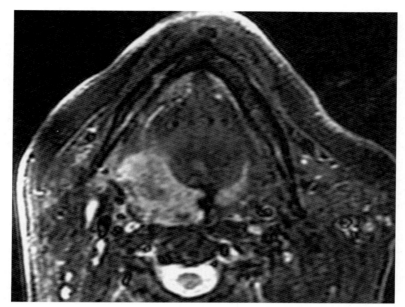

Figure 20-1

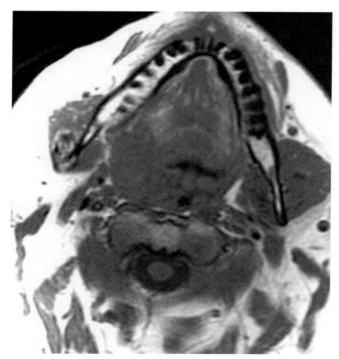

Figure 20-2

HISTORY: An older man with a 25–pack-year smoking history has lost 20 pounds of weight in 6 months.

1. Which of the following is the single best diagnosis?
   A. Squamous cell carcinoma of the floor of mouth
   B. Oral cavity cancer
   C. Retromolar trigone cancer
   D. Squamous cell carcinoma of the tonsil

2. Which is the most common direction of spread of tonsil cancer?
   A. Across the midline to the contralateral tonsil
   B. Across the midline via the posterior pharyngeal wall
   C. Across the midline via the buccal space
   D. Across the midline via the base of the tongue

3. What is the most common risk factor for tonsil squamous cell carcinoma in a 35-year-old?
   A. Smoking cigarettes
   B. Smoking marijuana
   C. Chewing tobacco
   D. Oral sex

4. Why is the prognosis for tonsil cancer worse than the prognosis for floor-of-mouth cancer?
   A. Higher rate of coincidental presence of a second primary cancer
   B. Higher rate of human papillomavirus (HPV) cancers
   C. Higher rate of mandibular involvement
   D. Increased rate of nodal spread

CASE 20

Squamous Cell Carcinoma of the Tonsil

1. **D.** Squamous cell carcinoma of the tonsil. The location of the lesion is in the tonsil, which is a part of the oropharynx.

2. **D.** Across the midline via the base of the tongue. When tonsillar cancer crosses the midline, it usually does so via the tongue base rather than via the contralateral tonsil, posterior pharynx, or buccal space.

3. **D.** Oral sex. HPV exposure increases with the number of sexual partners with whom a person has oral sex. This is a risk factor for oropharyngeal carcinoma.

4. **D.** Increased rate of nodal spread. The high incidence of nodal spread by oropharyngeal cancer dramatically affects the prognosis because nodal disease decreases the rate of 5-year survival by 50%. HPV-positive cancers have a better prognosis than do HPV-negative cancers.

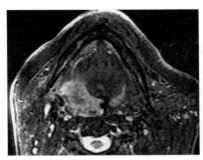

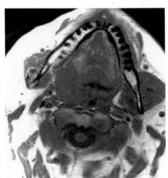

Comment

HPV-Positive Oropharyngeal Cancer

The incidence of tonsil cancer has risen dramatically in a younger age group that is not smoking or drinking excessively. This is thought to be due to HPV-positive squamous cell carcinomas of the oropharynx predominately affecting the tongue base and tonsil. Whereas oral cavity and laryngeal cancers have been declining with the lower incidence of smoking, tonsil cancers have been rising in prevalence. The increase has been attributed to increased oral sex engaged in at younger ages and with multiple partners. The spread of HPV may be abated with the vaccination against HPV in teenage males and females.

HPV Types

There are different HPV types that have high and low risks:

- High-risk HPV types: 16, 18, 31, 33, 35, 52, 58, 59, 68, 73, 82
- Low-risk HPV types: 6, 11, 40, 42, 43, 44, 54, 61, 70, 72, 81

HPV 16 is the most prevalent and, unfortunately, the most virulent type observed with oropharyngeal cancer. More men than women are affected. The disease spreads more readily to nodes, which are more commonly cystic. HPV type 16 tumors are, however, more responsive to all therapeutic maneuvers than are other types.

Risk Factors for HPV-Positive Cancers

The risk factors include higher numbers of sex partners for vaginal intercourse (>26) and for oral sex (>6) and intercourse with a sexual partner known to have a history of HPV-associated cancer. These factors increase the risk for subsequent HPV-positive cancer. Anal-oral sex, sexual intercourse with a partner with an abnormal finding on Papanicolaou smear, and HPV type 16 oral infection are also risk factors.

References

Corey AS, Hudgins PA. Radiographic imaging of human papillomavirus related carcinomas of the oropharynx. *Head Neck Pathol.* 2012; 6(suppl 1):S25-S40.

D'Souza G, Kreimer AR, Viscidi R, et al. Case-control study of human papillomavirus and oropharyngeal cancer. *N Engl J Med.* 2007; 356(19):1944-1956.

Cross-Reference

Neuroradiology: THE REQUISITES, 4th ed, p 461.

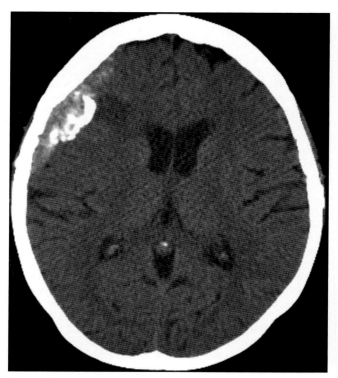

Figure 21-1

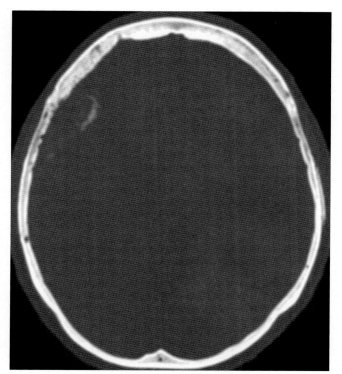

Figure 21-2

HISTORY: Headache.

1. Which of the following is included in the differential diagnosis for a calcified extra-axial mass?
   A. Acute hemorrhage
   B. Meningioma
   C. Initial presentation of lymphoma
   D. Astrocytoma

2. What finding on magnetic resonance imaging (MRI) or computed tomography (CT) would help identify an extra-axial mass?
   A. Cerebral edema
   B. Intralesional hemorrhage
   C. Buckling of the gray matter
   D. Avid enhancement

3. Approximately what percentage of these masses have calcification?
   A. 5%
   B. 15%
   C. 25%
   D. 35%

4. What percentage of these masses undergo cystic or fatty degeneration?
   A. Less than 25%
   B. 25% to 50%
   C. 50% to 75%
   D. More than 75%

CASE 21

Meningioma

1. **B.** Meningioma. This is an extra-axial partially calcified mass. Acute blood and lymphoma without treatment would not be calcified. Astrocytomas are intra-axial.

2. **C.** Buckling of the gray matter. Characteristics of extra-axial masses include a cleft or "pseudocapsule" (composed of cerebrospinal fluid, dura, or vessels) that separates the mass from the brain (as in this case); buckling of the gray matter; and a mass that is broad-based against a dural surface.

3. **B.** 15%.

4. **A.** Less than 25%.

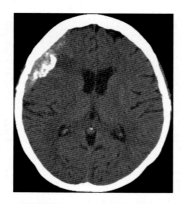

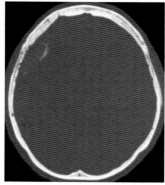

Comment

Meningiomas are the most common intracranial, extra-axial neoplasm. Although there are a variety of histologies, including fibroblastic, angioblastic, syncytial, and transitional types, prognosis does not primarily depend on the histology but rather on the location of the meningioma. Large meningiomas occurring over the cerebral convexities may be treated with embolization when necessary, followed by surgery without neurologic deficit; in contrast, meningiomas as small as 1 cm involving the cavernous sinus may be very symptomatic and present a more challenging treatment dilemma. Meningiomas occur most commonly in middle-aged women; however, they are also often found in men. Most meningiomas are sporadic, isolated lesions. Multiple meningiomas may be familial or may be seen in patients with a history of radiation therapy to the brain, neurofibromatosis type 2, and basal cell nevus (Gorlin-Goltz) syndrome.

On unenhanced CT, more than 50% of meningiomas are hyperdense as in this case (Figure 21-1). Approximately 20% to 25% are associated with calcification or a reaction in the adjacent bone (hyperostosis is more common than osteolysis). The bone window in this patient shows that the mass is calcified, but close inspection of the inner cortical table shows secondary "blistering" (Figure 21-2). On MRI, meningiomas are often isointense to gray matter on T1-weighted and T2-weighted sequences; however, they may be hyperintense on T2-weighted imaging. Meningiomas typically have avid, homogeneous enhancement. The most important clue to making the diagnosis of a meningioma is in establishing that the mass is extra-axial. One finding consistent with an extra-axial location is the presence of a pseudocapsule, which can represent cerebrospinal fluid, dura, or vessels along the pia-arachnoid. Although the presence of an enhancing dural tail is highly suggestive of meningioma, this is a nonspecific finding and may be seen in other disease processes.

References

Alvernia JE, Sindou MP. Preoperative neuroimaging findings as a predictor of the surgical plane of cleavage: prospective study of 100 consecutive cases of intracranial meningioma. *J Neurosurg.* 2004;100:422-430.

Sheporaitis LA, Osborn AG, Smirniotopoulos JG, et al. Intracranial meningioma. *AJNR Am J Neuroradiol.* 1992;13:29-37.

Cross-Reference

Neuroradiology: THE REQUISITES, 4th ed, pp 41-44, 370.

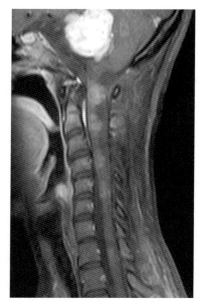

Figure 22-1

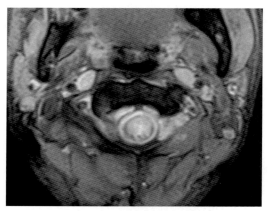

Figure 22-2

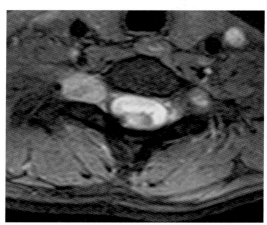

Figure 22-3

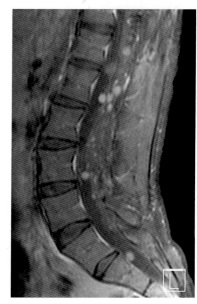

Figure 22-4

HISTORY: A 23-year-old woman presents with a history of deafness and multiple spinal tumors.

1. Which of the following should be included in the differential diagnosis?
   A. Neurofibromatosis type 1 (NF1)
   B. Neurofibromatosis type 2 (NF2)
   C. Multiple meningiomas
   D. Metastasis

2. What is the most common tumor associated with NF2?
   A. Ependymoma
   B. Meningioma
   C. Vestibular schwannoma
   D. Trigeminal nerve schwannoma

3. What is the most likely diagnosis for the intramedullary lesion in this patient with NF2?
   A. Astrocytoma
   B. Meningioma
   C. Hemangioblastoma
   D. Ependymoma

4. Which of the following imaging studies could be diagnostic?
   A. Computed tomography (CT) scan of the abdomen
   B. Ultrasound of the kidneys
   C. Magnetic resonance imaging (MRI) of the internal auditory canals
   D. CT scan of the temporal bones

CASE 22

Neurofibromatosis Type 2

1. **B.** Neurofibromatosis type 2. MISME: *m*ultiple *i*nherited *s*chwannomas, *m*eningiomas, and *e*pendymomas. NF1 is not associated with vestibular schwannomas.

2. **C.** Vestibular schwannoma.

3. **D.** Ependymoma.

4. **C.** MRI of the internal auditory canals. Bilateral vestibular schwannomas are diagnostic for NF2 (see image below).

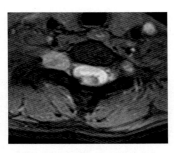

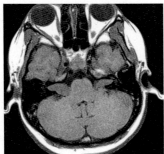

Image refers to Question 4.

Comment

Background

NF2 is an inherited autosomal dominant syndrome characterized by the development of various tumors of the central and peripheral nervous systems. The mnemonic *MISME* (*m*ultiple *i*nherited *s*chwannomas, *m*eningiomas, and *e*pendymomas) is widely used to remember the disease.

Histopathology

The genetic defect responsible for NF2 is a deletion of a portion of chromosome 22. The NF2 gene product serves as a tumor suppressor, and decreased function or production of this protein results in a predisposition to tumor development.

Imaging

Imaging findings in NF2 include bilateral vestibular schwannomas, meningiomas, and schwannomas involving the cranial nerves. Spinal manifestations include meningiomas, ependymomas (Figures 22-1 and 22-2), and nerve sheath tumors (Figures 22-3 and 22-4). Contrast-enhanced MRI of the brain and entire spine is the modality of choice in screening for NF2. Contrast agent administration is important for detecting small schwannomas (see Figure 22-4) and intraparenchymal ependymomas (see Figures 22-1 and 22-2). High-resolution fast spin echo T2 cisternography can aid in evaluation of the cranial nerves.

Management

Surgical resection of tumors is the mainstay of treatment; more recent advances in surgery and stereotactic radiosurgery permit preservation of hearing and facial nerve function. Resection of spinal cord tumors is often difficult, and complete resection is not always possible. The risks and benefits of surgery must be considered on an individual basis.

References

Mautner VF, Tatagiba M, Lindenau M, et al. Spinal tumors in patients with neurofibromatosis type 2: MR imaging study of frequency, multiplicity, and variety. *AJR Am J Roentgenol.* 1995;165(4): 951-955.

Selch MT, Pedroso A, Lee SP, et al. Stereotactic radiotherapy for the treatment of acoustic neuromas. *J Neurosurg.* 2004;101(Suppl 3):362-372.

Cross-Reference

Neuroradiology: THE REQUISITES, 4th ed, pp 292-295.

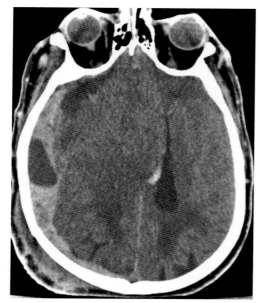

Figure 23-1

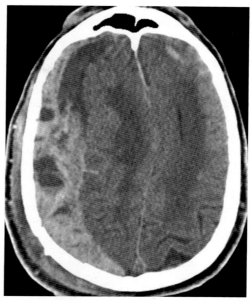

Figure 23-2

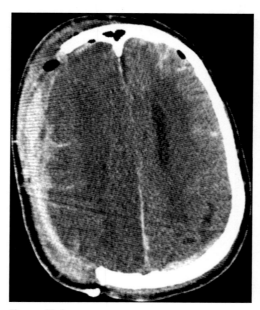

Figure 23-3

HISTORY: Patient found down.

1. Which of the following is the single best diagnosis for this particular case?
   A. Subdural hematoma
   B. Epidural hematoma
   C. Metastases
   D. Contusion

2. What is the imaging finding in subfalcine herniation?
   A. Displacement of the septum pellucidum
   B. Displacement of the falx
   C. Contralateral ventricular entrapment
   D. Displacement of the cingulate gyrus beneath the free edge of the interhemispheric falx

3. What new finding is evident on this patient's postevacuation head computed tomography (CT) scan (Figure 23-3), obtained 6 hours later?
   A. Acute infarct in the left middle cerebral artery (MCA) territory
   B. Acute infarct in the right posterior cerebral artery (PCA) territory
   C. Acute infarct in the right anterior cerebral artery (ACA) territory
   D. Acute infarct in the left ACA territory

4. Aside from nonaccidental trauma and coagulopathy, what is the next most recognized cause of subdural hematoma in neonates?
   A. Birth injury
   B. Germinal matrix hemorrhage
   C. Acute infarct
   D. Venous thrombosis

CASE 23

Acute Actively Bleeding Subdural Hematoma—Subfalcine Herniation and Infarct

1. **A.** Subdural hematoma.

2. **D.** Displacement of the cingulate gyrus beneath the free edge of the interhemispheric falx.

3. **C.** Acute infarct in the right ACA territory. There is loss of gray-white differentiation in the right medial frontal lobe consistent with acute ischemia secondary to compression of the ACA from subfalcine herniation.

4. **A.** Birth injury. Germinal matrix hemorrhage and acute infarct do not cause subdural hematomas. Venous thrombosis may be associated with subdural hematoma but that occurrence is rare.

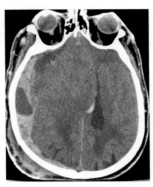

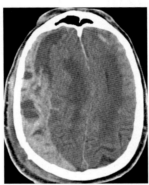

Comment

Acute subdural hematomas in young patients are usually the result of closed head injury (e.g., motor vehicle accident), as in this case. This case shows a large right convexity, acute, actively bleeding subdural hematoma with right-to-left subfalcine herniation (Figures 23-1 and 23-2) complicated by an acute right ACA infarct (Figure 23-3) resulting from compression of this vessel. The heterogeneous "swirling" appearance within the subdural hematoma signifies active bleeding in this case, but such an appearance can also be related to leakage of serum from the clot in coagulopathic patients or patients receiving anticoagulation therapy. Also noted is subarachnoid blood and left frontal contusion (see Figure 23-2).

Subdural hematomas are typically caused by tearing of the bridging veins that cross the subdural compartment, extending from the pia to the venous sinuses. Tearing of these veins is caused by motion of the brain relative to the fixed dural sinuses. Most subdural hematomas are located along the supratentorial convexities; however, they can also occur in the posterior fossa and along the tentorium cerebelli.

Imaging features of subdural hematomas on CT scans depend on their age. Acute (hours to days old) hematomas are typically hyperdense crescentic extracerebral collections. Subacute (days to weeks old) hematomas tend to be isodense to gray matter; therefore, it is easy to miss them on a quick glance at a CT scan. To avoid missing this finding, compare the size of the sulci over the left and right cerebral convexities. Absence of sulci or asymmetric sulci should raise suspicion. Always check that the sulci extend to the inner table of the calvarium, and evaluate the gray-white matter interface for inward buckling. Chronic (weeks to months old) hematomas are usually hypodense. Fluid levels within these hematomas may be caused by interval bleeding. Calcification along the dural membrane can also occur.

References

Gentry LR, Godersky JC, Thompson B, Dunn VD. Prospective comparative study of intermediate-field MR and CT in the evaluation of closed head trauma. *AJR Am J Roentgenol.* 1988;150:673-682.

Rooks VJ, Eaton JP, Ruess L, et al. Prevalence and evolution of intracranial hemorrhage in asymptomatic term infants. *Am J Neuroradiol.* 2008;29:1082-1089.

Cross-Reference

Neuroradiology: THE REQUISITES, 4th ed, pp 154-158.

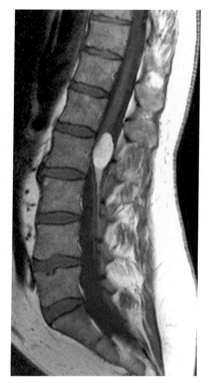

Figure 24-1

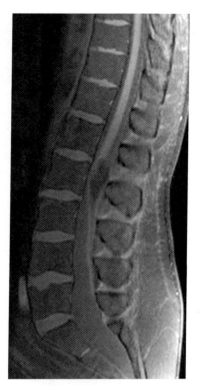

Figure 24-2

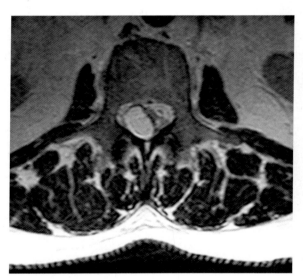

Figure 24-3

HISTORY: A 30-year-old man has a 2-year history of low back pain.

1. What is the best diagnosis?
   A. Schwannoma
   B. Arachnoid cyst
   C. Lipoma
   D. Meningioma

2. What is the most common location of intradural lipomas?
   A. Cervical spine
   B. Thoracic spine
   C. Lumbar spine
   D. Sacral spine

3. Which of the following is *typically* hypointense on T1-weighted images?
   A. Subacute blood
   B. Melanin
   C. Proteinaceous fluid
   D. Coarse calcifications

4. Which of the following statements regarding spinal lipomas is true?
   A. The clinical presentation of spinal lipomas is mainly related to tethered spinal cord.
   B. There is often a dural defect related to the lipoma.
   C. Chiari II malformations are related to spinal lipomas.
   D. Spinal lipomas are *not* affected by hormonal changes or weight gain.

CASE 24

Lipoma of the Conus Medullaris

1. **C.** Lipoma. This is the most likely fat-containing intradural mass.

2. **B.** Thoracic spine. Most intradural lipomas are found in the thoracic region, probably only because by volume/space available, this is the largest region.

3. **D.** Coarse calcifications are typically hypointense on T1-weighted images. Hyperintense T1 signal is seen with subacute blood (methemoglobin), melanin, and protein-aceous fluid.

4. **B.** There is often a dural defect related to the lipoma. The relationship to the lipoma is variable, although a defect is often found. Lipomas are due to mass effect, infrequently tethering. Chiari II is associated with myelomeningoceles. Lipomas may grow as a patient does and are affected by hormonal changes such as during pregnancy.

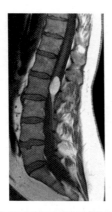

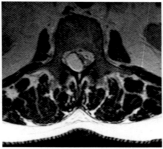

Comment

Background

Lipomas of the conus medullaris without spinal dysraphism in adults are rare. Most patients have symptoms for more than 2 years before the diagnosis. Although spinal lipomas are often discussed in the context of the tethered spinal cord, the clinical presentation of intradural spinal lipoma is mainly related to the mass effect with resulting displacement of the conus or crowding of the nerve roots.

Histopathology

Although lipomas of the conus may appear intradural, these tumors usually have some connection with the dorsal thecal sac and are not completely intradural. Chapman and colleagues (1999) proposed an anatomic classification of lumbosacral lipomas based on the relationship of the lipoma to the conus medullaris. Dorsal lipomas are located entirely on the dorsal aspect of the lower spinal cord and always spare the conus. Caudal types are attached to the termination of the spinal cord and involve the tip of the conus. A transitional type represents a complex malformation that extends inferiorly from the dorsum of the terminal spinal cord to involve both the conus and elements of the cauda equina. This latter type is frequently complicated further by rotation of the neural placode to one side or the other, resulting in forward displacement and apparent shortening of the nerve roots. The dura mater is typically deficient dorsally and occasionally laterally where the lipoma erupts through the spinal defect.

Imaging

Magnetic resonance imaging (MRI) is the best diagnostic modality to evaluate spinal lipoma and delineate the adjacent neural structures (Figures 24-1 through 24-3). The fat component can be confirmed easily with fat suppression images (see Figure 24-2).

Management

The goal of surgery is to release the tethered neural elements and remove the bulk of the lipoma, while preserving neurologic functions. Because the dorsal roots sometimes exit through the lateral aspect of the lipoma, a distinct plane between tumor and spinal cord may not be present, precluding complete resection of the tumor.

References

Chapman P, Stieg PE, Magge S, et al. Spinal lipoma controversy. *Neurosurgery*. 1999;44(1):186-192, discussion 192-193.

Hsieh CT, Sun JM, Liu MY, et al. Lipoma of conus medullaris without spinal dysraphism in an adult. *Neurol India*. 2009;57(6):825-826.

Wykes V, Desai D, Thompson DN. Asymptomatic lumbosacral lipomas—a natural history study. *Childs Nerv Syst*. 2012;28(10):1731-1739.

Cross-Reference

Neuroradiology: THE REQUISITES, 4th ed, pp 578, 581.

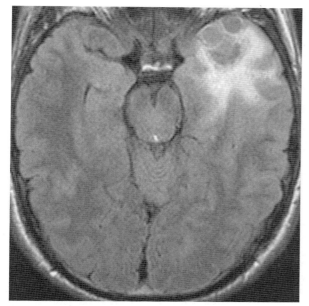

Figure 25-1

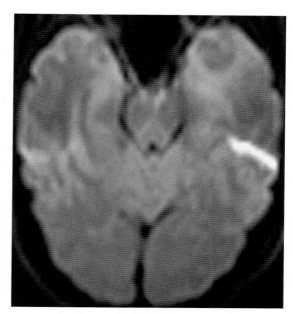

Figure 25-2

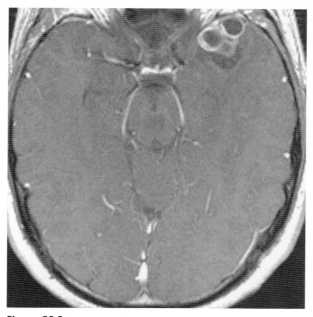

Figure 25-3

HISTORY: New-onset seizures.

1. The T2-FLAIR (fluid-attenuated inversion recovery) signal abnormality in the white matter is likely related to which of the following?
   A. Acute infarct
   B. Infiltrating tumor
   C. Infection
   D. Demyelination

2. In this case, the restricted diffusion is likely related to which of the following?
   A. Cytotoxic edema
   B. T2 shine-through
   C. Lymphocytic infiltration
   D. Hypercellularity

3. In cases of treated glioma, what imaging sequence would be best to differentiate treatment-related changes from progression or recurrence of tumor?
   A. Diffusion
   B. Susceptibility
   C. Perfusion
   D. Contrast-enhanced T1-weighted imaging

4. Which one of the following is *not* a World Health Organization (WHO) subtype of infiltrating astrocytic neoplasm?
   A. Astrocytoma
   B. Anaplastic astrocytoma
   C. Oligo-astrocytoma
   D. Glioblastoma
   E. All of the above are subtypes of infiltrating astrocytic neoplasm.

51

CASE 25

Infiltrating Astrocytoma: Low Grade

1. **B.** Infiltrating tumor. Although this "peritumoral" signal is frequently attributed to vasogenic edema, in cases of infiltrative gliomas, there are often infiltrative tumor cells in the white matter that have been found to correlate to the region of signal abnormality.

2. **D.** Hypercellularity. Restricted diffusion in the setting of infiltrative neoplasms is attributed to hypercellular tumors with high nuclear-cytoplasm ratios.

3. **C.** Perfusion. Areas of new increased perfusion are most likely recurrent or progressive neoplasm. Diffusion and contrast enhancement may be positive in both scenarios. Hemorrhage, resulting in susceptibility-weighted imaging (SWI) positivity, can also be seen in treated or progressing tumor.

4. **C.** Oligo-astrocytoma. This is not a subtype of infiltrating astrocytic neoplasm. In fact, recent literature on using genetic profiling suggests that there is very rarely, if ever, this mixed tumor, and a tumor should be characterized based on genetics more reliably than on imaging.

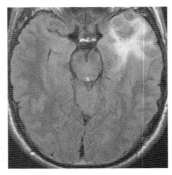

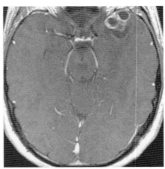

Comment

According to the WHO classification, infiltrating astrocytic tumors may be divided into three subtypes: astrocytoma, anaplastic astrocytoma, and glioblastoma (GBM). The histologic criteria for these subdivisions depend on many factors, including cellular density, number of mitoses, presence of necrosis, nuclear or cytoplasmic pleomorphism, and vascular endothelial proliferation. GBM typically has all of these histologic features, whereas the lower-grade astrocytomas might only demonstrate minimal increased cellularity and cellular pleomorphism. The presence of necrosis and vascular endothelial proliferation in particular favor GBM, the most malignant of the glial neoplasms.

Astrocytomas are central nervous system neoplasms in which the predominant cell type is derived from an astrocyte. Two classes of astrocytic tumors are recognized: those with narrow zones of infiltration (e.g., pilocytic astrocytoma, subependymal giant cell astrocytoma, pleomorphic xanthoastrocytoma) and those with diffuse zones of infiltration (e.g., low-grade astrocytoma, anaplastic astrocytoma, GBM). The latter group can diffusely infiltrate contiguous and distant central nervous system structures, regardless of histologic stage, and they have a tendency to progress to more advanced grades. Regions of a tumor demonstrating the greatest degree of anaplasia are used to determine the histologic grade of the tumor. On imaging, glioblastomas manifest with infiltrative T2-FLAIR signal abnormalities (Figure 25-1) more extensive than the rim-enhancing centrally necrotic area (Figure 25-3) and can show areas of restricted diffusion indicating high cellularity (Figure 25-2). Nonenhancing areas are likely lower grade than the area of enhancement and necrosis.

Low-grade infiltrating astrocytomas correspond to WHO grade II, and they grow slowly compared with their malignant counterparts, anaplastic astrocytomas. Several years can intervene between initial symptoms and establishment of the diagnosis of low-grade astrocytoma. Seizures, often generalized, are the initial presenting symptom in approximately one half of patients with low-grade astrocytoma.

References

Bagley LJ, Grossman RI, Judy KD, et al. Gliomas: correlation of magnetic susceptibility artifact with histologic grade. *Radiology*. 1997;202:511-516.

Preul C, Kuhn B, Lang EW, et al. Differentiation of cerebral tumors using multi-section echo planar MR perfusion imaging. *Eur J Radiol*. 2003;48:244-251.

Sahm F, Reuss D, Koelsche C, et al. Farewell to oligoastrocytoma: in situ molecular genetics favor classification as either oligodendroglioma or astrocytoma. *Acta Neuropathol*. 2014;128:551-559.

Cross-Reference

Neuroradiology: THE REQUISITES, 4th ed, pp 57-58.

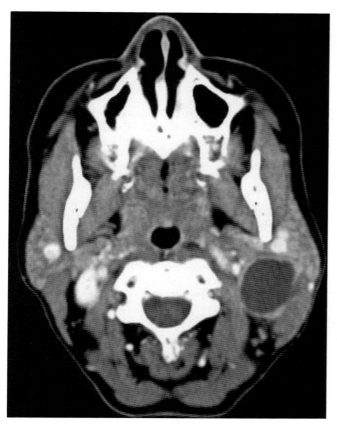

Figure 26-1

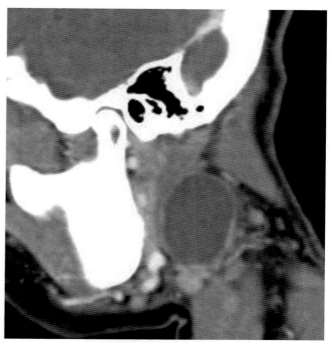

Figure 26-2

HISTORY: A young patient has a long history of left-sided neck swelling.

1. In addition to this diagnosis, what other diagnosis should be considered?
   A. Thyroglossal duct cyst
   B. Cystic nodal mass
   C. Jugular lymphatic sac
   D. Tornwaldt cyst

2. Which primary tumor is most commonly associated with a cystic lymph node?
   A. Papillary carcinoma of the thyroid
   B. Lymphoma
   C. Human papillomavirus (HPV)–negative squamous cell carcinoma of the larynx
   D. Melanoma

3. Where is a Bailey type 3 second branchial cleft cyst (BCC) located?
   A. Deep to the sternocleidomastoid muscle (SCM)
   B. Superficial to the SCM
   C. Deep to the carotid sheath
   D. Insinuating in the carotid bifurcation, like a carotid body tumor

4. Which neck cyst has a strong predilection for the left side of the neck?
   A. Thyroglossal duct cyst
   B. Second BCC
   C. Jugular lymphatic sac
   D. Zenker diverticulum

CASE 26

Second Branchial Cleft Cyst

1. **B.** Cystic nodal mass. This cystic mass may be a BCC or a cystic nodal mass. Tornwaldt cysts occur in the nasopharynx, and jugular lymphatic sacs occur in the lower neck. Thyroglossal duct cysts are closely associated with the hyoid and near midline.

2. **A.** Papillary carcinoma of the thyroid. Thyroid cancer and tonsil cancers, particularly ones that are HPV positive, have a strong association with cystic nodes.

3. **D.** Insinuating in the carotid bifurcation, like a carotid body tumor. Bailey type 1 second BCCs are superficial to the SCM, type 2 are between the SCM and the carotid bifurcation, type 3 insinuate between the carotid arteries, and type 4 are deep to the carotid bifurcation.

4. **C.** Jugular lymphatic sac and thymopharyngeal cysts have a predilection for the lower left side of the neck.

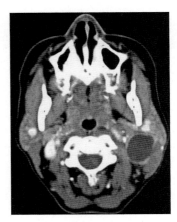

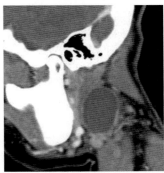

Comment

Bailey Classification of Second Branchial Cleft Cysts

Bailey classified second BCCs in 1929. He defined them as follows:

> Type I: along the anterior surface of the SCM, deep to the platysma muscle
> Type II: along the anterior margin of the SCM, deep to it, and posterior to the submandibular gland
> Type III: invaginating into the carotid bifurcation
> Type IV: deep to the carotid bifurcation along the lateral pharyngeal wall or parapharyngeal space

Appearance of Second Branchial Cleft Cysts

Second BCCs usually develop in the second and third decades of life with an enlarging neck mass (Figures 26-1 and 26-2). The mass may be traumatized or infected, which may lead to a less-than-pure cystic anechoic ultrasound appearance. In fact, in more than half the cases reported by Ahuja and colleagues (2000), there was internal debris, a complex heterogeneous echo pattern, or a uniformly homogeneous pseudosolid appearance. Thick walls were present in 12% of cases.

Differential Diagnosis

The differential diagnosis includes cystic nodal disease, which also is uncommonly anechoic. Lymphatic low-flow malformations and cystic hygromas may simulate second BCCs when they are lower in location in the neck. Lymphatic malformations tend to appear in the posterior triangle and axilla and manifest earlier in life.

Reference

Ahuja AT, King AD, Metreweli C. Second branchial cleft cysts: variability of sonographic appearances in adult cases. *AJNR Am J Neuroradiol.* 2000;21(2):315-319.

Cross-Reference

Neuroradiology: THE REQUISITES, 4th ed, pp 504-505.

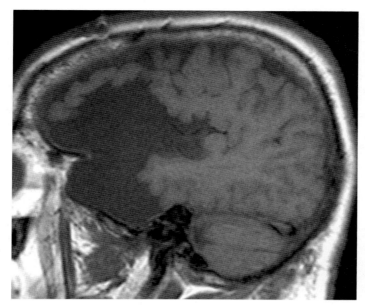

Figure 27-1

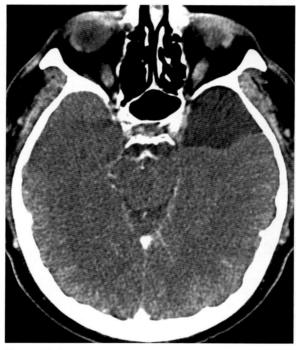

Figure 27-2

HISTORY: Incidental findings in asymptomatic patients.

1. What would be the best diagnosis if on magnetic resonance imaging (MRI) this lesion demonstrated restricted diffusion?
   A. Epidermoid
   B. Arachnoid cyst
   C. Abscess
   D. Cystic glioma

2. Which one of the following is a feature of an intra-axial mass rather than an extra-axial mass?
   A. Buckling of the gray and white matter
   B. Cortical expansion
   C. Cerebrospinal fluid (CSF) cleft
   D. Smooth remodeling of the overlying bone

3. From what structure do these lesions derive?
   A. Meninx primitiva
   B. Neuroectoderm
   C. Antoni A and B tissue
   D. Arachnoid rests

4. What is the most common cause of an arachnoid cyst?
   A. Acquired
   B. Post-traumatic
   C. Congenital
   D. Neoplastic

CASE 27

Arachnoid Cyst

1. **A.** Epidermoid. These may appear similar to arachnoid cysts on both computed tomography (CT) and MRI, although they tend to have slightly "dirty" CSF signal on MRI and demonstrate restricted diffusion.

2. **B.** Cortical expansion. The other answers are all characteristics of extra-axial masses such as this arachnoid cyst.

3. **A.** Meninx primitiva. This envelops the developing CSF. Arachnoid rests give rise to meningiomas.

4. **C.** Congenital.

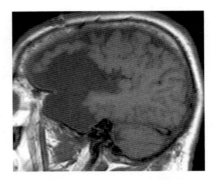

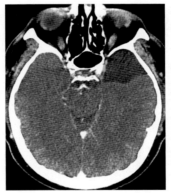

Comment

Most intracranial arachnoid cysts are congenital and are derived from the meninx primitiva, which envelops the developing central nervous system. As CSF fills the subarachnoid spaces, the meninx is resorbed. At the same time, a cleft can develop between layers of the arachnoid membrane and can behave as a one-way ball-valve mechanism. There is preferential flow of CSF into this cleft, resulting in formation of a cyst. Less commonly, arachnoid cysts may be acquired as a result of adhesions in the subarachnoid space related to a previous inflammatory process or hemorrhage.

The most common location for an arachnoid cyst is the middle cranial fossa. Other common locations include the cerebral convexities (most commonly, the frontal convexity), the basal cisterns (suprasellar, cerebellopontine angle, and quadrigeminal), and the retrocerebellar region. On CT and MRI, arachnoid cysts usually follow the density or intensity of CSF, respectively (Figure 27-1). When large enough, cysts can cause smooth remodeling of the inner table of the bony calvarium and osseous expansion. There may also be hypogenesis of the underlying brain parenchyma, most commonly described in the temporal lobe with middle cranial fossa cysts (Figure 27-2). Calcification is unusual, and enhancement should not be present.

The major differential consideration is an epidermoid cyst. On unenhanced T1-weighted images, an internal matrix, although subtle, is typically evident in epidermoid cysts. On fluid-attenuated inversion recovery (FLAIR) images, arachnoid cysts follow the signal intensity characteristics of CSF, whereas epidermoid cysts tend to be hyperintense relative to CSF. In addition, on diffusion-weighted images, arachnoid cysts are hypointense (similar to the CSF in the ventricles), resulting from an increased apparent diffusion coefficient, whereas epidermoid cysts do not have an increased apparent diffusion coefficient.

Reference

Sze G. Diseases of the intracranial meninges: MR imaging features. *AJR Am J Roentgenol.* 1993;160:727-733.

Cross-Reference

Neuroradiology: THE REQUISITES, 4th ed, pp 287-288.

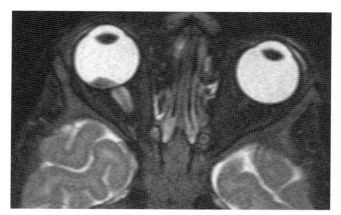

Figure 28-1

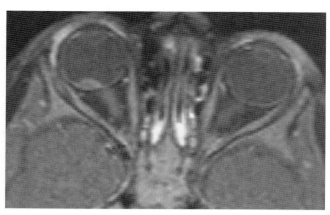

Figure 28-2

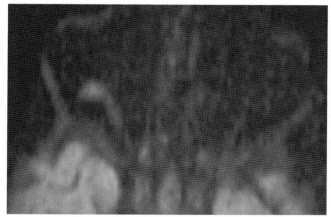

Figure 28-3

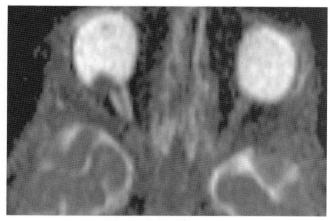

Figure 28-4

HISTORY: Leukocoria and strabismus.

1. What is the single best diagnosis in this case?
   A. Retinoblastoma
   B. Persistent hyperplastic primary vitreous (PHPV)
   C. Toxocaral endophthalmitis
   D. Coat disease

2. Where is the typical histology and location of the third tumor in trilateral retinoblastoma?
   A. Pituicytoma—Pituitary gland
   B. Retinoblastoma—Optic chiasm
   C. Primitive neuroectodermal tumor—Pineal gland
   D. Retinoblastoma—Pineal gland

3. How often are retinoblastomas bilateral?
   A. 1%
   B. 10%
   C. 30%
   D. 70%

4. What is the most common clinical presentation of retinoblastoma?
   A. Strabismus
   B. Severe vision loss
   C. Leukocoria
   D. Proptosis

CASE 28

Retinoblastoma

1. **A.** Retinoblastoma. There is an enhancing mass with restricted diffusion at the retina.

2. **C.** Primitive neuroectodermal tumor (PNET)—Pineal gland. The third tumor occurring in the autosomal dominant pattern of retinoblastoma is a pineoblastoma, which is a primitive neuroectodermal tumor, occurring in the pineal gland.

3. **C.** 30%.

4. **C.** Leukocoria. Approximately 50% to 60% of retinoblastomas manifest with leukocoria before vision loss. The other answer options are usually later findings.

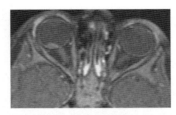

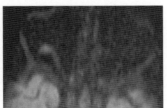

Comment

Presentation

Retinoblastoma represents the most common intraocular tumor in childhood. The typical clinical presentation is leukokoria, an abnormal pupillary reflex characterized by a "white" pupil. Other common clinical presentations include strabismus, decreased visual acuity, and eye pain (which may be related to glaucoma). The majority of retinoblastomas (98%) occur before 3 years of age. Retinoblastomas most commonly represent isolated sporadic tumors; however, they may be heritable in an autosomal dominant pattern. Up to 30% to 40% of patients with retinoblastoma have bilateral tumors; familial disease should be considered in these cases.

Imaging

Because the radiologic hallmark of retinoblastoma is the presence of intraocular calcification before the age of 3 years, computed tomography (CT) remains the best imaging modality for the detection of retinoblastoma. CT is also important in assessing the other eye for small calcifications. Magnetic resonance imaging (MRI) is not as sensitive in detecting calcification. This case shows a small retinoblastoma of the right eye with restricted diffusion (Figures 28-3 and 28-4). Not all retinoblastomas (particularly small ones) have calcification, so the absence of calcification does not exclude the possibility of retinoblastoma. Calcifications present as T2 hypointense foci in the posterior globe (Figure 28-1) and retinoblastoma will enhance with contrast (Figure 28-2). MRI plays an important role in assessing these patients because retinoblastoma can spread along the nerves and vessels to the retrobulbar orbit, and there may be subarachnoid seeding. Both modes of transmission can result in intracranial dissemination of disease. Therefore, patients with retinoblastoma should be evaluated with MRI to determine the extent of disease. A small percentage (<5%) of patients with bilateral retinoblastomas also have a pineoblastoma/PNET of the pineal gland (trilateral).

References

Brisse HJ, Lumbroso L, Freneaux PC, et al. Sonographic, CT, and MR imaging findings in diffuse infiltrative retinoblastoma: report of two cases with histological comparison. *AJNR Am J Neuroradiol.* 2001;22:499-504.

Tateishi U, Hasegawa T, Miyakawa K, et al. CT and MRI features of recurrent tumors and second primary neoplasms in pediatric patients with retinoblastoma. *AJR Am J Roentgenol.* 2003;181: 879-884.

Cross-Reference

Neuroradiology: THE REQUISITES, 4th ed, pp 318-319.

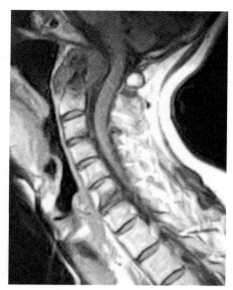

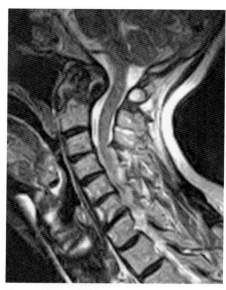

Figure 29-1 Patient A.

Figure 29-2 Patient A.

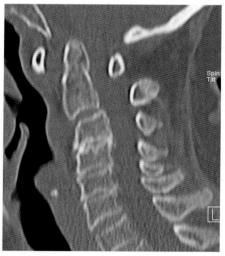

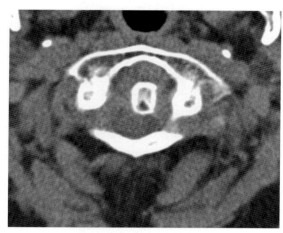

Figure 29-3 Patient B.

Figure 29-4 Patient B.

HISTORY:

Patient A: A 62-year-old woman with a 3-year history of progressive hand numbness and weakness presents with increased limitations with head rotation, stabbing neck pain, and occipital pain for the past 2 months.

Patient B: A 70-year-old woman presents with neck pain, Lhermitte sign, and upper extremity numbness.

1. Considering all of the imaging findings and *both* patient histories, what is the single best diagnosis?
   A. Chordoma
   B. Rheumatoid arthritis
   C. Plasmacytoma
   D. Hangman fracture

2. Which magnetic resonance imaging (MRI) sequence is most helpful in distinguishing between joint effusion and pannus in patients with this process in the craniocervical region?
   A. Proton density
   B. T2
   C. T2*GRE
   D. Post-contrast T1

3. In adults, what is the upper limit of normal for the atlanto-dental interval?
   A. 1 mm
   B. 2 mm
   C. 3 mm
   D. 4 mm

4. What is the appropriate recommendation regarding imaging for a clinician suspecting this disease in a patient?
   A. Obtain MRI. It is the appropriate first step.
   B. Discography may help differentiate inflammatory from proliferative arthritis.
   C. Bone scan is helpful to evaluate for metastatic disease.
   D. Radiographs should be obtained before using other imaging modalities.

CASE 29

Rheumatoid Arthritis

1. **B.** Rheumatoid arthritis. Although rheumatoid arthritis has a higher incidence, if calcium pyrophosphate deposition disease (CPPD) had been offered as an answer option, it would be an acceptable answer. Chordoma should appear as a hyperintensity on T2-weighted imaging. In the setting of diffuse arthritis, and the history, plasmacytoma is a less appealing choice. There is no fracture.

2. **D.** Post-contrast T1. Pannus enhances avidly.

3. **C.** 3 mm. The upper limit of normal for children is 4 mm.

4. **D.** Radiographs should be the first imaging examination following a good clinical examination. MRI should be obtained only after radiographs. Discography and bone scans have little if any role in the evaluation of arthritis.

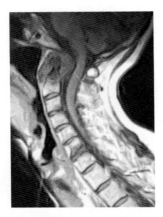

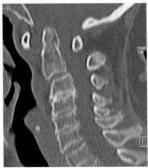

Comment

Background

Rheumatoid arthritis is a chronic systemic inflammatory disease; the cause is unknown. It is characterized by proliferative, hypervascularized synovitis, resulting in bone erosion, cartilage damage, and joint destruction. The atlantoaxial joint is commonly involved because it contains multiple synovial joints, resulting in erosion of the stabilizing ligaments of the atlantoaxial articulation, producing instability leading to spinal cord compromise. Pannus may also erode the bone and produce compression of the thecal sac and spinal cord. Facet joints may be involved as well, leading to instability within the spinal axis.

Histopathology

Proliferative synovitis (rheumatoid pannus) is the earliest pathologic abnormality in rheumatoid arthritis. Pannus is an inflammatory exudate overlying the lining layer of synovial cells on the inside of a joint; however, histologic findings in rheumatoid patients with inflamed synovium may vary from a fibrinous fluid collection in the joint space, to granulation tissue with abundant vessels, to dense fibrous tissue without proliferating vessels or edema.

Imaging

Lateral flexion and extension plain radiographs are initially used to evaluate the anterior atlantodental interval (posterior margins of the anterior C1 arch to the anterior aspect of the odontoid) and obtain an initial assessment to the classification of arthritis if rheumatoid arthritis is suspected. An interval of more than 3 mm in adults and 4 mm in children is considered abnormal. A computed tomography scan (Figures 29-1 and 29-2) is performed to obtain more accurate measurement in patients with abnormal radiographs. MRI (Figures 29-3 and 29-4) is performed to visualize the pannus better and to evaluate for spinal cord compression or spinal cord signal changes. There are four classifications of pannus on the basis of enhancement patterns: joint effusion, hypervascular pannus, hypovascular pannus, and fibrous pannus. These patterns have been detected even when plain radiographs are negative. Thickening of the ligaments and dura may also contribute to the mass-like appearance of pannus.

Management

Treatment goals are to avoid irreversible neurologic deficit and prevent sudden death (reported in 10% of patients). In asymptomatic patients, early aggressive medical management is important because cervical spine involvement correlates with disease activity. Symptomatic patients often require surgery to relieve compression and establish stability. Patients with atlantoaxial subluxation who are asymptomatic may be observed. In symptomatic patients, posterior atlantoaxial fusion can be performed if the subluxation is reducible. Patients with irreducible deformity can be treated with C1 laminectomy and transarticular stabilization.

References

Karhu JO, Parkkola RK, Koskinen SK. Evaluation of flexion/extension of the upper cervical spine in patients with rheumatoid arthritis: an MRI study with a dedicated positioning device compared to conventional radiographs. *Acta Radiol.* 2005;46(1):55-66.

Stiskal MA, Neuhold A, Szolar DH, et al. Rheumatoid arthritis of the craniocervical region by MR imaging: detection and characterization. *AJR Am J Roentgenol.* 1995;165(3):585-592.

Cross-Reference

Neuroradiology: THE REQUISITES, 4th ed, pp 498, 599.

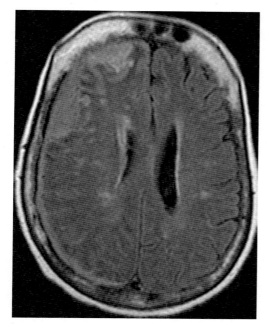

Figure 30-1

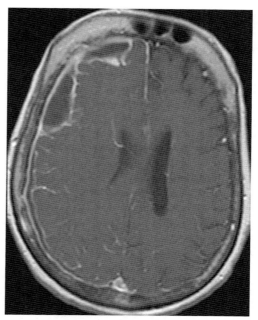

Figure 30-2

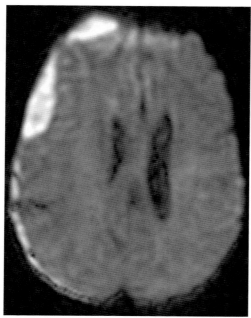

Figure 30-3

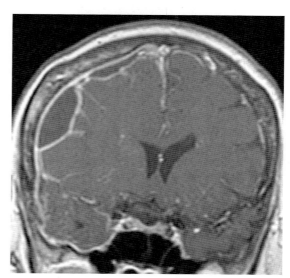

Figure 30-4

HISTORY: Fever and meningismus.

1. What is the best diagnosis of the extra-axial collections?
   A. Subdural empyema
   B. Cerebritis
   C. Meningitis
   D. Epidural abscess

2. Which one of the following is more commonly seen with epidural abscess rather than subdural empyema?
   A. Cerebritis
   B. Brain abscess
   C. Sinusitis
   D. Venous sinus thrombosis

3. What other process is present in this patient?
   A. Acute infarct
   B. Arachnoid cyst
   C. Ventriculitis
   D. Cerebritis

4. Which one of the following is the standard treatment for subdural empyema?
   A. Supportive care
   B. Decompressive craniotomy
   C. Surgical drainage and antibiotic therapy
   D. Antiobiotic treatment only

CASE 30

Subdural Empyema—Complicated by Cerebritis

1. **A.** Subdural empyema. There are peripherally enhancing subdural collections with restricted diffusion.

2. **C.** Sinusitis. A complication of sinusitis includes epidural abscess rather than subdural empyema. The other answer options would more likely be associated with subdural empyema.

3. **D.** Cerebritis. There is enhancement and T2-FLAIR (fluid-attenuated inversion recovery) signal abnormality in the brain parenchyma adjacent to the subdural empyema.

4. **C.** Surgical drainage and antibiotic therapy. These are the accepted treatment for subdural empyema.

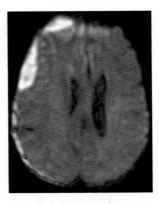

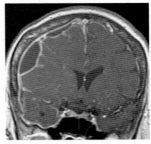

Comment

Interruption of the arachnoid meningeal barrier by infection leads to the formation of subdural empyemas. Mechanisms by which subdural empyemas can develop include rupture of a distended arachnoid villus into the subdural compartment, thrombophlebitis of a bridging cortical vein, hematogenous spread, and direct spread of an extracranial infection (sinusitis, otomastoiditis, osteomyelitis). These serious infections can also occur as a complication after craniotomy or in patients with meningitis. Epidural abscesses are most commonly caused by direct extension of infection from the paranasal sinuses or mastoid air cells. Of conditions affecting the paranasal sinuses, frontal sinusitis is probably the most common cause of intracranial epidural abscesses and subdural empyemas.

On imaging, these lesions share the common appearance of other extracerebral collections. Epidural abscesses (like hematomas) are contained by the cranial sutures and can cross the midline. In contrast, subdural hematomas do not spread across the midline because they are confined by the falx, allowing differentiation from epidural collections. On magnetic resonance imaging, these extracerebral infections are usually hypointense to isointense on T1-weighted imaging (depending on the protein concentration and the cellular content (Figures 30-2 and 30-4) and hyperintense relative to the brain on FLAIR and T2-weighted imaging (Figure 30-1). Empyemas typically are hyperintense on diffusion-weighted imaging (DWI) and have low apparent diffusion coefficients (ADCs), as in this case, whereas sterile subdural effusions are hypointense on DWI (Figure 30-3). There is usually prominent enhancement of thickened dura or a dural membrane (see Figures 30-2 and 30-4). Epidural and subdural empyemas may be complicated by cerebritis (as in this case, Figure 30-1) and intraparenchymal abscess formation (see Figures 30-1 through 30-4). In addition, dural venous or cortical vein thrombosis with venous infarction can occur. In the presence of suspected epidural abscess or subdural empyema, the radiologist (and the clinician!) should search for a site of origin of the infection, as well as its contiguous spread into the intracranial compartment.

Reference

Fountas KN, Duwayri Y, Kapsalaki E, et al. Epidural intracranial abscess as a complication of frontal sinusitis: case report and review of the literature. *South Med J.* 2004;97:279-282.

Cross-Reference

Neuroradiology: THE REQUISITES, 4th ed, pp 175-180.

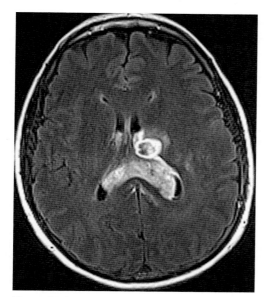

Figure 31-1

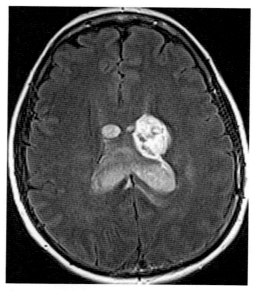

Figure 31-2

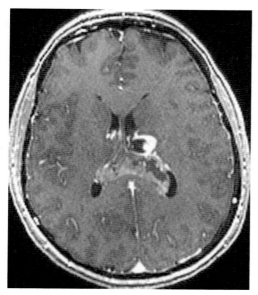

Figure 31-3

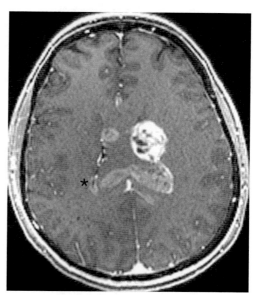

Figure 31-4

HISTORY: Mental status changes and new-onset seizure.

1. Included in the accepted treatment of this disease, which intravenous drug works by alkylating/methylating DNA and is often used concurrently with radiation?
   A. Erlotinib
   B. Carmustine wafers
   C. Temozolomide
   D. Bevacizumab

2. Which of the following is the *best* explanation for the corpus callosum's relative resistance to edema?
   A. White matter tracts are resistant to edema.
   B. Spread of edema is less facilitated in the horizontal direction.
   C. The orientation and compact nature of the white matter tract forming the corpus callosum limits edema.
   D. The location of the corpus callosum is less accessible to edema.

3. Regarding high-grade tumor monitoring, magnetic resonance imaging (MRI) perfusion has which of the following?
   A. High specificity to determine radiation necrosis
   B. High sensitivity to determine radiation necrosis
   C. High negative predictive value to determine tumor progression
   D. High positive predictive value to determine tumor progression and recurrence

4. Which of the following *best* describes the imaging findings of gliomatosis cerebri?
   A. Extensive enhancement
   B. Cortically based mass with associated calcification
   C. Extensive infiltrating glioma with gray and white matter involvement of more than two lobes and minimal or no enhancement
   D. Involves only gray matter

CASE 31

Glioblastoma of the Corpus Callosum: Butterfly Glioma

1. **C.** Temozolomide. This is an alkylating agent. Erlotinib is a tyrosine kinase inhibitor. Carmustine is an alkylating agent, but the wafers are used within the surgical resection cavity, not intravenously. Bevacizumab is an antiangiogenic agent.

2. **C.** The orientation and compact nature of the white matter tract forming the corpus callosum limits edema.

3. **D.** High positive predictive value to determine tumor progression and recurrence. If there is an increase in relative cerebral blood volume (rCBV), there is tumor present.

4. **C.** Extensive infiltrating glioma with gray and white matter involvement of more than two lobes and minimal or no enhancement.

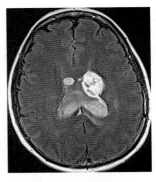

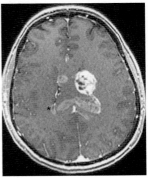

Comment

This case demonstrates findings characteristic of a butterfly glioma. There is a complex extensive mass with expansion of the splenium and body of the corpus callosum. Abnormal signal intensity and multiple more defined areas of necrotic mass are noted (Figures 31-1 and 31-2). Enhanced images better reveal the marked necrosis of certain portions of the tumor (Figures 31-3 and 31-4). Ventricular ependymal enhancement is shown.

Multicentric gliomas are uncommon, occurring in 1% to 5% of cases of glioblastoma (GBM). They can represent true separate lesions; however, more often they represent contiguous spread of tumor (which is the case in this patient). Multicentric gliomas may be synchronous (multiple lesions detected at the time of presentation) or metachronous (occurring at different times and pathologically discontinuous). Occasionally it is difficult to distinguish such gliomas from metastases on imaging. When separate lesions are identified, it is important to evaluate for the presence of continuity between the separate lesions on the basis of abnormal T2-weighted signal intensity. However, the connection might not be apparent on imaging and may be seen only on pathologic evaluation. There is an increased association of multicentric gliomas in neurofibromatosis type 1. In this case, a thin rind of ependymal enhancement is present along the body of the right lateral ventricle just medial to the asterisk (Figure 31-4). Of the infiltrative astrocytic tumors, GBM is most commonly associated with subependymal and ependymal spread.

Perfusion

Differentiating tumor recurrence from radiation necrosis is difficult. One process rarely occurs in isolation. Therefore progressive disease may also have necrosis. Tumor usually has increased perfusion, specifically rCBV. Necrosis has decreased perfusion. MRI perfusion has a high positive predictive value in detecting the presence of high-grade malignancy. If there is new increased perfusion after treatment, tumor is present.

Reference

Rees JH, Smirniotopoulos JG, Jones RV, Wong K. Glioblastoma multiforme: radiologic-pathologic correlation. *Radiographics*. 1996;16: 1413-1438.

Cross-Reference

Neuroradiology: THE REQUISITES, 4th ed, pp 59-62.

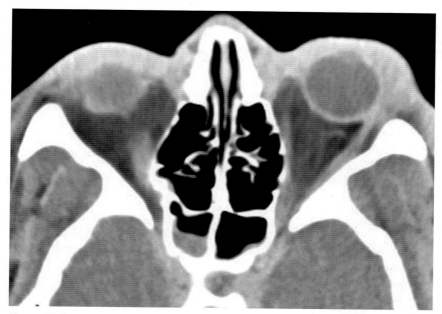

Figure 32-1

HISTORY: A young patient presents with a 1-week history of left eye swelling after an insect bite.

1. Which of the following is the single best diagnosis for the imaging findings presented?
   A. Periorbital cellulitis
   B. Orbital cellulitis
   C. Periorbital abscess
   D. Periosteal abscess

2. What is the structure that distinguishes periorbital cellulitis from orbital cellulitis?
   A. The globe
   B. The periosteum
   C. The sclera
   D. The septum

3. Which of the following is more common in periorbital cellulitis than in orbital cellulitis?
   A. Ophthalmoplegia
   B. Eyelid swelling
   C. Loss of vision
   D. Pain on eye movement

4. Why is distinguishing periorbital from orbital cellulitis important?
   A. Periorbital cellulitis increases the risk for optic neuritis.
   B. Orbital cellulitis may lead to periorbital cellulitis.
   C. Orbital cellulitis is a disease that must be treated surgically with incision and drainage, whereas periorbital cellulitis is not treated surgically.
   D. Orbital cellulitis must be treated with intravenous antibiotics, whereas periorbital cellulitis is treated with oral antibiotics.

CASE 32

Preseptal Cellulitis

1. **A.** Periorbital cellulitis. The inflammation is limited to the superficial tissues around the left eye.

2. **D.** The septum. The orbital septum is the structure that is violated when a periorbital cellulitis spreads to become an orbital cellulitis. Once the orbital septum has been violated, the infection is much more dangerous.

3. **B.** Eyelid swelling. Ophthalmoplegia, visual loss, pain on eye movement, and ischemic optic neuropathy may complicate orbital cellulitis.

4. **D.** Orbital cellulitis must be treated with intravenous antibiotics, whereas periorbital cellulitis is treated with oral antibiotics.

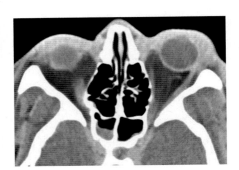

Comment

Symptoms of Periorbital Cellulitis

Periorbital cellulitis is best termed *preseptal cellulitis* to indicate that the infection remains anterior to the orbital septum (Figure 32-1). Orbital cellulitis, or *postseptal cellulitis,* is a more dangerous infection that can infiltrate the intraconal structures, including the optic nerve and sheath, and can lead to vascular complications as well. Visual loss, ophthalmoplegia, pain on eye movement, and proptosis may be clinical indications of orbital cellulitis, whereas periorbital cellulitis may manifest with eyelid swelling, superficial pain, and erythema.

Causes of Periorbital Cellulitis

The orbital septum is usually a fairly good barrier to the spread of infection. It is a membranous septum of fibrous tissue that is continuous with the periosteum in both a transverse direction and a craniocaudal direction. Periorbital cellulitis is usually caused by superficial pathogens such as puncture wounds, insect bites, dog bites, trauma, dermatitis, acne, or conjunctivitis, whereas the most common cause of orbital cellulitis is sinusitis. Sinusitis also occasionally causes periorbital cellulitis.

Treatment of Periorbital Cellulitis

Periorbital cellulitis is nearly 10 times more common than orbital cellulitis and is a milder infection, usually treated with oral antibiotics. The antibiotics prescribed cover the most common pathogens, usually *Staphylococcus aureus* (including methicillin-resistant *S. aureus* [MRSA]), *Streptococcus pneumoniae,* other streptococci, and anaerobes. If the patient does not respond in 24 to 48 hours after administration of antibiotics, imaging may be necessary to confirm or rule out spread from a preseptal location.

Complications of Sinusitis

This is the Chandler classification of orbital infections (derived from complications of sinusitis):

> Group I: preseptal cellulitis
> Group II: orbital cellulitis
> Group III: subperiosteal abscess
> Group IV: orbital abscess
> Group V: cavernous sinus thrombosis

Reference

Botting AM, McIntosh D, Mahadevan M. Paediatric pre- and post-septal peri-orbital infections are different diseases. A retrospective review of 262 cases. *Int J Pediatr Otorhinolaryngol.* 2008;72:377-383.

Cross-Reference

Neuroradiology: THE REQUISITES, 4th ed, p 338.

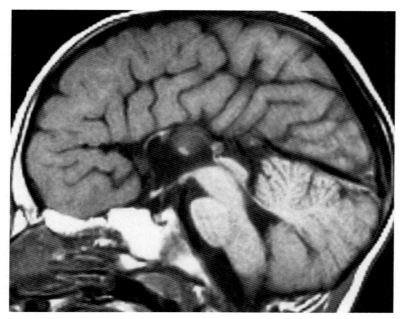

Figure 33-1

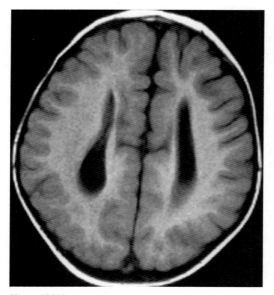

Figure 33-2

HISTORY: Developmental delay and seizures.

1. What is the single best diagnosis of the choices provided?
   A. Agenesis of the corpus callosum
   B. Hypoplasia of the corpus callosum
   C. Stretched corpus callosum
   D. Dandy-Walker syndrome

2. What structure is most often absent in association with this abnormality?
   A. Gyrus rectus
   B. Cingulate gyrus
   C. Posterior commissure
   D. Parahippocampal gyrus

3. Which of the following congenital anomalies is *least* likely associated with this entity?
   A. Lipomas
   B. Hemimegalencephaly
   C. Chiari malformation
   D. Dandy-Walker syndrome

4. What is conventionally thought of as the last part of the corpus callosum to form?
   A. Splenium
   B. Body
   C. Genu
   D. Rostrum

CASE 33

Agenesis of the Corpus Callosum

1. **A.** Agenesis of the corpus callosum. Parallel orientation of the lateral ventricles and presence of Probst bundles are seen. No ventriculomegaly or posterior fossa cystic space is identified.

2. **B.** Cingulate gyrus. Although multiple different malformations of gyration, sulcation, and migration can occur in patients with dysgenesis or agenesis of the corpus callosum, the most frequently affected structure is the cingulate gyrus.

3. **B.** Hemimegalencephaly. There is no association between hemimegalencephaly and callosal dysgenesis or agenesis. Lipomas, migrational abnormalities, Dandy-Walker syndrome, Chiari malformations, holoprosencephaly, and many others are associated with it.

4. **D.** Rostrum. This is thought to be the last part to form, although there is some debate as to the convention of ordered formation. Almost all patients with dysgenesis have some form of rostral abnormality.

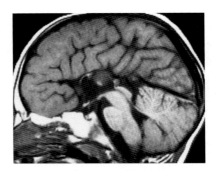

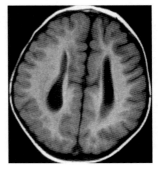

Comment

Axons arising from the right and left cerebral hemispheres grow into the lamina reuniens (the dorsal aspect of the lamina terminalis), giving rise to the corpus callosum (and the hippocampal commissures). The corpus callosum develops between the eleventh and twentieth gestational weeks in an organized manner, with formation of the anterior genu first, followed in order by the anterior body, posterior body, splenium, and rostrum. Given this pattern of development, in partial dysgenesis of the corpus callosum, the anterior portion is formed and partial dysgenesis affects the posterior portions (posterior body, splenium) and rostrum. In cases in which the splenium is very small or is not visualized, partial dysgenesis of the corpus callosum can be readily distinguished from an insult to a previously fully developed splenium by checking for the presence of the rostrum. If the rostrum is absent, the splenial abnormality corresponds to partial dysgenesis. However, if the rostrum is present, given that it forms after the splenium, a splenial abnormality must have occurred on the basis of an insult, resulting in secondary atrophy or volume loss.

Imaging findings in complete agenesis of the corpus callosum include lack of convergence of the lateral ventricles, which are displaced laterally and oriented in a vertical fashion (Figure 33-2); a high-riding third ventricle (which can form an interhemispheric cyst; Figure 33-1), and ex vacuo enlargement of the occipital and temporal horns (colpocephaly) related to deficient white matter. The Probst bundles are the white matter tracts that were destined to cross the corpus callosum (see Figure 33-2). The axons that would usually cross from right to left in the corpus callosum instead form tracts that run anterior to posterior along the medial walls of the lateral ventricles parallel to the interhemispheric fissure.

References

Lee SK, Mori S, Kim DJ, et al. Diffusion tensor MR imaging visualizes the altered hemispheric fiber connection in callosal dysgenesis. *AJNR Am J Neuroradiol.* 2004;25:25-28.

Quigley M, Cordes D, Turske P, et al. Role of the corpus callosum in functional connectivity. *AJNR Am J Neuroradiol.* 2003;24:208-212.

Cross-Reference

Neuroradiology: THE REQUISITES, 4th ed, pp 263-285.

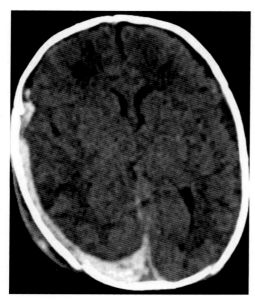

Figure 34-1

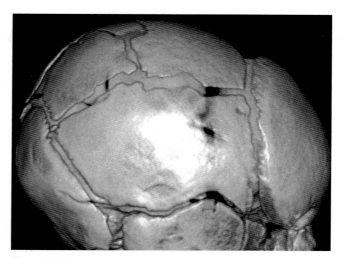

Figure 34-2

HISTORY: Irritable child.

1. What is the single best diagnosis?
   A. Vascular malformation
   B. Protein C deficiency
   C. Nonaccidental trauma
   D. Medulloblastoma

2. Which of the following cranial findings is often present in nonaccidental trauma?
   A. Lacerations of the scalp
   B. Skull fractures
   C. Dural venous sinus thrombosis
   D. Single vascular territory infarct

3. What finding in the eyes is characteristic of nonaccidental trauma?
   A. Retinal detachment
   B. Globe rupture
   C. Retinal hemorrhage
   D. Corneal tear

4. Which of the following is the most likely cause of a leptomeningeal cyst?
   A. Congenital malformation
   B. Calvarial fracture and dural tear
   C. Epidural hematoma and parenchymal laceration
   D. Subarachnoid hemorrhage

CASE 34

Nonaccidental Trauma: Child Abuse

1. **C.** Nonaccidental trauma. In the setting of subdural hematoma and skull fractures, this is the best answer choice.

2. **B.** Skull fractures. These are often depressed, potentially multiple, and potentially of different ages.

3. **C.** Retinal hemorrhage. Depending on the exact mechanism, each of the answer choices may be present, although the common mechanism including violent shaking results in retinal hemorrhage.

4. **B.** Calvarial fracture and dural tear. Cyst is a misnomer; this is actually evagination of (usually) encephalomalacic brain through the fracture in the calvarium, propagated by cerebrospinal fluid pulsations, and resulting in a lytic appearance.

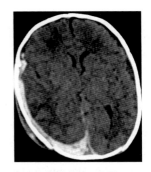

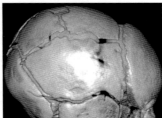

Comment

The presence of skull fractures or intracranial hemorrhage, particularly in children younger than 2 years, in the absence of known trauma to explain such injuries, should raise the suspicion of child abuse (nonaccidental trauma). More than 1 million cases of child abuse are reported each year, and closed head injury is among the leading causes of morbidity and death in these children. Approximately 10% of neurologic developmental delays can be attributed to nonaccidental trauma. Brain injury may be the result of direct trauma, aggressive shaking, or strangulation or suffocation. There is often little or no evidence of external trauma.

The most common type of intracranial hemorrhage in the setting of child abuse is a subdural hematoma (Figure 34-1), although subarachnoid hemorrhage, epidural hematoma, intraventricular hemorrhage, hemorrhagic cortical contusion, and diffuse axonal injury are all manifestations of nonaccidental trauma. Bilateral retinal hemorrhages are highly suggestive of child abuse (shaken baby syndrome). In the absence of significant head trauma, the presence of skull fractures (especially bilateral, depressed, or occipital fractures), which are found in as many as 45% of nonaccidental trauma cases, should raise suspicion for child abuse (Figure 34-2). Because it is not fully developed, the infant skull is extremely pliable and relatively resistant to fracture. In the worst case, diffuse cerebral edema resulting in mass effect and herniation can occur in nonaccidental trauma. Cerebral infarction can result from strangulation or anoxic-hypoxic injury, and vascular compromise may be caused by intracranial mass effect. Infarctions in multiple vascular territories should be viewed with suspicion.

The radiologist plays an important role in identifying nonaccidental head trauma. The clinical presentation can be nonspecific. The radiologist is sometimes in a position to suggest the possibility of child abuse. It is therefore important to know the spectrum of sometimes subtle imaging findings that may be encountered. Computed tomography (CT) of the head is regularly used. Repeat or serial imaging may be necessary. Brain magnetic resonance imaging (MRI) can contribute to the diagnostic work-up, particularly in the absence of characteristic CT findings.

References

Demaerel P, Casteels I, Wilms G. Cranial imaging in child abuse. *Eur Radiol.* 2002;12:849-857.

Mogbo KI, Slovis TL, Canady AI, et al. Appropriate imaging in children with skull fractures and suspicion of abuse. *Radiology.* 1998;208:521-524.

Cross-Reference

Neuroradiology: THE REQUISITES, 4th ed, pp 165-166.

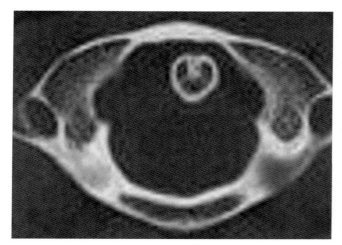

Figure 35-1

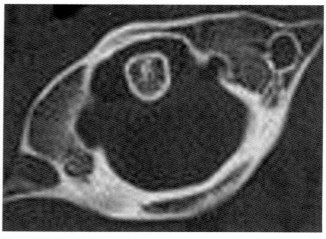

Figure 35-2

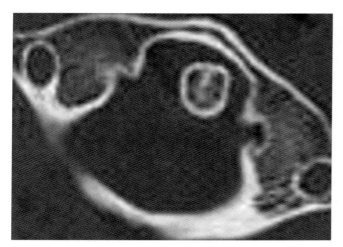

Figure 35-3

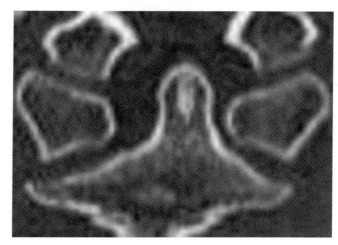

Figure 35-4

HISTORY: Neck pain.

1. What is the best diagnosis for the images provided?
   A. Jefferson fracture
   B. Atlantoaxial dislocation
   C. Atlantoaxial rotatory subluxation
   D. Hangman fracture

2. Which imaging technique is recommended for establishing the diagnosis of atlantoaxial rotatory fixation?
   A. Magnetic resonance imaging (MRI) with head rotation
   B. Computed tomography (CT) with head rotation
   C. Radiography
   D. Ultrasound

3. Which of the following is not a cause of acquired, nondystonic torticollis?
   A. Atlantoaxial rotatory subluxation
   B. Anterior atlantoaxial dislocation
   C. C2-C3 rotatory dislocation
   D. Cranial settling

4. What is Grisel syndrome?
   A. Atlantoaxial rotatory deformity resulting from trauma
   B. Atlantoaxial rotatory deformity associated with hemihypertrophy
   C. Atlantoaxial rotatory deformity resulting from infection
   D. Atlantoaxial rotatory deformity and mental retardation

CASE 35

Atlantoaxial Rotatory Deformity

1. **C.** Atlantoaxial rotatory subluxation. There is no fracture or dislocation.

2. **B.** CT with head rotation. Low-dose CT with head in a neutral position and with rotation maximally to each side is recommended.

3. **D.** Cranial settling. This is not a cause for nondystonic torticollis.

4. **C.** Atlantoaxial rotatory deformity resulting from infection. Grisel syndrome classically results from nasopharyngeal infection.

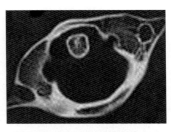

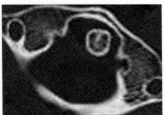

Comment

Background

Atlantoaxial rotatory deformity (Figures 35-1 through 35-4) is a spectrum of disorders. Atlantoaxial rotatory dislocation generally refers to complete dislocation of the C1-C2 facet joints. Rotational deformity of the C1-C2 joints within the physiologic range of motion has been referred to as atlantoaxial rotatory displacement by Fielding and Hawkins (other authors prefer the term *rotary subluxation*). In this deformity, the joints are not dislocated. If this condition persists and becomes fixed (refractory to nonoperative management), it is referred to as atlantoaxial rotatory fixation.

Pathophysiology

Rotatory deformity may result from infection, trauma, and other conditions, or it may arise spontaneously (as in this case).

Imaging

Recognizing the importance of transverse ligament integrity in determining the degree of canal compromise that can accompany rotational deformities, Fielding and Hawkins described four types of rotatory fixation, as follows:

> Type I: Rotatory fixation with no anterior displacement (see Figures 35-1 through 35-4). The transverse ligament is intact, and the odontoid acts as the pivot.
> Type II: Rotatory fixation with anterior displacement of 3 to 5 mm. The transverse ligament is mildly deficient or lax, and one facet acts as the pivot.
> Type III: Rotatory fixation with anterior displacement of more than 5 mm. The transverse ligament and alar ligaments are deficient.
> Type IV: Rotatory fixation with posterior displacement. This is rare; the only case reported by Fielding and Hawkins was in an adult with rheumatoid arthritis and absence of the dens because of erosion.

Management

Nonoperative treatment includes soft collar and antiinflammatory medications. If subluxation persists, head traction may be required. Operative treatment (posterior C1-C2 fusion) is considered when subluxation persists more than 3 months or if neurologic deficit is present.

References

Currier BL. Atlantoaxial rotatory deformities. In: Levine AM, Eismont FJ, Garfin SR, et al., eds. *Spine Trauma*. Philadelphia: Saunders; 1998:249-267.

Eran A, Yousem DM, Izbudak I. Asymmetry of the odontoid lateral mass interval in pediatric trauma CT: do we need to investigate further? *AJNR Am J Neuroradiol.* 2016;37:176-179.

Fielding JW, Hawkins RJ. Atlanto-axial rotatory fixation. Fixed rotatory subluxation of the atlanto-axial joint. *J Bone Joint Surg Am.* 1977; 59:37-44.

Kowalski HM, Cohen WA, Cooper P, et al. Pitfalls in the CT diagnosis of atlantoaxial rotary subluxation. *AJR Am J Roentgenol.* 1987; 149(3):595-600.

Cross-Reference

Neuroradiology: THE REQUISITES, 4th ed, p 598.

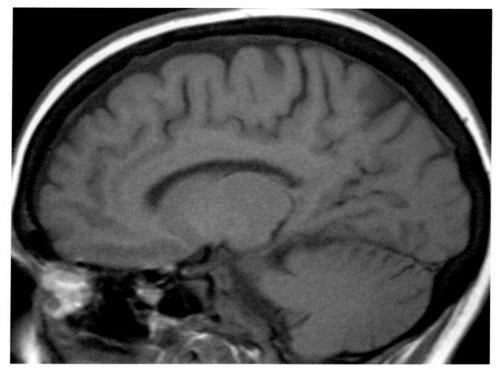

Figure 36-1

HISTORY: Chronic renal failure with fatigue.

1. What would be the *least* likely diagnosis for these imaging findings?
   A. Chronic anemia
   B. Diffuse metastasis
   C. Hematologic malignancies
   D. Radiation changes

2. In children with sickle cell disease, what noninvasive test is often used to monitor for changes in the intracranial vasculature?
   A. Magnetic resonance angiography (MRA)
   B. Computed tomographic angiography (CTA)
   C. Transcranial Doppler (TCD)
   D. Electromyography (EMG)

3. Aside from signal changes in the marrow spaces, what other structural change may occur?
   A. Development of paraspinal masses
   B. Decreased size of the spleen
   C. Thinning of the calvarium
   D. Elongation of long bones

4. What is the cause of hypointense marrow on T1-weighted imaging in chronic anemia?
   A. Infiltrative neoplastic cells
   B. Increased fat content within the marrow
   C. Hematopoietic marrow in response to chronic blood loss
   D. Renal osteodystrophy

CASE 36

Chronic Anemia: Diffuse Replacement of Fat in the Calvarial Marrow

1. **D.** Radiation changes. This would cause T1 hyperintense marrow signal due to fatty replacement of the marrow. T1 hypointense marrow signal is a nonspecific finding and can be seen with hematologic processes such as chronic anemia, primary hematologic malignancies, myelofibrosis, granulomatous diseases such as sarcoid, and neoplastic processes such as metastasis.

2. **C.** TCD. Transcranial Doppler is a noninvasive examination that measures velocities and resistance of blood flow within the intracranial arteries. This is an indirect measure of luminal caliber and therefore predictive of vascular insults. It guides the practice of transfusion therapy.

3. **A.** Development of paraspinal masses. This is a manifestation of extramedullary hematopoiesis.

4. **C.** Hematopoietic marrow in response to chronic blood loss. The marrow in this chronic anemia case appears hypointense on T1-weighted imaging. In contrast, increased fat content causes marrow to appear hyperintense on T1-weighted images.

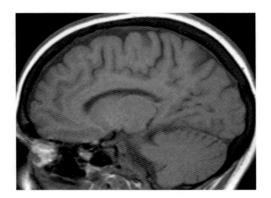

Comment

The normal signal intensity of marrow is dependent on the ratio of cells, fat, and water. In children, hematopoietic (red) marrow has a high cell-to-fat ratio and appears hypointense on imaging (Figure 36-1). As we age, the amount of fat increases such that by early adulthood the marrow has undergone fatty conversion (yellow marrow), and on T1-weighted images, it appears isointense to hyperintense to white matter. Unenhanced T1-weighted imaging is probably the best way to assess for marrow abnormalities, especially because it is part of all standard brain magnetic resonance imaging protocols.

Hematopoietic (red) marrow is composed of approximately 40% fat, 40% water, and 20% protein; in contrast, inactive fatty (yellow) marrow contains approximately 80% fat, 10% to 15% water, and 5% to 10% protein. On unenhanced T1-weighted images, yellow marrow shows high signal intensity relative to that of muscle; it approaches the intensity of subcutaneous fat. Cellular red marrow has intermediate signal intensity and may be isointense or slightly hyperintense relative to muscle. Marrow conversion represents a normal process in which yellow marrow gradually replaces red marrow. At birth, marrow is predominantly red in both the appendicular and axial skeletons. In the appendicular skeleton, most of the marrow has undergone conversion by the time a person is 21 years of age. Residual red marrow is found in the proximal metaphyses of the femurs and humeri. In the axial skeleton in adults, a larger portion of the marrow remains hematopoietic compared with marrow in the appendicular skeleton.

In severe cases of anemia, especially those anemias causing failure of erythropoiesis in the marrow, extramedullary hematopoiesis may occur. This usually manifests as hepatosplenomegaly although it can affect many more organs. Development of paraspinal masses may occur as hematopoietic centers. When this occurs, there is usually marked expansion of the ribs.

The differential diagnosis of diffuse replacement of the fatty marrow with hypointense tissue (cells or water) includes hematologic malignancies (lymphoma, leukemia, and myeloma); granulomatous disease (sarcoid and tuberculosis); chronic anemias, such as thalassemia, sickle cell disease, or chronic blood loss; and AIDS (hypointense marrow has been attributed to several factors, including chronic anemia and low CD4 counts). Metastases can diffusely replace the marrow (most common with breast carcinoma in women and prostate carcinoma in men). More often, metastatic disease occurs with multiple focal lesions.

References

Loevner LA, Tobey JD, Yousem DM, et al. MR imaging characteristics of cranial bone marrow in adults with underlying systemic disorders compared with healthy controls. *Am J Neuroradiol.* 2002;23:248-254.

Ricci C, Cova M, Kang YS, et al. Normal age-related patterns of cellular and fatty bone marrow distribution in the axial skeleton: MR imaging study. *Radiology.* 1990;177:83-88.

Cross-Reference

Neuroradiology: THE REQUISITES, 4th ed, p 538.

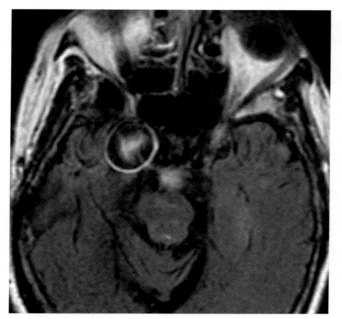

Figure 37-1

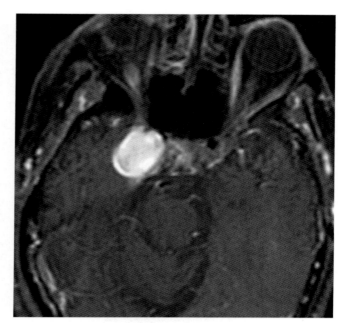

Figure 37-2

HISTORY: Right-sided cranial nerve palsy and painful ophthalmoplegia.

1. What is the single best diagnosis of the case?
   A. Giant aneurysm
   B. Glioma
   C. Meningioma
   D. Schwannoma

2. What location for aneurysm occurrence, all other variables controlled, has the lowest mortality?
   A. Cavernous internal carotid artery
   B. Tip of the basilar artery
   C. Posterior communicating artery
   D. Anterior communicating artery

3. What is the definition of a giant aneurysm?
   A. >1 cm
   B. >1.5 cm
   C. >2 cm
   D. >2.5 cm

4. What is a clinical presentation of unruptured cavernous internal carotid artery aneurysms?
   A. Painful ophthalmoplegia
   B. Blindness
   C. Subarachnoid hemorrhage
   D. Cavernous-carotid fistula

CASE 37

Giant Aneurysm: Middle Cerebral Artery

1. **A.** Giant aneurysm. Large flow void on the T1-weighted sequence, which enhances after contrast administration, is in keeping with a large right cavernous sinus aneurysm.

2. **A.** Cavernous internal carotid artery. The extradural location results commonly in a cavernous carotid fistula rather than subarachnoid hemorrhage.

3. **D.** >2.5 cm. This is considered a giant aneurysm.

4. **A.** Painful ophthalmoplegia. This and cranial nerve palsies are typical presentations of cavernous carotid artery aneurysms. Cavernous-carotid fistula occurs when ruptured. Blindness is not attributed to the cavernous segment aneurysms.

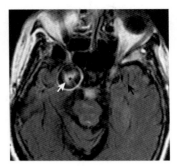

Figure S37-1

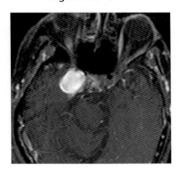

Comment

The middle cerebral artery bifurcation or trifurcation has a propensity for the development of giant aneurysms. Giant aneurysms can manifest with subarachnoid hemorrhage or symptoms caused by mass effect (nausea, vomiting, focal neurologic deficits) related to aneurysm size or intraparenchymal rupture or hematoma.

A thrombus can form within large aneurysms and may be a source of distal emboli. Unenhanced computed tomography (CT) can show the giant aneurysm as a hyperdense mass. At its periphery, there may be heterogeneous density related to the presence of thrombus. On magnetic resonance imaging, giant aneurysms have a characteristic appearance, as in this case. Findings include signal void consistent with flow in the patent lumen (Figure S37-1, *asterisk*); phase artifact related to arterial pulsation, as is seen in this case (Figure S37-1, *black arrow*); and heterogeneous signal intensity representing thrombi of varying ages (Figure S37-1, *white arrow*). Postcontrast images show enhancement of the aneurysm, but presence of pulsation (phase) artifact argues against a neoplasm (Figure 37-2).

Recent investigations with CT angiography in the setting of subarachnoid hemorrhage have shown detection rates for all aneurysms as high as 96%. False-negative findings may be related to CT angiography technique, aneurysm size (especially those <3 mm), and aneurysm location. Aneurysms originating from the posterior communicating artery, the infraclinoid internal carotid artery, and the ophthalmic artery that are in close proximity to bone now are readily detected because bone subtraction techniques have been improved. Advantages of CT angiography include its rapidity, noninvasiveness, ability to provide information about potential neuroangiographic intervention, and ability to provide preoperative information about the relationship of an aneurysm to adjacent bony landmarks. Catheter angiography is still the most commonly used technique and the accepted standard in the assessment of acute subarachnoid hemorrhage. Although angiography will adequately assess the patent lumen, it cannot evaluate the true size of these aneurysms because the thrombosed portions are not visualized. Combining angiographic images with dynamic CT utilizing modern flat panel fluoroscopic equipment yields higher specificity when interrogating intracranial aneurysms and may allow for improved pre-treatment planning. Magnetic resonance angiography (MRA) is also a widely used technique for the evaluation of intracranial aneurysms. This can be performed without or with contrast.

Reference

Jayaraman MV, Mayo-Smith WW, Tung GA, et al. Detection of intracranial aneurysms: multi-detector row CT angiography compares with DSA. *Radiology.* 2004;230:510-518.

Cross-Reference

Neuroradiology: THE REQUISITES, 4th ed, pp 366-367.

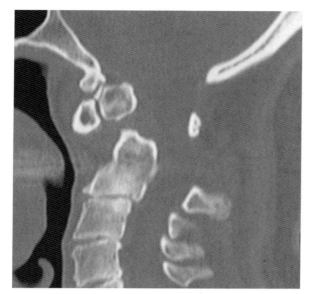

Figure 38-1

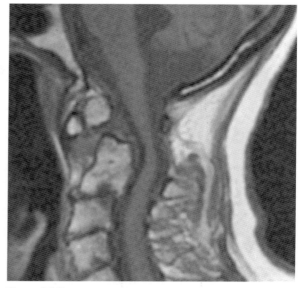

Figure 38-2

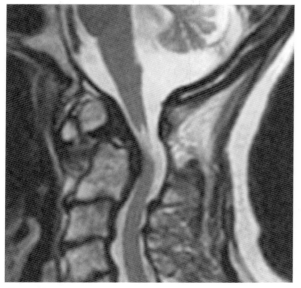

Figure 38-3

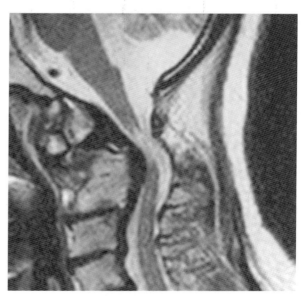

Figure 38-4

HISTORY: A 66-year-old woman presents with a history of neck pain for the past 2 months and a fall 3 years prior.

1. What is the most likely diagnosis for this entity?
   A. Klippel-Feil syndrome
   B. Atlantoaxial subluxation
   C. Odontoid nonunion
   D. Persistent ossiculum terminale

2. Which of the following is the most common type of odontoid fracture based on the Anderson and D'Alonzo classification?
   A. Type I
   B. Type II
   C. Type III
   D. Type IV

3. Which of the following is a risk factor for odontoid fracture nonunion in adults?
   A. Young age of patient
   B. Adequate halo immobilization
   C. Ability to reduce the fracture
   D. Increased displacement or angulation of fracture fragments

4. Which of the following statements regarding odontoid fracture is true?
   A. Type III fractures are usually stable.
   B. In asymptomatic older adult patients, surgical treatment is recommended.
   C. Type I fractures are the most common.
   D. Nonunion occurs most frequently with type I fracture.

CASE 38

Odontoid Nonunion

1. **C.** Odontoid nonunion. Posttraumatic changes related to an os odontoideum would also be within the differential. There are no bony changes that are characteristic of Klippel-Feil, and the atlantoaxial interval is maintained. An ossiculum terminale is not associated with any instability.

2. **B.** Type II. Type I is the least common, and there is no type IV.

3. **D.** Increased displacement or angulation of fracture fragments. The other answers are good prognostic characteristics for union.

4. **A.** Type III fractures are usually stable. Type I fractures are usually stable as well. Type II fractures are usually unstable, which is why nonunion occurs most frequently in Type II.

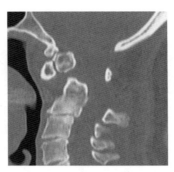

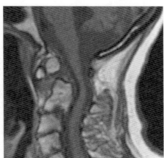

Comment

Background

Odontoid fractures account for 10% to 15% of all cervical spine fractures. In elderly patients, odontoid fracture can be caused by minimal trauma. The incidence of odontoid fracture nonunion following conservative treatment may be 63%. Nonunion may predispose to a myelopathy secondary to the resultant instability of the atlantoaxial joint.

Pathophysiology

The Anderson and D'Alonzo classification of odontoid fractures describes three types of fractures: type I, an oblique fracture through the upper portion of the odontoid; type II, a transverse fracture through the base of the odontoid; and type III, a fracture through the body of the axis. The importance of the classification is that type II fractures, which are the most common, may be unstable, whereas type III fractures are usually stable and heal with conservative treatment. Nonunion occurs most frequently with type II fractures. Atlantoaxial subluxation may occur with or without odontoid displacement.

Imaging

Plain radiography can be used to assess atlantoaxial subluxation and stability. Computed tomography scan (Figure 38-1) can provide information on the chronicity of the fracture, the size of the gap between the fracture fragment and odontoid, and the presence of atlantoaxial subluxation. Magnetic resonance imaging can evaluate for spinal cord compression, spinal cord signal changes, and the presence or absence of mechanical compression during flexion and extension (Figures 38-2 through 38-4). Posttraumatic fracture fragment and congenital os odontoideum may be indistinguishable if the fracture is old and has smooth sclerotic margins similar to the ossicle. In patients with os odontoideum, hypoplasia of the dens is almost always present, and often there is a wide gap between the dens and the ossicle. Additional findings that favor the diagnosis of os odontoideum are hypertrophy of the anterior arch of C1, which may be associated with clefting and absence of the posterior arch of C1.

Management

Odontoid nonunion is a potentially hazardous complication that can lead to neurologic deficits months or years later. In general, odontoid nonunion should be managed surgically.

References

Blacksin MF, Avagliano P. Computed tomographic and magnetic resonance imaging of chronic odontoid fractures. *Spine (Phila Pa 1976)*. 1999;24(2):158-161.

Koivikko MP, Kiuru MJ, Koskinen SK, et al. Factors associated with nonunion in conservatively-treated type-II fractures of the odontoid process. *J Bone Joint Surg Br*. 2004;86(8):1146-1151.

Cross-Reference

Neuroradiology: THE REQUISITES, 4th ed, p 601.

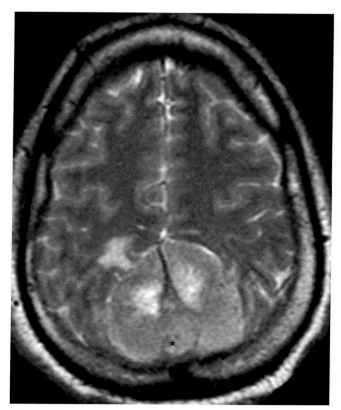

Figure 39-1

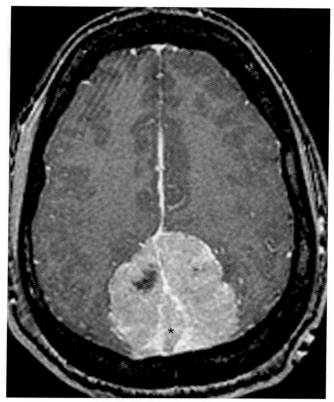

Figure 39-2

HISTORY: Headaches and papilledema.

1. What should *not* be included in the differential diagnosis of the case?
   A. Glioblastoma
   B. Lymphoma with dural venous sinus invasion
   C. Hemangiopericytoma
   D. Metastasis

2. What is a potential imaging finding related to intracranial hypertension?
   A. Bulging of the diaphragma sellae
   B. Tortuosity of the optic nerve–sheath complex
   C. Enlarged extra-axial spaces
   D. Dural enhancement

3. The *least* advantageous vascular imaging technique for assessing superior sagittal sinus patency is which of the following?
   A. Two-dimensional time-of-flight magnetic resonance angiography (MRA) in the coronal plane
   B. Two-dimensional time-of-flight MRA in the sagittal plane
   C. Contrast-enhanced magnetic resonance venogram (MRV)
   D. Two-dimensional phase-contrast MRV

4. Tumor control for this diagnosis utilizing stereotactic radio-surgery is advocated for which of the following?
   A. Tumors larger than 3 cm
   B. Convexity tumors
   C. Skull-base tumors
   D. Younger patients

CASE 39

Parafalcine Meningioma Invading the Superior Sagittal Sinus

1. **A.** Glioblastoma. The differential for an extra-axial dural-based mass would include meningioma, metastasis, hemangiopericytoma, and lymphoma.

2. **B.** Tortuosity of the optic nerve–sheath complex. Additionally, partially empty sella, papilledema, or flattening of the optic disc, and venous sinus stenosis are potential imaging findings of intracranial hypertension.

3. **B.** Two-dimensional time-of-flight MRA in the sagittal plane. This technique is most susceptible to dephasing of signal in the imaging slice acquired. To view the superior sagittal sinus, if performing the two-dimensional time-of-flight technique, it should be performed in the coronal plane to avoid transverse dephasing. The other techniques are better options for imaging of the superior sagittal sinus.

4. **C.** Skull-base tumors. Gamma knife or stereotactic radiosurgery is currently advocated primarily for tumor control or for small tumors at the skull base and in other patients who are at high operative risk. Surgery for resection is the mainstay of treatment.

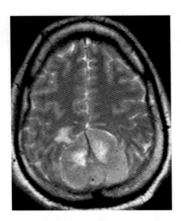

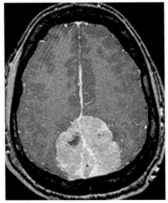

Comment

This case shows a well-demarcated extra-axial mass (cerebrospinal fluid [CSF] cleft separating the mass from the brain on T2-weighted image; Figure 39-1) in the posterior interhemispheric fissure along the falx cerebri. The mass is predominantly isointense to gray matter (because of its cellularity; see Figure 39-1) and enhances avidly (Figure 39-2), with the exception of a few small areas of cystic degeneration (T2-weighted hyperintense region on Figure 39-1, nonenhancing regions on Figure 39-2). Enhancing tumor obliterates the superior sagittal sinus.

In trying to determine the cause of this lesion, it is important to view the remainder of the brain as well as the calvaria to look for other abnormalities. This is because the vast majority of malignant extra-axial neoplasms are caused by bone metastases. Destructive or infiltrative lesions within the calvaria that can affect the inner and outer cortical tables should be sought. In addition, metastases may be associated with extraosseous soft tissue masses within the scalp. The finding of multiple lesions within the calvaria suggests the presence of metastatic disease. Additional malignant extra-axial masses include metastases and lymphoma (which can involve the leptomeninges, dura, or bone). Finally, the absence of significant associated vasogenic edema in this case makes a malignant process unlikely. The opposite is not true, however; the presence of significant vasogenic edema would support meningioma or a more aggressive neoplasm (e.g., metastases, lymphoma).

The most common cause of an extra-axial neoplasm in adults is meningioma. Although meningiomas can demonstrate changes along the inner table of the skull (hyperostosis and, less commonly, lysis), a dural-based mass in the absence of disease involving the diploic space or the outer table of the skull still favors meningioma (as do statistics).

References

Takeguchi T, Miki H, Shimizu T, et al. The dural tail of intracranial meningiomas on fluid-attenuated inversion-recovery images. *Neuroradiology.* 2004;46:130-135.

Tsuchiya K, Katase S, Yoshino A, Hachiay J. MR digital subtraction angiography in the diagnosis of meningiomas. *Eur J Radiol.* 2003;46:130-138.

Cross-Reference

Neuroradiology: THE REQUISITES, 4th ed, pp 41-42.

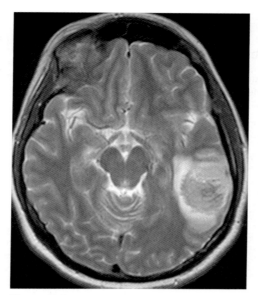

Figure 40-1

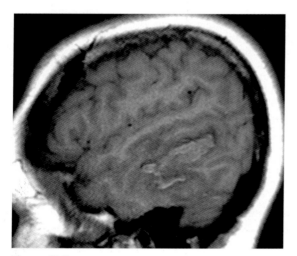

Figure 40-2

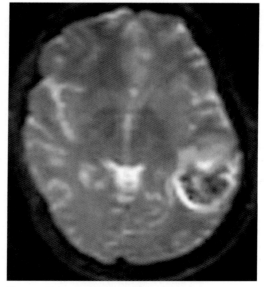

Figure 40-3

HISTORY: Headaches and focal neurologic deficit.

1. What is the *least* favorable disease process in the differential diagnosis of the case?
   A. Venous infarct
   B. Aneurysm hemorrhage
   C. Hemorrhagic contusion
   D. Amyloid
   E. Cavernoma

2. In hypercoagulable states related to antiphospholipid antibodies, are cerebral arterial or venous infarcts more common?
   A. Arterial infarct
   B. Venous infarct
   C. They are equally common.
   D. Neither is associated with a hypercoagulable state.

3. What kidney disorder is associated with a hypercoagulable state?
   A. Nephritic syndrome
   B. Chronic renal failure
   C. Polycystic kidney disease
   D. Nephrotic syndrome

4. The contrast in Figure 40-1, a T2-weighted image, is formed predominately from which of the following?
   A. Regrowth of longitudinal magnetization after a radiofrequency (RF) pulse
   B. Decay of longitudinal magnetization after an RF pulse
   C. Regrowth of transverse magnetization after an RF pulse
   D. Decay of transverse magnetization after an RF pulse

CASE 40

Hemorrhagic Venous Infarction

1. **B.** Aneurysm hemorrhage. Intraparenchymal hemorrhage from aneurysm is rare, less common than the other answer choices, especially in this location.

2. **A.** Arterial infarct. This is more common than venous infarct in antiphospholipid antibody syndrome.

3. **D.** Nephrotic syndrome. The hypercoagulable state is multifactorial and includes the combined effects of endothelial injury, platelet hyperaggregability, and abnormalities in the coagulation cascade (such as protein C or S deficiency).

4. **D.** Decay of transverse magnetization after an RF pulse. After one T2-weighted period, 63% of magnetization has decayed as a result of spin-spin relaxation properties. In spin echo techniques, transverse magnetization is 99% decayed after five T2-weighted times.

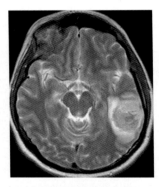

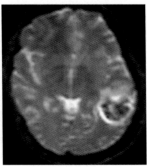

Comment

This case illustrates a hemorrhagic venous infarction in the left temporal lobe (Figures 40-1 through 40-3). Unlike arterial infarctions, the anatomic territories for venous occlusive disease are less consistent than with the territory supplied by arteries. Several findings should raise the suspicion of a venous infarct: the presence of hemorrhage, especially in the white matter or at the gray-white matter interface (see Figure 40-2); the presence of an abnormality that is not in a single arterial distribution; and an infarct in a young patient. This patient had acute thrombosis of the vein of Labbé and the distal left transverse sinus. The hemorrhagic infarct in the left temporal lobe is in the territory drained by the vein of Labbé.

Symptoms of venous occlusion are related to the rate at which collateral venous drainage is established, the location of the clot, and the rate of clot formation. Because of the network of venous collaterals in the brain, if the venous occlusive process is slow enough to allow time for collateral circulation to develop, the patient might remain asymptomatic. However, in the setting of acute occlusion of a large vein or dural venous sinus, venous congestion will result in back-pressure that extends to the capillary bed, where the flow will be diminished such that there is ischemia and, if the diminished flow is severe enough, infarction.

Before magnetic resonance imaging and computed tomographic (CT) venography, the diagnosis of venous occlusive disease was more difficult, and a high index of suspicion was necessary. Many conventional CT findings have been described (including the delta sign, in which there is enhancement around the clot or filling defect in the sinus, and the cord sign, in which high density is seen in a venous sinus or vein); however, they are inconsistent.

References

Hashemi RH, Bradley WG Jr, Lisanti CJ. T1, T2, and T2*. In: *MRI: The Basics*. 3rd ed. Philadelphia: Lippincott Williams & Wilkins; 2010:40-47.

Tong KA, Ashwal S, Obenaus A, et al. Susceptibility-weighted MR imaging: a review of clinical applications. *Am J Neuroradiol*. 2008;29:9-17.

Cross-Reference

Neuroradiology: THE REQUISITES, 4th ed, pp 137, 146.

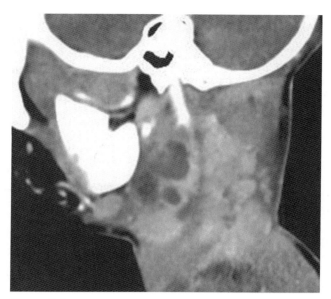

Figure 41-1

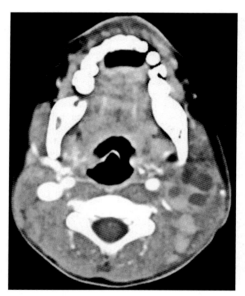

Figure 41-2

HISTORY: A child presents with fever, neck swelling, and tenderness.

1. Which of the following should *not* be included in the differential diagnosis for the imaging findings and clinical presentation?
   A. Necrotizing adenitis
   B. Infected lymphatic malformation
   C. Abscess
   D. Rhabdomyosarcoma

2. What percentage of lymphatic malformations manifest before age 3?
   A. Less than 25%
   B. 26% to 50%
   C. 51% to 75%
   D. More than 75%

3. In children, for which space in the neck do lymphatic malformations have a predilection?
   A. Submandibular space
   B. Visceral space
   C. Posterior triangle
   D. Masticator space

4. In which infection do lymph nodes commonly become necrotic?
   A. Epstein-Barr virus (EBV)
   B. Cat scratch disease
   C. Toxoplasmosis
   D. Tuberculosis

CASE 41

Necrotizing Adenitis

1. **D.** Rhabdomyosarcoma. All of the other lesions could cause an inflamed multiloculated "mass" in a child. In an adult, the differential diagnosis would probably not include a lymphatic malformation.

2. **D.** More than 75%. The classical teaching is that 90% of lymphatic malformations manifest before the age of 2. Some are being diagnosed through fetal magnetic resonance imaging (MRI).

3. **C.** Posterior triangle. Lymphatic malformations tend to develop in the posterior triangle and the axilla. They also develop in the orbits.

4. **D.** Tuberculosis. Tuberculosis is the infection that classically causes necrotic infectious adenopathy. However, any of the mycobacterial infections can also do so. Because staphylococcal and streptococcal infections are more common than tuberculosis in the United States, they are also common sources of necrotizing adenitis.

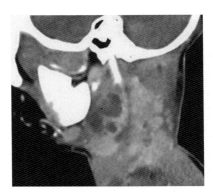

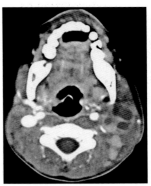

Comment

Types of Necrotic Masses

In a child with a necrotic mass in the soft tissues of the neck that is unassociated with the mucosa or the Waldeyer ring and that appears to be inflammatory, the clinician should consider several entities. The most common lesion is necrotizing adenitis. Children have a propensity for necrotic adenopathy, which is often seen with pharyngitis and classically may be located in the retropharyngeal space. Staphylococcal and streptococcal infections, by virtue of being so common, are the pathogens most commonly associated with necrotic adenopathy. Nonetheless, the clinician should also assess for mycobacterial and fungal infections, which cause a high rate of lymph node necrosis.

Differential Diagnosis

In this case, the debate was whether this infection had an underlying lesion because of the multiloculated nature of the process. The clinician should consider underlying lymphatic malformation, although most such malformations are located in the posterior triangle of the neck or extend to the axilla (Figures 41-1 and 41-2). Another alternative would be an infected second branchial cleft cyst (BCC), but necrotic adenopathy usually has more solid tissue associated with it than classic Bailey type 2 BCC. To call this an abscess with associated lymphadenopathy is not wrong, but it does not clarify the source. Most pediatric abscesses are associated with pharyngitis, tonsillitis, dental lesions, or puncture wounds; otherwise, there is no reason for an infection to develop de novo in the soft tissues of the neck. The clinician should therefore investigate the possibility of an underlying lesion unless there is a puncture wound, a fistula, or a dermal appendage infection, for example. That is why most of these infections are thought to represent necrotizing adenitis.

Lymphatic Malformations

Of all lymphatic malformations, 90% manifest before the age of 3. Microcytic and macrocytic (spaces >2 cm) varieties exist. Treatment of the macrocytic varieties may include sclerotherapy with bleomycin, alcohol (which can be painful), doxycycline, or OK-432. Laser therapy and radiofrequency ablation may also be an option. In some cases, surgery is the best option and is curative. Radiofrequency ablation has also been tried for the microcytic varieties.

Reference

Perkins JA, Manning SC, Tempero RM, et al. Lymphatic malformations: current cellular and clinical investigations. *Otolaryngol Head Neck Surg.* 2010;142(6):789-794.

Cross-Reference

Neuroradiology: THE REQUISITES, 4th ed, pp 446, 510.

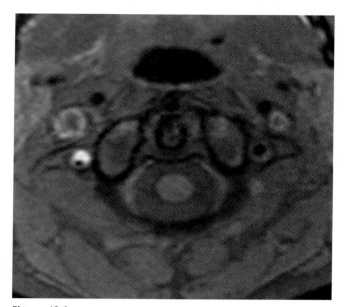

Figure 42-1

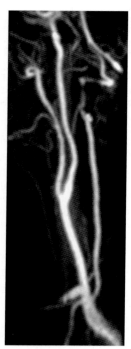

Figure 42-2

HISTORY: Neck pain and transient ischemic attack.

1. What is the single best diagnosis of the case?
   A. Vertebral artery dissection
   B. Vertebral artery occlusion
   C. Vertebral arteriovenous fistula
   D. Vertebral artery transection

2. What segment of the vertebral artery is most prone to traumatic injury in adults?
   A. V1
   B. V2
   C. V3
   D. V4

3. What is indicated by the *hyperintense* T1 signal associated with the vertebral artery on Figure 42-1?
   A. Flowing blood in the artery lumen
   B. Hematoma in the vessel lumen
   C. Subintimal/intramural hematoma
   D. Extravascular hematoma

4. What is the function of shim coils in magnetic resonance (MR) scanners?
   A. To improve signal homogeneity in spin echo sequences
   B. To reduce chemical shift artifacts
   C. To reduce B1 inhomogeneities
   D. To reduce B0 inhomogeneities

CASE 42

Vertebral Artery Dissection: Spontaneous

1. **A.** Vertebral artery dissection. There is a pseudoaneurysm in the distal right V2 segment and narrowing of the V3 segment on the maximum intensity projection (MIP) (Figure 42-2). There is T1 hyperintense intramural hematoma at the skull base (Figure 42-1). The constellation of findings is in keeping with right vertebral artery dissection and pseudoaneurysm formation.

2. **B.** V2. Most traumatic injuries occur in the V2 segments, probably related to the tight association of the artery with the spine as it courses through the foramen transversaria. In children, injuries commonly occur in the upper V2 and V3 segments, possibly associated with ligament laxity in the upper spine and at the skull base.

3. **C.** Subintimal/intramural hematoma. There is nonflowing blood within the vessel wall.

4. **D.** To reduce B0 inhomogeneities. Shimming makes the magnetic field as homogenous as possible. It does not affect chemical shift artifacts. Refocusing pulses in SE sequences reduce field inhomogeneities.

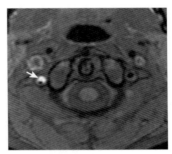

Figure S42-1

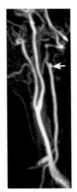

Figure S42-2

Comment

These MR images show narrowing of the lumen of the distal extracranial right vertebral artery (Figure 42-2) with surrounding mural hematoma (*arrow,* Figure S42-1) that is hyperintense on the fat-suppressed unenhanced T1-weighted image. Vascular dissections may be asymptomatic. When they are symptomatic, the symptoms can occur days to weeks after the actual injury. As a result, dissections often escape clinical detection. In addition, symptomatic lesions can be overlooked or masked by other injuries in patients with acute injuries. Therefore, the key to making the diagnosis is considering it in the appropriate clinical scenario. Although computed tomography is not a sensitive study for detecting vascular injuries, it can identify patients at increased risk (those with skull base fractures or fractures of the vertebral bodies extending through the foramen transversarium, which houses the cervical vertebral artery). It is also important to recognize that vertebral artery dissections may be spontaneous (no clear cause, minor trauma) and can occur in association with excessive vomiting, coughing, and excessive straining.

The combination of MR imaging and MR angiography is sensitive for detecting vascular injuries because these assess the vascular lumen, the vessel wall, and tissues around the vessel. MR imaging findings include intramural hematoma, which is typically hyperintense on unenhanced T1-weighted images (as in this case), and narrowing and compromised flow in the arterial lumen (a narrowed but patent vessel can usually be distinguished from one that is occluded). Pseudoaneurysms can also be detected. The conventional angiographic appearance of a dissection can vary and includes spasm, segmental tapering related to intramural hematoma (the hematoma is not visualized on angiography), aneurysmal dilation of the vessel, vascular occlusion, intimal flap, or retention of contrast material in the vessel wall.

References

Hashemi RH, Bradley WG Jr, Lisanti CJ. Basic principles of MRI. In: *MRI: The Basics.* 3rd ed. Philadelphia: Lippincott Williams & Wilkins; 2010:16-30.

Naggara O, Oppenheim C, Toussaint JF, et al. Asymptomatic spontaneous acute vertebral artery dissection: diagnosis by high-resolution magnetic resonance images with a dedicated surface coil. *Eur Radiol.* 2007;17:2434-2435.

Cross-Reference

Neuroradiology: THE REQUISITES, 4th ed, p 162.

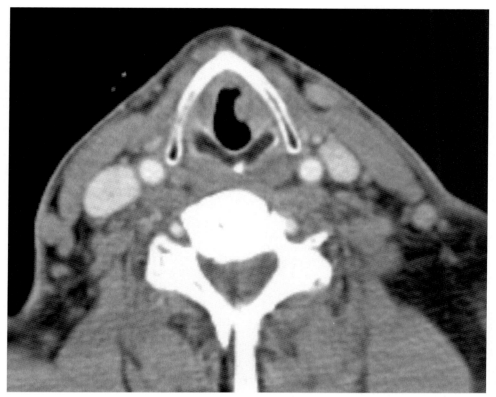

Figure 43-1

HISTORY: The patient presents with a change in voice after a smoking history of 40 pack-years.

1. Which of the following is the best diagnosis for the imaging findings presented?
   A. Chondrosarcoma of the cricoid cartilage
   B. Rhabdomyosarcoma
   C. Squamous cell carcinoma
   D. Minor salivary gland tumor

2. Of what part of the head and neck is the retromolar trigone?
   A. Supraglottic larynx
   B. Oral cavity
   C. Oropharynx
   D. Glottic larynx

3. What is the significance of the anterior commissure involvement by this mass?
   A. It means the tumor is transglottic.
   B. It means the patient's options are limited to a total laryngectomy.
   C. It means the staging is T3b.
   D. It means the surgery required may be an extended vertical hemilaryngectomy.

4. What structure must be tumor free if a supracricoid laryngectomy is to be performed?
   A. The vocal cords
   B. The thyroid cartilage
   C. The epiglottis
   D. The interarytenoid area

Larynx Squamous Cell Carcinoma

1. **C.** Squamous cell carcinoma. There is a soft tissue mass that affects the true vocal cord. There is no chondroid matrix or involvement of the cricoid cartilage. Rhabdomyosarcomas occur in children and not in older patients. Minor salivary gland tumor should not occur here.

2. **B.** Oral cavity. The oral cavity includes the lips, oral tongue, floor of mouth, alveolar ridges, and retromolar trigone.

3. **D.** It means the surgery required may be an extended vertical hemilaryngectomy. This procedure allows removal of one third of the contralateral vocal cord but preserves voice.

4. **D.** The interarytenoid area. The arytenoids must be mobile for the larynx to function. If the arytenoids are immobilized by tumor, a total laryngectomy is the only surgical option.

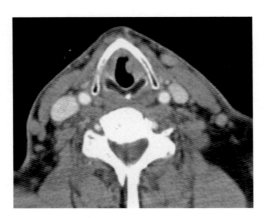

Comment

Management

This is a glottic cancer that has spread from the left true vocal cord to the anterior commissure. Once the anterior commissure has become involved, possible spread may occur anteriorly through the soft tissues to the strap muscles, to the top of the thyroid cartilage, and to the Delphian node anterior to the larynx and trachea. It also means that the surgeon cannot perform a *simple* vertical hemilaryngectomy, which is one of the preferred procedures for bulky cancers of the true vocal cord that are not amenable to primary laser or cordectomy surgery or to radiation therapy. However, the *extended* vertical hemilaryngectomy, in which a sizable portion of the contralateral vocal cord is resected, would still be an option for this patient. If the arytenoids are mobile, and if the cricoid cartilage, the base of the tongue, and the hyoid bone are free of tumor, another surgical option is the supracricoid laryngectomy with cricohyoidopexy. Because of the valve-like effect of the epiglottis, it would be preferable for the epiglottis to be incorporated into the reconstruction, in a cricohyoidoepiglottopexy, but this is not essential.

Tumor Staging of Glottis Cancer

Glottis cancer is staged as follows:

> **T1:** Tumor is limited to one or both vocal cords (may involve anterior or posterior commissure) with normal mobility.
> **T1a:** Tumor is limited to one vocal cord.
> **T1b:** Tumor involves both vocal cords.
> **T2:** Tumor extends to supraglottis and/or subglottis, with or without impaired vocal cord mobility.
> **T3:** Tumor is limited to the larynx with vocal cord fixation and/or invades paraglottic space, with or without minor erosion of the thyroid cartilage (e.g., inner cortex).
> **T4a:** Tumor invades through the thyroid cartilage and/or invades tissue beyond the larynx (e.g., trachea; soft tissues of the neck, including the deep extrinsic muscle of the tongue, strap muscles, thyroid, or esophagus).
> **T4b:** Tumor invades prevertebral space, encases carotid artery, or invades mediastinal structures.

References

Edge SB, Byrd DR, Compton CC, et al., eds. *AJCC Cancer Staging Manual*. 7th ed. New York: Springer; 2010:57-67.
Tufano RP. Organ preservation surgery for laryngeal cancer. *Otolaryngol Clin North Am*. 2002;35(5):1067-1080.

Cross-Reference

Neuroradiology: THE REQUISITES, 4th ed, pp 466-472.

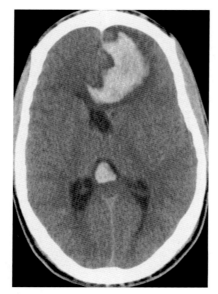

Figure 44-1

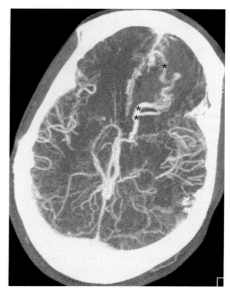

Figure 44-2

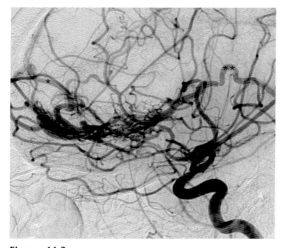

Figure 44-3

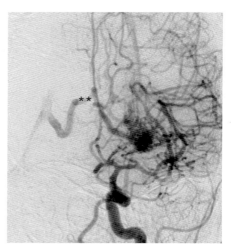

Figure 44-4

HISTORY: Headache and focal neurologic deficit.

1. What is the single best diagnosis of the case?
   A. Hemorrhage into underlying neoplasm
   B. Hemorrhagic transformation of infarct
   C. Hemorrhage into an underlying vascular malformation
   D. Amyloid angiopathy

2. In children with this entity, what extracranial pathology often occurs?
   A. Hemihypertrophy
   B. Hepatic failure
   C. Renal insufficiency
   D. Cardiac failure

3. What does the radiation unit of absorbed dose measure?
   A. Amount of energy absorbed per unit mass from ionizing radiation
   B. Amount of energy absorbed from noncharged particles
   C. Amount of energy absorbed from photoelectric effects
   D. Amount of energy absorbed through Compton scatter

4. In Figures 44-2 and 44-3, what is the anatomic structure marked with a single asterisk?
   A. Draining vein to deep venous system
   B. Draining vein to the superficial venous system
   C. Feeding artery
   D. Nidus

CASE 44

Spontaneous Cerebral Hematoma: Ruptured Cerebral Arteriovenous Malformation

1. **C.** Hemorrhage into an underlying vascular malformation. Differential considerations for a nontraumatic intraparenchymal hemorrhage include hemorrhage into an underlying tumor, hemorrhage into an underlying vascular malformation (ruptured arteriovenous malformation [AVM], cavernoma), venous infarct, vasculitis, hemorrhagic arterial infarct, substance abuse (cocaine), and amyloid angiopathy.

2. **D.** Cardiac failure. High-flow AVMs are left-right shunts and may cause high-output cardiac failure. This can be markedly reduced upon treatment of a shunting lesion.

3. **A.** Amount of energy absorbed per unit mass from ionizing radiation. This quantifies the energy from all types of radiation without distinction. The SI unit for absorbed dose is J/Kg, or Gy.

4. **B.** Draining vein to the superficial venous system. It connects the nidus of this AVM with the superior sagittal sinus.

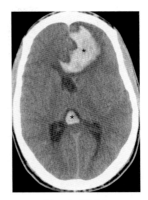

Figure S44-1

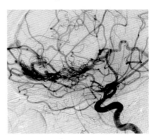

Figure S44-3

Comment

This case shows a nontraumatic spontaneous hematoma in the left frontal lobe with surrounding hypodensity (Figure S44-1, *black asterisk*), consistent with edema and early clot retraction. There is local mass effect with sulcal effacement and mild posterior displacement of the frontal horn of the left lateral ventricle. There is blood in a persistent cavum vergae (Figure 44-1). In this case, the hematoma is caused by a ruptured AVM. The vascular nidus is noted in the left frontal lobe (Figures 44-2 through 44-4). An AVM represents a vascular nidus made up of a core of entangled vessels fed by one or more enlarged feeding arteries. Blood is shunted from the nidus to enlarged draining veins that terminate in the deep or superficial venous system. In this case, there is superficial venous drainage (*single asterisk* in Figures 44-2, 44-3, and S44-3) in the left frontal region that drains to the superior sagittal sinus, and there is deep venous drainage (*double asterisk* in Figures 44-2 and 44-4) to the internal cerebral veins.

On unenhanced computed tomography, the vascular nidus of an AVM and enlarged draining veins are usually isodense or hyperdense to gray matter as a result of pooling of blood. Calcification may be present. AVMs enhance and have characteristic serpentine flow voids on magnetic resonance (MR) imaging related to fast flow in dilated arteries. In lesions associated with an acute parenchymal hemorrhage, phase-contrast MR angiography best demonstrates the AVM (it subtracts out the signal intensity of the blood products in the hematoma, in contrast to time-of-flight MR angiography). Cerebral angiography shows enlarged feeding arteries, the vascular nidus, and early draining veins. In cases of very small AVMs, early venous filling should be sought on careful evaluation of the angiographic images.

References

Cloft HJ, Joseph GJ, Dion JE. Risk of cerebral angiography in patients with subarachnoid hemorrhage, cerebral aneurysm, and arteriovenous malformation. *Stroke.* 1999;30:317-320.

Spetzler RF, Martin NA. A proposed grading system for arteriovenous malformations. *J Neurosurg.* 1986;65:476-483.

Cross-Reference

Neuroradiology: THE REQUISITES, 4th ed, pp 154, 298.

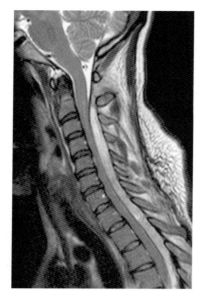

Figure 45-1

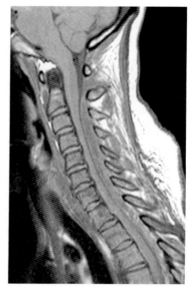

Figure 45-2

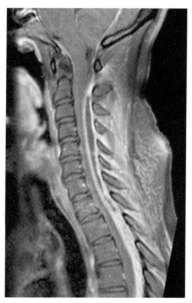

Figure 45-3

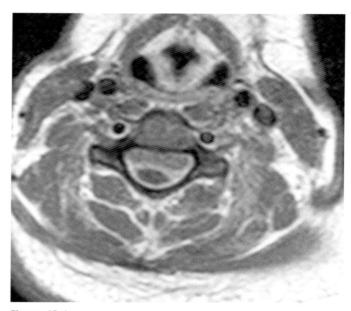

Figure 45-4

HISTORY: A 34-year-old woman presents with fever, headaches, and neck pain for the past 4 days and myelopathy on physical examination.

1. What is the single most likely diagnosis considering the imaging findings and the clinical presentation?
   A. Epidural abscess
   B. Ependymoma
   C. Lymphoma
   D. Epidural hematoma

2. What is the next step in the imaging evaluation of this patient?
   A. Gallium scan
   B. Computed tomography (CT) myelography
   C. Magnetic resonance imaging (MRI) of the thoracic and lumbar spine
   D. Radiolabeled leukocyte scan

3. What organism is most likely to cause an epidural abscess?
   A. *Staphylococcus aureus*
   B. *Mycobacterium tuberculosis*
   C. *Escherichia coli*
   D. *Salmonella*

4. Which of the following is *not* a risk factor for the development of epidural abscess?
   A. Intravenous drug abuse
   B. Alcoholism
   C. Spinal surgery
   D. Disc herniation

CASE 45

Epidural Abscess

1. **A.** Epidural abscess. A rim-enhancing epidural collection in a patient with fever should raise the suspicion for an abscess. Ependymoma is intramedullary. Lymphoma would tend to enhance homogenously. A hematoma may enhance and look similar, but the clinical presentation makes this less likely.

2. **C.** MRI of the thoracic and lumbar spine. The full extent of the process must be identified before surgery. Gallium scanning is useful for the evaluation of osteomyelitis of the spine, but there is no role for it here. CT myelography is relatively contraindicated, wouldn't add much information, and could spread infection. White blood cell scanning would delay treatment and not add much helpful information.

3. **A.** *Staphylococcus aureus.* This is the cause in 45% of cases.

4. **D.** Disc herniation. This is not a risk factor. Intravenous drug abuse, alcoholism, and surgery are all risk factors for epidural abscess.

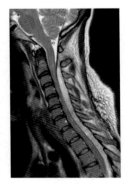

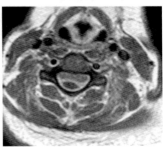

Comment

Background

The peak incidence for spinal epidural abscess is between 60 and 70 years old, and it is most often caused by *S. aureus* infection. The signs and symptoms of epidural abscess are nonspecific and can range from low back pain to frank sepsis. Neurologic dysfunction is often disproportionate to the observed degree of compression of the cord and nerve roots by the extradural mass. This disproportion has been attributed to edema and inflammation, affecting the epidural venous plexus, compromising circulation, and resulting in cord ischemia. Both compressive and ischemic mechanisms may contribute to neurologic dysfunction in such cases.

Histopathology

Most epidural abscesses are located posteriorly in the thoracic or lumbar canal and are thought to originate from hematogenous spread from a distant focus, such as a skin infection, pharyngitis, or dental abscess. Anterior epidural abscesses are commonly associated with discitis osteomyelitis.

Imaging

Epidural abscess is typically hyperintense on T2-weighted images (Figure 45-1) and isointense to hypointense on T1-weighted images (Figure 45-2). Enhancement after contrast administration demonstrates one of the following patterns: homogeneous enhancement representing a phlegmon, peripheral enhancement representing a mature abscess (Figures 45-3 and 45-4), or heterogeneous enhancement representing a combination of both. Diffusion imaging shows the same findings of restricted diffusion and corresponding low apparent diffusion coefficient values that have been reported for pyogenic abscesses in the brain.

Management

Treatment consists of both medical and surgical therapy. Empiric antibiotic coverage should include an antibiotic effective against methicillin-resistant *S. aureus,* which was the organism found in this case. Emergency surgical decompression of the spinal cord with drainage of the abscess is the usual surgical treatment.

References

Chao D, Nanda A. Spinal epidural abscess: a diagnostic challenge. *Am Fam Physician.* 2002;65(7):1341-1346.

Numaguchi Y, Rigamonti D, Rothman MI, et al. Spinal epidural abscess: evaluation with gadolinium-enhanced MR imaging. *Radiographics.* 1993;13(3):545-559, discussion 559-560.

Rigamonti D, Liem L, Sampath P, et al. Spinal epidural abscess: contemporary trends in etiology, evaluation, and management. *Surg Neurol.* 1999;52(2):189-196, discussion 197.

Cross-Reference

Neuroradiology: THE REQUISITES, 4th ed, pp 174-175.

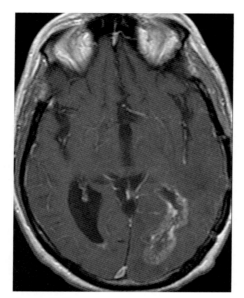

Figure 46-1

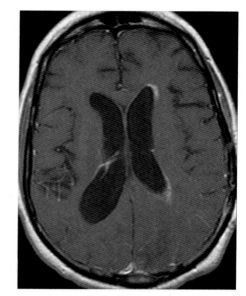

Figure 46-2

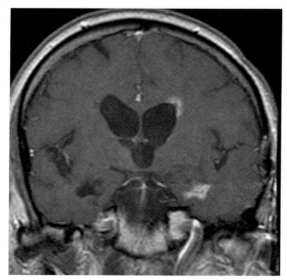

Figure 46-3

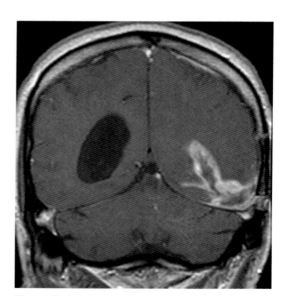

Figure 46-4

HISTORY: Seizure and neurologic deficit.

1. What is the single best diagnosis of the case?
   A. Subependymal spread of neoplasm
   B. Metastatic disease
   C. Sarcoidosis
   D. Abscess

2. Which of the following correlates to a higher grade and aggressiveness of primary glial neoplasm?
   A. Decreased lactic acid on magnetic resonance (MR) spectroscopy
   B. Less avid enhancement following radiation
   C. Larger extent of intratumoral necrosis
   D. Decreased tumor blood volume

3. What best accounts for pathologic intraparenchymal enhancement?
   A. Necrosis
   B. Breakdown or absence of the blood-brain barrier
   C. Lymphocytic infiltration
   D. Tumor blood volume

4. In a patient with AIDS, what is the most likely cause of subependymal enhancement?
   A. Sarcoidosis
   B. Glioblastoma
   C. Infectious ventriculitis
   D. Lymphoma

CASE 46

Glioblastoma: Subependymal Spread

1. **A.** Subependymal spread of neoplasm. The histologic grade of these aggressive neoplasms in adults progresses with age. Other imaging features that correlate with higher grades include enhancement, extensive mass effect, intratumoral necrosis, hemorrhage, vascularity and elevated relative cerebral blood volume, and elevated lactic acid on MR spectroscopy.

2. **C.** Larger extent of intratumoral necrosis. This would correlate with elevated lactic acid. The increased enhancement and tumor blood volume also have been shown to correlate with grade.

3. **B.** Breakdown or absence of the blood-brain barrier. This is the overall principle used to assess pathology when administering contrast at MR imaging. Areas of tumor infiltration, demyelination, infection, and infarct (subacute) all show enhancement with contrast.

4. **D.** Lymphoma. It is the most likely cause of subependymal enhancement in a patient with AIDS.

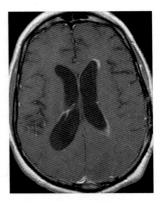

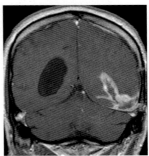

Comment

Glioblastoma (GBM) classically manifests with an ill-defined necrotic brain mass. The histologic grade of these aggressive neoplasms in adults progresses with age: the older the patient is, the higher the histologic grade will be. Other imaging features that correlate with higher grades include enhancement, extensive mass effect, intratumoral necrosis, hemorrhage, vascularity and elevated relative cerebral blood volume, and elevated lactic acid on MR spectroscopy. GBMs infiltrate the brain parenchyma, and this is manifested as T2-weighted hyperintensity; however, there is little doubt that these neoplasms have also infiltrated into areas of the brain that appear normal on current diagnostic MR studies. Most GBMs enhance and usually demonstrate heterogeneity because of the presence of necrosis or hemorrhage. Enhancement can extend into the adjacent white matter. These tumors often cross the corpus callosum and the anterior or posterior commissures to spread to the contralateral cerebral hemisphere. Of the astrocytomas in adults, GBMs most commonly are associated with hemorrhage and subarachnoid seeding (2% to 5%) of neoplasm. Occasionally, at presentation, GBMs coat the subependyma or ependyma of the ventricles (Figures 46-1 through 46-4). However, it is important to recognize that although overall long-term survival rates in patients with GBM are still very poor, patients are living longer and, in some instances, with improved quality of life as a result of changes in treatment protocols and of clinical trials looking at a spectrum of chemotherapeutic agents. Hence, in these patients, less typical patterns of disease progression on imaging, such as coating of the ventricles from subependymal tumor spread, will become more common, as in this case.

In a newly identified brain tumor in which biopsy is anticipated, regions of enhancement correlate with regions of solid tumor on pathology and have the best diagnostic yield. In addition, enhanced images can identify tumor spread to regions that otherwise would not be noticed on unenhanced images, such as the leptomeninges, subarachnoid space, or subependymal region along the ventricular margins, as in this case. In the postoperative setting, contrast can help to distinguish surgical change from residual tumor.

Reference

Christoforidis GA, Grecula JC, Newton HB, et al. Visualization of microvascularity in glioblastoma multiforme with 8-T high-spatial-resolution MR imaging. *AJNR Am J Neuroradiol.* 2002;23: 1553-1556.

Cross-Reference

Neuroradiology: THE REQUISITES, 4th ed, pp 51-52, 59.

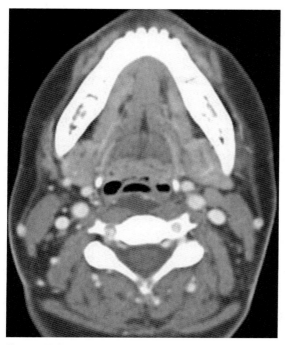

Figure 47-1

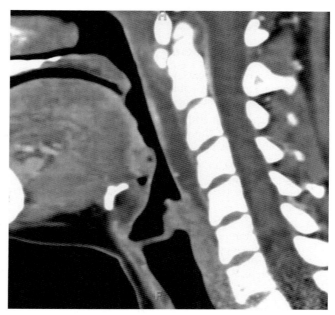

Figure 47-2

HISTORY: A young adult presented with a 24-hour history of neck pain and stiffness.

1. Which of the following is the single best diagnosis for the imaging findings presented?
   A. Normal
   B. Longus colli tendinitis
   C. Edema
   D. Abscess

2. Which of the following is most likely to cross the midline?
   A. Retropharyngeal course of carotid arteries
   B. Necrotizing retropharyngeal adenitis
   C. Tonsil cancer
   D. Retropharyngeal abscess

3. How is a retropharyngeal abscess distinguished from phlegmon or edema?
   A. Degree/character of enhancement
   B. Density of collection
   C. Crossing of the midline
   D. Necrotizing adenitis

4. What is not a cause of retropharyngeal edema?
   A. Lymphoma
   B. Calcific longus tendonitis
   C. Radiation therapy
   D. Pharyngitis

CASE 47

Retropharyngeal Edema

1. **C.** Edema. In the absence of peripheral enhancement, the choices generally are phlegmon versus retropharyngeal edema, although the former may show faint enhancement.

2. **D.** Retropharyngeal abscess. Nodes and vessels very rarely cross the midline. The abscess may cross the midline if it represents coalescent adenitis, or it may develop de novo.

3. **A.** Degree/character of enhancement. Edema, phlegmon, and abscesses may cross the midline and have low density, but abscesses typically exhibit peripheral well-defined enhancement.

4. **A.** Lymphoma. Lymphoma does not present as low-density edema (but the other entities might). It appears as a solid mass that may occur in the retropharyngeal space either as a primary tumor or as a metastasis from the aerodigestive system lymphoid tissue.

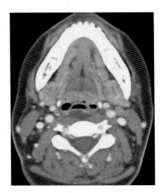

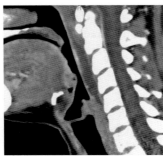

Comment

Distinction between Retropharyngeal Edema and Other Lesions

The distinction among the four entities of retropharyngeal edema, retropharyngeal phlegmon, necrotizing retropharyngeal adenitis, and retropharyngeal abscess is a difficult one that many head and neck radiologists ponder. Although this may be a personal approach, two lesions can be ruled out for the following reasons:

1. A patient with unilateral abnormalities that are in the expected location of the medial or lateral retropharyngeal lymph nodes without extension across the midline probably has necrotizing adenitis. The patient should have an intact nodal capsule. Whether those necrotic, purulent nodes need to be drained depends on early response to therapy and surgical philosophy.

2. A patient with a ring-enhancing collection that crosses the midline and shows mass effect has a retropharyngeal abscess. This probably necessitates percutaneous or surgical drainage, although for small abscesses in older patients, antibiotics may be tried for 24 to 48 hours.

The following two entities are more difficult to determine:

3. An amorphous collection without enhanced, well-defined borders is phlegmon, with adjacent edema and inflammatory changes in the nearby tissues.

4. Retropharyngeal edema usually has no inflammatory component evident, crosses the midline, and is not drainable. It is usually symmetric and fills the space as in this case (Figures 47-1 and 47-2).

Gray Zones

Unfortunately there *are* abscesses that do not enhance in a rim manner. If a large collection has distinct borders without enhancement, it is probably a purulent drainable collection (i.e., abscess). Some phlegmons are as drainable as abscesses and may show faint rim enhancement. Sometimes necrotizing adenitis coalesces and, in fact, may be the cause of the abscess. Pharyngitis and longus tendinitis, both inflammatory conditions, may cause retropharyngeal edema.

Reference

Hoang JK, Branstetter BF 4th, Eastwood JD, Glastonbury CM. Multiplanar CT and MRI of collections in the retropharyngeal space: is it an abscess? *AJR Am J Roentgenol.* 2011;196(4):W426-W432.

Cross-Reference

Neuroradiology: THE REQUISITES, 4th ed, pp 446, 512.

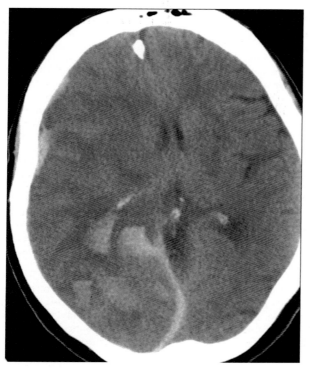

Figure 48-1

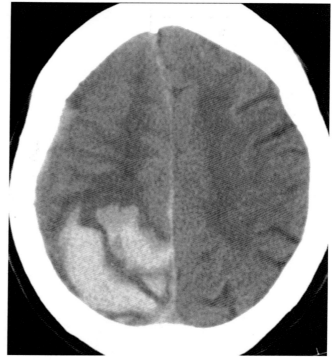

Figure 48-2

HISTORY: Headaches and focal neurologic deficit.

1. What is the most common presentation of cerebral amyloid angiopathy?
   A. Infarct
   B. Lobar hematoma
   C. Brainstem hematoma
   D. Extra-axial hematoma

2. What is the most common cause of nontraumatic intraparenchymal hemorrhage in adults?
   A. Hypertension
   B. Amyloid angiopathy
   C. Arteriovenous malformation
   D. Aneurysm rupture

3. What is a major risk factor for amyloid angiopathy?
   A. Age >60 years
   B. Anticoagulation
   C. Hypertension
   D. History of radiation

4. What region of the brain is typically involved in amyloid angiopathy?
   A. Basal ganglia
   B. Brainstem
   C. Deep white matter
   D. Gray-white junction

CASE 48

Amyloid Angiopathy

1. **B.** Lobar hematoma. These hematomas mostly occur in the periphery of the cerebral hemispheres.

2. **A.** Hypertension. Hypertension accounts for more than 75% of nontraumatic intraparenchymal hemorrhages.

3. **A.** Age >60 years. This is the single major risk factor. There is likely a genetic component, as family history is also a strong risk factor.

4. **D.** Gray-white junction. The gray-white junction is often involved in amyloid angiopathy, whereas the basal ganglia, brainstem, deep white matter, and cerebellum are often spared.

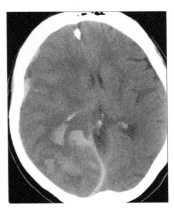

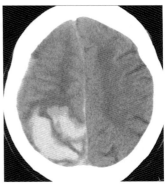

Comment

Central nervous system amyloid angiopathy results from deposition of β-pleated proteins within the media and adventitia of small- and medium-sized vessels of the superficial layers of the cortex and leptomeninges. Amyloid deposition increases with age and results in loss of elasticity of the walls of involved vessels. On pathologic examination, microaneurysms and fibrinoid degeneration are often present. Amyloid stains intensely with Congo red dye (previously referred to as congophilic angiopathy) and demonstrates yellow-green birefringence under polarized light.

On computed tomography (CT) and magnetic resonance imaging (MRI), hemorrhages are characteristically lobar in location, and they most commonly occur in the frontal and parietal lobes (Figure 48-2). Multiple hemorrhages of different ages, as well as multiple simultaneous hemorrhages, are often present. Subarachnoid and subdural blood may be present owing to perforation of blood through the pia arachnoid or involvement of superficial blood vessels with amyloid deposition (Figure 48-1). MRI, including gradient echo images or similar techniques such as susceptibility-weighted images (SWI), may be especially useful for demonstrating the full extent of intracranial involvement. (CT readily shows acute hemorrhage, as in this case; however, regions of old blood products are often occult.) Patients can have numerous small subcortical regions of focal hypointensity (multiple hypointense foci may also be related to cavernomas or microhemorrhages, as is seen in hypertension). Importantly, there is no association of hypertension with the development of amyloid angiopathy.

Reference

Walker DA, Broderick DF, Kotsenas AL, Rubino FA. Routine use of gradient-echo MRI to screen for cerebral amyloid angiopathy in elderly patients. *Am J Roentgenol.* 2004;182:1547-1550.

Cross-Reference

Neuroradiology: THE REQUISITES, 4th ed, pp 133-135.

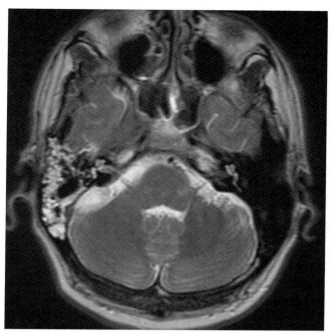

Figure 49-1

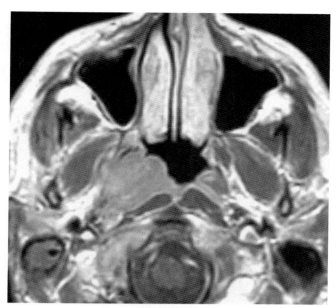

Figure 49-2

HISTORY: The patient presents with right-sided hearing loss and a sensation of fullness in the right ear.

1. Which of the following is the single best diagnosis?
   A. Nasopharyngeal carcinoma
   B. Malignant otitis externa
   C. Calcific tendinitis of the longus colli musculature
   D. Otomastoiditis

2. Which of the following is most likely to occur?
   A. A mucosal lesion of the nasopharynx growing into the skull base
   B. A skull base tumor growing into the nasopharynx
   C. A sinonasal tumor growing into the nasopharynx
   D. A temporal bone lesion growing into the nasopharynx

3. Through which orifice might this lesion spread into the cavernous sinus and/or Meckel cave?
   A. The foramen ovale
   B. The pterygoid canal
   C. The eustachian tube
   D. The fonticulus frontalis

4. Which of the following is *not* a World Health Organization (WHO) 2005 histologic subtype of nasopharyngeal carcinoma?
   A. Keratinizing squamous cell carcinoma
   B. Nonkeratinizing carcinomas
   C. Basaloid squamous cell carcinoma
   D. Lymphoepithelioma

CASE 49

Nasopharyngeal Carcinoma

1. **A.** Nasopharyngeal carcinoma. There is a mass in the posterolateral right nasopharynx.

2. **A.** A mucosal lesion of the nasopharynx growing into the skull base is more likely to occur.

3. **A.** The foramen ovale. Nasopharyngeal carcinoma may spread directly with contiguous tumor growth or along the nerves. The route to the cavernous sinus and/or Meckel cave may be most common through the foramen ovale.

4. **D.** Lymphoepithelioma. The WHO recognizes keratinizing squamous cell carcinoma, nonkeratinizing carcinoma (differentiated and undifferentiated types), and basaloid squamous cell carcinoma. The term *lymphoepithelioma* is no longer used.

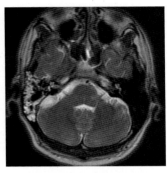

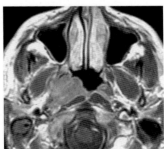

Comment

Incidence of Nasopharyngeal Carcinoma

The incidence of nasopharyngeal carcinoma in the native or immigrant Asian population is about 20 times greater than in the white U.S. population. Polymerase chain reaction with the Epstein-Barr virus is positive in the nonkeratinizing carcinoma and undifferentiated carcinomas but not in the keratinizing squamous cell tumors and adenocarcinomas. Smoking and alcohol use do not appear to be significant risk factors. Nasopharyngeal carcinoma is not treated surgically; a cure relies on radiation therapy, chemotherapy, or both. Once disease has spread intracranially or outside the nasopharynx, the prognosis is poor, mainly because of the higher incidence of hematogenous metastases and poor local control rates.

Imaging Findings after Treatment

After radiotherapy (and chemotherapy), fibrotic changes that resemble persistent tumor often occur. The presence of a defined mass and enhancing focal tissue, rather than mucosal asymmetry, suggests persistent or recurrent disease. Lobulation is an ominous sign; smoothness is benign. Magnetic resonance imaging (MRI) is superior to computed tomography for both the initial and the follow-up evaluations of nasopharyngeal carcinoma (Figures 49-1 and 49-2). Because nasopharyngeal tumors often burrow submucosally, imaging and nasopharyngoscopy play complementary roles in evaluation. For diagnosing spread to the lymph nodes (retropharyngeal lymph nodes in 50% of cases), imaging is superior to clinical evaluation. The mechanism of spread through the skull base may be through the fascial planes and bone or via perineural extension.

The Sinus of Morgagni

The sinus of Morgagni lies between the superior pharyngeal constrictor muscle and the skull base. It is a defect in the pharyngobasilar fascia through which the eustachian tube and levator veli palatini muscle gain access to the nasopharynx. It is a route for the spread of carcinoma from the nasopharynx to the skull base, especially via the mandibular nerve through foramen ovale. Trotter syndrome (also called sinus of Morgagni syndrome) consists of a clinical triad of unilateral deafness, trigeminal neuralgia, and soft palate dysmotility.

Reference

Hyare H, Wisco JJ, Alusi G, et al. The anatomy of nasopharyngeal carcinoma spread through the pharyngobasilar fascia to the trigeminal mandibular nerve on 1.5 T MRI. *Surg Radiol Anat.* 2010;32(10): 937-944.

Cross-Reference

Neuroradiology: THE REQUISITES, 4th ed, pp 458-461.

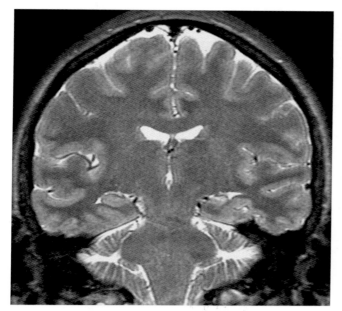

Figure 50-1   Patient A.

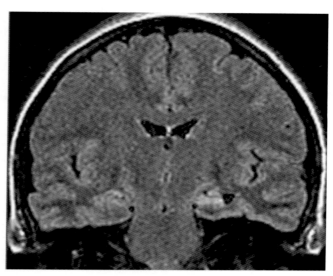

Figure 50-2   Patient A.

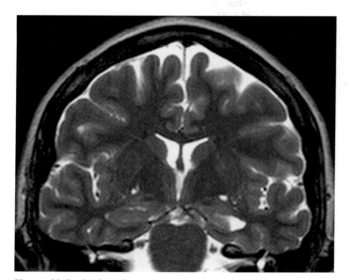

Figure 50-3   Patient B.

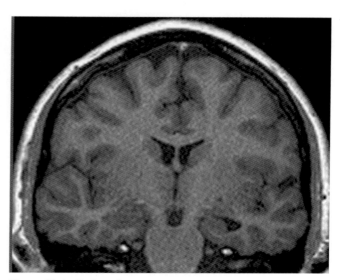

Figure 50-4   Patient B.

HISTORY: Withheld.

1. What is the single best diagnosis of these cases?
    A. Mesial temporal sclerosis
    B. Low-grade glioma
    C. Cortical dysplasia
    D. Ganglioglioma

2. What is the patient's clinical presentation?
    A. Complex partial seizure
    B. Sleep disturbance
    C. Memory loss
    D. Focal neurologic deficit

3. Which additional structure(s) often shows volume loss in the setting of this disease?
    A. Pituitary gland
    B. Optic nerves
    C. Mammillary bodies
    D. Vermis

4. What condition in infancy has been associated with mesial temporal sclerosis?
    A. Jaundice
    B. Talipes equinus varus
    C. Rapidly involuting congenital hemangioma
    D. Complex infantile febrile seizures

CASE 50

Mesial Temporal Sclerosis

1. **A.** Mesial temporal sclerosis (MTS). Volume loss and T2 hyperintensity of the left hippocampus are present. Tumors are usually associated with enlargement, and there is no evidence of cortical dysplasia.

2. **A.** Complex partial seizure. Almost all patients with MTS have seizures, usually complex partial.

3. **C.** Mammillary bodies. Although this may be seen as a congenital variation or in other disease settings such as Wernicke encephalopathy, ipsilateral mammillary body and forniceal atrophy is seen in association with MTS.

4. **D.** Complex infantile febrile seizures. Patients with complex febrile seizures have an increased incidence of mesial temporal sclerosis.

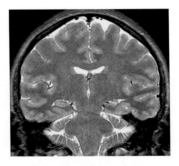

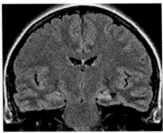

Comment

Temporal lobe epilepsy is the most common epilepsy syndrome in adults. Seizures usually begin in late childhood or adolescence. Virtually all patients have complex partial seizures. In most patients, the epileptogenic focus involves the structures of the mesial temporal lobe. These structures include the hippocampus, amygdala, and parahippocampal gyrus. The histologic substrate in approximately two thirds of cases is mesial temporal sclerosis. The hippocampal formation located in the mesial temporal lobe protrudes into the medial temporal horn and is roofed by the choroidal fissure. It is a complex structure composed of the hippocampus proper, subiculum, dentate gyrus, parahippocampal gyrus, fimbria, and fornix. The hippocampus proper (or cornu ammonis) can be subdivided into four subfields, CA1 though CA4, depending on the appearance of pyramidal neurons. Neuronal loss is accompanied by fibrillary gliosis, leading to hippocampal atrophy. In mesial temporal sclerosis, gliosis can also affect the amygdala, uncus, and parahippocampal gyrus.

The differential diagnosis for hippocampal sclerosis includes cortical dysplasias and primary brain neoplasm. Mesial temporal sclerosis is usually radiologically characteristic. Magnetic resonance imaging (MRI) using high-resolution thin-section coronal fluid-attenuated inversion recovery (FLAIR) and T2-weighted and T1-weighted gradient volumetric sequences is the imaging modality of choice for evaluating patients with seizure disorders. These cases illustrate the classic MRI appearance of hippocampal sclerosis in which there is atrophy of the left hippocampal in both cases as well as mild ipsilateral dilation of the adjacent temporal horn (Figures 50-1 through 50-4). Patient A also shows T2-weighted hyperintensity in the abnormal hippocampus that is believed to reflect gliosis (see Figures 50-1 and 50-2).

Whether mesial temporal sclerosis is the cause or the result of temporal lobe epilepsy is controversial. Some studies have shown a relationship between complex infantile febrile seizures and mesial temporal sclerosis. Patients with complex febrile seizures (duration longer than 15 minutes, convulsive activity, or more than three seizures within 24 hours) have an increased incidence of mesial temporal sclerosis.

References

Briellmann RS, Syngeniotis A, Fleming S, et al. Increased anterior temporal lobe T2 times in cases of hippocampal sclerosis: a multi-echo T2 relaxometry study at 3T. *Am J Neuroradiol.* 2004;25:389-394.

Hogan RE, Wang L, Bertrand ME, et al. MRI-based high dimensional hippocampal mapping in mesial temporal lobe epilepsy. *Brain.* 2004;127:1731-1740.

Ozturk A, Yousem DM, Mahmood A, El Sayed S. Prevalence of asymmetry of mammillary body and fornix size on MR imaging. *AJNR Am J Neuroradiol.* 2008;29:384-387.

Cross-Reference

Neuroradiology: THE REQUISITES, 4th ed, pp 308-310.

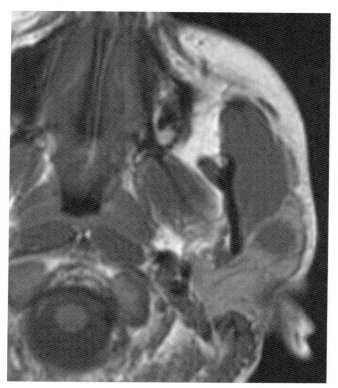

Figure 51-1

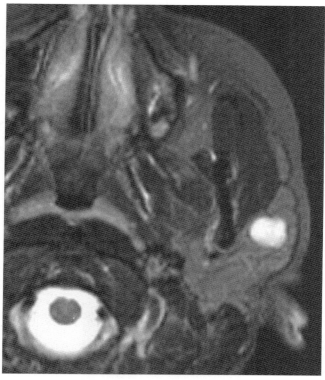

Figure 51-2

HISTORY: A 34-year-old woman was being evaluated for a headache.

1. Which of the following should *not* be included in the differential diagnosis?
   A. Warthin tumor
   B. Pleomorphic adenoma
   C. Lymph node
   D. Low-grade mucoepidermoid carcinoma

2. What percentage of pleomorphic adenomas dedifferentiate into carcinoma?
   A. 0% to 25%
   B. 26% to 50%
   C. 51% to 75%
   D. More than 75%

3. What is the typical appearance of a pleomorphic adenoma on dynamic enhancement?
   A. Early rapid wash-in and rapid wash-out
   B. Early rapid wash-in and delayed wash-out
   C. Gradual increase over time, plateau, and maintenance of the plateau
   D. Late persistent enhancement

4. What percentage of parotid tumors are pleomorphic adenomas?
   A. 20% to 40%
   B. 41% to 60%
   C. 61% to 80%
   D. More than 80%

CASE 51

Pleomorphic Adenoma

1. **A.** Warthin tumor. Warthin tumors rarely occur in patients this young. They have a predilection for the tail of the parotid gland.

2. **A.** 0% to 25%. Carcinoma ex pleomorphic adenoma occurs in only a small percentage of tumors because the masses are usually removed electively. However, the natural history of the tumor, if it is left untreated, is malignant degeneration in 25% of cases in 20 years.

3. **C.** Gradual increase over time, plateau, and maintenance of the plateau. Enhancement increases gradually over time, plateaus, and then is sustained on delayed images with pleomorphic adenomas.

4. **C.** 61% to 80%. According to the 80% rule, 80% of parotid masses are benign, and 80% of those are pleomorphic adenomas; thus, pleomorphic adenomas represent 64% of tumors.

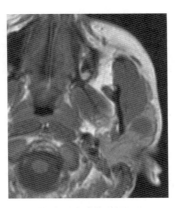

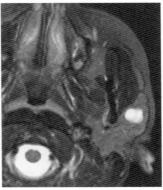

Comment

Imaging Findings

The most common benign tumor of the salivary glands, the pleomorphic adenoma, has very high signal intensity on T2-weighted images (Figures 51-1 and 51-2). Benign cysts (mucous retention cyst, lymphoepithelial cyst, first branchial cleft cyst, ranula, sialocele, and pseudocyst) may also appear hyperintense on T2-weighted image. Gadolinium is employed to distinguish a pleomorphic adenoma from a cyst: Cysts do not enhance, or if they do, it is only on their periphery, whereas pleomorphic adenomas enhance throughout and thus appear solid.

Incidence of Malignant Salivary Gland Tumors

The smaller the salivary gland is, the higher the rate of malignancy will be in salivary gland tumors. The malignancy rate of salivary gland tumors is 20% to 25% in the parotid gland, 40% to 50% in the submandibular gland, and 50% to 81% in the sublingual glands and minor salivary glands.

Implications of Parotid Pleomorphic Adenoma

Pleomorphic adenomas, also known as *benign mixed tumors,* occur most commonly in middle-aged women. They are the most common parotid mass, representing approximately 65% to 70% of parotid masses and approximately 80% of the benign ones. Of all pleomorphic adenomas, 80% occur in the superficial lobe. Pleomorphic adenomas are the most common benign tumors in the submandibular gland, sublingual gland, and minor salivary glands.

In surgical treatment of a pleomorphic adenoma, the danger is the potential for seeding of the operative bed, which would lead to multifocal pleomorphic adenoma with the risk of malignant degeneration into an adenocarcinoma. Thus, these tumors are treated with wide local excision, with adequate attention to facial nerve preservation.

Reference

Yabuuchi H, Fukuya T, Tajima T, et al. Salivary gland tumors: diagnostic value of gadolinium enhanced dynamic MR imaging with histopathologic correlation. *Radiology.* 2003;226(2):345-354.

Cross-Reference

Neuroradiology: THE REQUISITES, 4th ed, pp 457-458, 488-490.

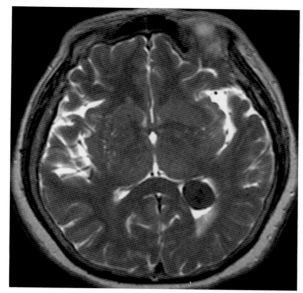

Figure 52-1 Patient A.

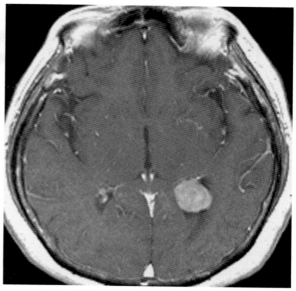

Figure 52-2 Patient A.

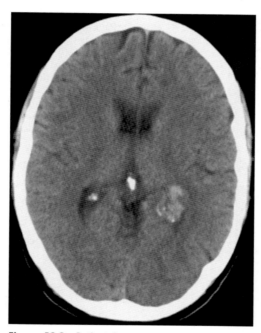

Figure 52-3 Patient B.

HISTORY: Incidental finding.

1. Regarding the correct diagnosis, which is the same for these two patients, what statement is correct?
   A. In adults, these masses occur in the ventricles more than 5% of the time.
   B. Males are more likely affected than females.
   C. In the pediatric population, one fifth of these masses occur in the ventricles.
   D. This is the most common intraventricular tumor in tuberous sclerosis.

2. This particular tumor most often arises in what ventricle in adults?
   A. Left lateral ventricle
   B. Right lateral ventricle
   C. Third ventricle
   D. Fourth ventricle

3. What is the most common presentation of these tumors?
   A. Headache
   B. Nausea
   C. Seizure
   D. Asymptomatic/incidental

4. In adults, choroid plexus papillomas most commonly occur in what ventricle? In children?
   A. Lateral ventricles for both children and adults
   B. Lateral and third ventricles, respectively
   C. Lateral and fourth ventricles, respectively
   D. Fourth and lateral ventricles, respectively

CASE 52

Intraventricular Meningioma

1. **C.** In the pediatric population, one fifth of these masses occur in the ventricles. Knowing the diagnosis is the hardest part of answering this question correctly. Less than 1% of meningiomas occur in the ventricles in adults, females are more often affected than males, and this is not a subependymal giant cell tumor.

2. **A.** Left lateral ventricle. This tumor is slightly more predominate in the left lateral ventricle than in the right lateral ventricle. Overall, the majority occur in the atria when in the lateral ventricles.

3. **D.** Asymptomatic/incidental. These tumors are most often an incidental finding with no symptoms attributed to them. The other symptoms may occur although not most commonly.

4. **D.** Fourth and lateral ventricles, respectively. In adults, choroid plexus papillomas are most often in the fourth ventricle, and in children, most often in the atria of the lateral ventricles.

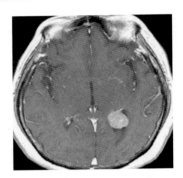

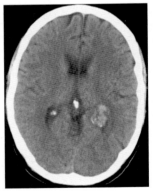

Comment

Patients A (Figures 52-1 and 52-2) and B (Figure 52-3) demonstrate well-demarcated mass lesions in the atria of the left lateral ventricle along the glomus of the choroid plexus, consistent with meningiomas. On T2-weighted imaging (see Figure 52-1), these tumors range from mildly hyperintense to the brain parenchyma (however, markedly hypointense to cerebrospinal fluid [CSF]) to hypointense to brain tissue in cases of very cellular or calcified tumors. After contrast administration, there is homogeneous avid enhancement (see Figure 52-2). In adults, this is the typical appearance of an intraventricular meningioma and the most common location for these neoplasms, which are speculated to arise from arachnoid rests within the choroid plexus. Like choroid plexus papillomas, intraventricular meningiomas occur slightly more often on the left, as illustrated in these cases. When large enough, intraventricular meningiomas can trap a particular segment of the lateral ventricle (usually the temporal or occipital horn), resulting in focal dilation and sometimes associated transependymal flow of CSF. When large enough, these tumors can compress the walls of the ventricles or grow through the ependyma, with resultant edema in the adjacent brain parenchyma. Their appearance on computed tomography (CT) imaging is similar to that of other intracranial meningiomas. On unenhanced CT images, these masses are often hyperdense with calcifications, as in Patient B (see Figure 52-3). They avidly enhance after contrast administration.

The differential diagnosis of a mass in this location in adults includes glial neoplasms (astrocytomas, ependymomas), metastasis to the choroid plexus, and vascular lesions such as hemangiomas and cavernomas. Choroid plexus papillomas can usually be eliminated as a diagnostic consideration because they occur most commonly in children and because in adults they are usually located within the fourth ventricle.

References

Jelinek J, Smirniotopoulos JG, Parisi JE, Kanzer M. Lateral ventricular neoplasms of the brain: differential diagnosis based on clinical, CT, and MR findings. *AJR Am J Roentgenol.* 1990;155:365-372.

Majos C, Cucurella G, Aguilera C, et al. Intraventricular meningiomas: MR imaging and MR spectroscopic findings in two cases. *AJNR Am J Neuroradiol.* 1999;20:882-885.

Cross-Reference

Neuroradiology: THE REQUISITES, 4th ed, pp 42-43.

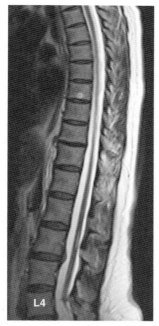

Figure 53-1

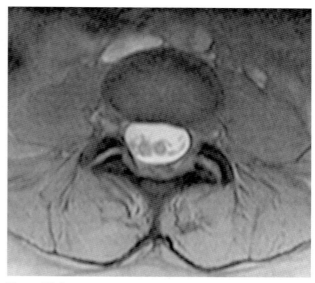

Figure 53-2

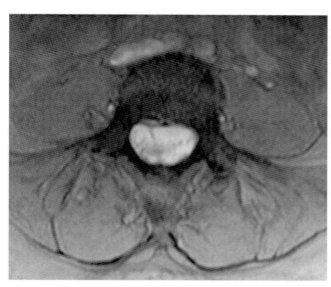

Figure 53-3

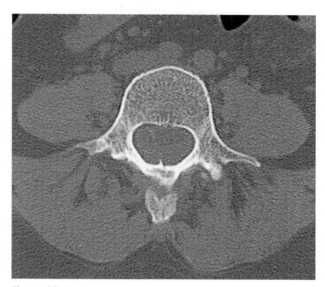

Figure 53-4

HISTORY: A 52-year-old woman presents with intractable low back pain, left leg numbness, and urinary incontinence.

1. What is the single best diagnosis?
   A. Chronic arachnoiditis
   B. Intradural lipoma
   C. Neurofibromatosis
   D. Diastematomyelia

2. Where along the spinal axis is a cleft in the cord most likely to be found?
   A. Upper cervical spine
   B. Upper thoracic spine
   C. Thoracolumbar spine
   D. Lower cervical spine

3. Which of the following abnormalities is *not* associated with diastematomyelia?
   A. Spina bifida
   B. Scoliosis
   C. Hemivertebra
   D. Short pedicles

4. Which of the following imaging studies would be the *least* helpful in further evaluation of this patient?
   A. Plain radiographs
   B. Bone scan
   C. Computed tomography (CT)
   D. Magnetic resonance imaging (MRI)

CASE 53

Diastematomyelia

1. **D.** Diastematomyelia. There are two hemicords. True duplication of the spinal cord, diplomyelia, may appear similarly.

2. **C.** Thoracolumbar spine. The cleft is located below T8 in 85% of cases.

3. **D.** Short pedicles. Short pedicles are associated with congenital spinal canal stenosis. There are associations of diastematomyelia with hemivertebra, spina bifida, and scoliosis.

4. **B.** Bone scan. This would yield no helpful information. Radiographs, CT, and MRI each contribute to diagnosis and management.

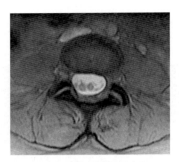

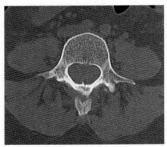

Comment

Background

Diastematomyelia is an uncommon congenital anomaly in which division of the spinal cord into two hemicords is present. Females are affected more than males, and the most common location is in the lower thoracic and upper lumbar spine. Most patients present in childhood, and presentation in adulthood is highly unusual. Symptoms may range from back pain to progressive neurologic deterioration and signs of spinal cord and cauda equina dysfunction. Patients often have midline cutaneous abnormalities associated with dysraphism, such as dimple and sinus tract. Vertebral anomalies are present in 85% of cases of diastematomyelia.

Histopathology

In diastematomyelia, spinal cord anatomy may range from a partial ventral or dorsal cleft to nearly complete duplication of the cord. Some authors have proposed that the spectrum of split cord entities be referred to as the split cord malformation syndrome, with two types of lesions. Type I lesions have a double dural sac and a double spinal canal with the two hemicords separated by an extradural bony or partially bony spur. This spur can be strictly anteroposterior in orientation and divide the canal and the cord into two symmetric halves, or it can be slanting in the axial plane and divide the canal asymmetrically (Figures 53-3 and 53-4). Type II lesions have one dural sac, one spinal canal, and two symmetric hemicords, between which there may be an anteroposterior fibrous intradural septum extending for no more than one or two vertebral segments in length. Type II split cord malformations account for 50% to 60% of all split cord malformations.

Imaging

MRI is the imaging modality of choice for assessing split cord malformations. MRI can demonstrate the conus position and the presence of hydromyelia and is very useful in detecting associated spinal abnormality commonly found in spinal dysraphism (Figures 53-1 through 53-3). CT may demonstrate the bony septum (see Figure 53-4) and is able to image anomalies of the vertebrae better.

Management

Asymptomatic patients do not require treatment. Surgical intervention is warranted in patients who present with new onset of neurologic signs and symptoms or have a history of progressive neurologic manifestations. Differentiation between types I and II split cord malformation has surgical importance because type I lesions are technically more difficult to correct and are associated with more surgical morbidity than type II lesions, especially if there is an oblique septum dividing the cord asymmetrically.

References

Lewandrowski KU, Rachlin JR, Glazer PA. Diastematomyelia presenting as progressive weakness in an adult after spinal fusion for adolescent idiopathic scoliosis. *Spine J.* 2004;4(1):116-119.

Pang D, Dias MS, Ahab-Barmada M. Split cord malformation. Part I: a unified theory of embryogenesis for double spinal cord malformations. *Neurosurgery.* 1992;31(3):451-480.

Cross-Reference

Neuroradiology: THE REQUISITES, 4th ed, pp 302-304.

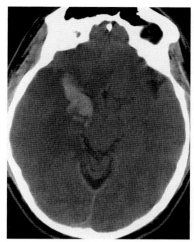

Figure 54-1

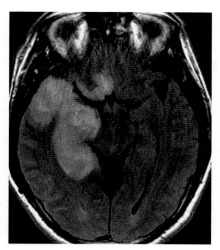

Figure 54-2

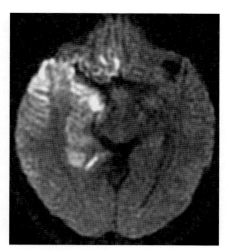

Figure 54-3

HISTORY: Headache, fever, and seizure.

1. What is the best management recommendation you can provide to the emergency department provider?
   A. Obtain magnetic resonance (MR) angiography to evaluate the vessels; this is likely acute infarct from arterial occlusion.
   B. Place this patient in isolation; this is likely Ebola encephalitis.
   C. Administer appropriate antiviral medications; this is likely herpes simplex virus type 1 (HSV-1) encephalitis.
   D. Perform a lumbar puncture to assess for bacteria; this is likely bacterial encephalitis.

2. What imaging findings are *not* typical for herpes simplex encephalitis?
   A. Involvement of the parietal lobe
   B. Involvement of the bilateral temporal lobes
   C. Asymmetric involvement of the inferomedial frontal lobes
   D. Cortical gyral enhancement

3. Among the following choices, which group of patients is at greatest risk for viral encephalitis?
   A. College students
   B. Females
   C. Males
   D. Immunocompromised

4. Which herpes simplex virus is responsible for neonatal infection?
   A. HSV-1
   B. HSV-2
   C. HSV-3
   D. HSV-1a

CASE 54

Herpes Simplex Encephalitis Type 1

1. **C.** Administer appropriate antiviral medications; this is likely HSV-1 encephalitis. This does not conform to an arterial distribution, Ebola is far less common and doesn't present with the same imaging findings, and a lumbar puncture should not postpone antiviral therapy.

2. **A.** Involvement of the parietal lobe. Asymmetric bilateral temporal and inferomedial frontal lobe involvement are common areas affected. Cortical gyral enhancement also occurs.

3. **D.** Immunocompromised. Immunocompromised populations are at the highest risk of reactivation related viral encephalitis and new infections. These populations include patients being treated for autoimmune diseases, chronic steroid users, chemotherapy patients, and transplant patients, to name a few.

4. **B.** HSV-2. This is the herpes virus most commonly affecting neonates, acquired either transplacentally or through the birth canal of a mother with genital herpes.

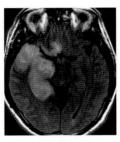

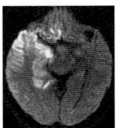

Comment

Type 1 herpes simplex virus produces necrotizing encephalitis in adults. The clinical presentation is varied, ranging from headache, fever, and seizures to coma. Radiologic evaluation often shows hypodensity with loss of gray-white matter differentiation in the temporal lobes and insular cortex on computed tomography (CT). Hemorrhage may also be present, as in this case (Figure 54-1). The CT appearance can simulate an infarct or a primary glial neoplasm. MR imaging findings in the acute stages of encephalitis show hyperintensity on T2-weighted images (Figure 54-2, T2-FLAIR) within involved brain (usually the temporal lobes and inferomedial frontal lobes). There often is local mass effect, which is manifest by gyral expansion and sulcal effacement. Restricted diffusion is possible, reflecting cerebritis or encephalitis (Figure 54-3).

Although bilateral disease is typical, herpes encephalitis usually involves the temporal lobes, insula, inferior frontal lobes, and cingulate gyrus in an asymmetric pattern, as in this case. A proposed explanation for this pattern of involvement is the presence of the latent virus within the gasserian ganglion in the Meckel cave. Reactivated virus can spread along the trigeminal nerve fibers, with subsequent spread along the meninges around the temporal lobes and the undersurface of the frontal lobes. Meningoencephalitis commonly results. Diagnosis can depend on brain biopsy with a positive viral culture or identification of viral inclusion bodies. A positive result on herpes simplex virus polymerase chain reaction testing is diagnostic, and results of this test are available before those from cultures. Cortical gyriform enhancement is often present and may be associated with meningeal enhancement.

A good outcome from herpes simplex encephalitis relies on early diagnosis, which of course depends on considering herpes as a diagnosis. Delay in therapy (acyclovir) or untreated herpes is associated with a high mortality rate (50% to 75%), with little chance of a full neurologic recovery.

Reference

Samann PG, Schlegel J, Muller G, et al. Serial proton MR spectroscopy and diffusion imaging findings in HIV-related herpes simplex encephalitis. *Am J Neuroradiol.* 2003;24:2015-2019.

Cross-Reference

Neuroradiology: THE REQUISITES, 4th ed, p 185.

Fair Game

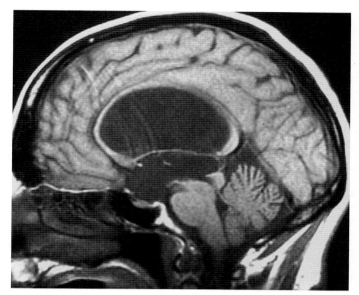

Figure 55-1

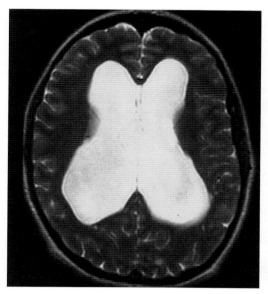

Figure 55-2

HISTORY: A 22-year-old male with headache, papilledema, and macrocephaly.

1. What is the single best diagnosis in this case?
   A. Congenital aqueductal stenosis
   B. Chiari malformation
   C. Extrinsic compression from infarct
   D. Meningitis

2. What is the level of ventricular obstruction in this case?
   A. Aqueduct of Sylvius
   B. Foramen of Monro
   C. Third ventricle
   D. Foramen of Luschka

3. In communicating hydrocephalus, where is the obstruction of cerebrospinal fluid (CSF) circulation?
   A. Aqueduct of Sylvius
   B. Foramen of Monro
   C. Fourth ventricle
   D. Arachnoid villi

4. What is the inheritance pattern in congenital aqueductal stenosis?
   A. Autosomal dominant
   B. Autosomal recessive
   C. X-linked dominant
   D. X-linked recessive

CASE 55

Aqueductal Stenosis

1. **A.** Congenital aqueductal stenosis. Considering the history and the answer options presented, this is the best answer. The abnormal morphology of the tectal plate is also suggestive of this diagnosis. In general, obstruction may be congenital (webs or diaphragms within the aqueduct or gliosis). Acquired aqueductal stenosis may be intrinsic, related to clot or adhesions from previous subarachnoid hemorrhage or infection (meningitis or ventriculitis), or from extrinsic compression of the aqueduct related to tumors (tectal gliomas, pineal tumors, cerebellar neoplasms) or cerebellar stroke. Chiari malformations may result in obstruction of CSF flow at the foramen magnum. Meningitis usually results in communicating hydrocephalus.

2. **A.** Aqueduct of Sylvius. The aqueduct of Sylvius, also known as the cerebral aqueduct, is the site of obstruction in this case. The abnormal morphology of the tectal plate and the normal size of the fourth ventricle are highly suggestive even if the patency of the aqueduct cannot be evaluated.

3. **D.** Arachnoid villi. Most commonly, the site of obstruction in communicating hydrocephalus is in the arachnoid villi, resulting in decreased resorption.

4. **D.** X-linked recessive. The inheritance pattern in congenital aqueductal stenosis is X-linked recessive.

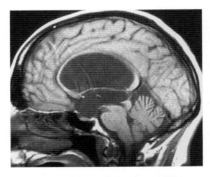

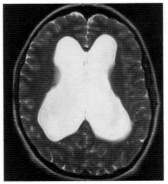

Comment

Congenital Aqueductal Stenosis

This case demonstrates the characteristic findings in congenital aqueductal stenosis. There is prominent dilation of the lateral (Figures 55-1 and 55-2) and third ventricles, with a relatively normal-sized fourth ventricle (see Figure 55-1). There is upward convexity or bowing of the corpus callosum related to the lateral ventricular dilation, and there is inferior bowing of the anterior recesses of the third ventricle, with depression of the optic chiasm (see Figure 55-1). Congenital aqueductal stenosis may be seen as an inherited X-linked recessive disorder in boys. Children can present with enlarging head circumference. Blockage of the aqueduct may be caused by webs, septa, or gliosis.

Acquired Aqueductal Stenosis

Aqueductal stenosis is often acquired secondary to previous subarachnoid hemorrhage, meningitis or ventriculitis, or extrinsic compression from a mass or tumor.

Imaging

Magnetic resonance imaging (MRI) is the modality of choice in evaluating affected patients; sagittal MRI is particularly useful in distinguishing intrinsic aqueductal abnormalities from extrinsic compression. The presence of aqueductal CSF flow may be evaluated using spin echo and gradient echo flow scans with gradient moment nulling. On spin echo images, hypointensity within the aqueduct (signal void) is consistent with flow, whereas on gradient echo imaging, the presence of high signal intensity within the aqueduct is consistent with flow.

Reference

Yoshimoto Y, Ochiai C, Kawamata K, et al. Aqueductal blood clot as a cause of acute hydrocephalus in subarachnoid hemorrhage. *AJNR Am J Neuroradiol.* 1996;17:1183-1186.

Cross-Reference

Neuroradiology: THE REQUISITES, 4th ed, pp 232, 286-287.

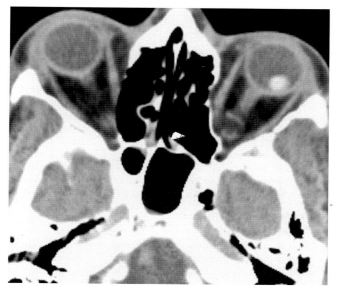

Figure 56-1 Patient A.

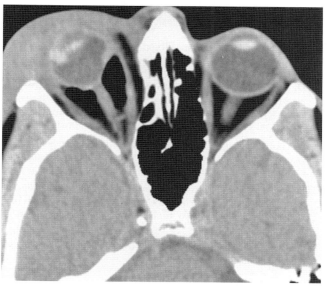

Figure 56-2 Patient B.

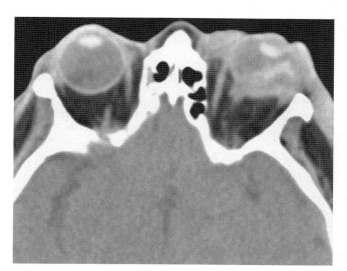

Figure 56-3 Patient C.

HISTORY: Trauma.

1. What abnormality is present in Figure 56-1?
   A. Retinoblastoma
   B. Retinal detachment
   C. Retrobulbar hematoma
   D. Traumatic lens dislocation

2. What abnormality is present in Figures 56-2 and 56-3?
   A. Traumatic lens dislocation
   B. Wood foreign bodies
   C. Post-septal hematoma
   D. Globe rupture

3. A patient was stabbed by a pine wood toothpick, and it is suspected that a retained fragment is present. What would the Hounsfield units (HU) of this retained foreign body most likely be?
   A. 500-750
   B. 250-499
   C. 1-249
   D. <0

4. What entity is associated with dislocation or subluxation of the lens?
   A. Kawasaki syndrome
   B. Ehlers-Danlos syndrome
   C. Maple syrup urine disease
   D. Glutaric aciduria

CASE 56

Ocular Trauma: Lens Dislocation and Globe Rupture

1. **D.** Traumatic lens dislocation. The lens is displaced from its normal anterior location. There is no hematoma in the conal tissues. The retina does not appear detached, and there is no retinal calcification as seen in retinoblastoma.

2. **D.** Globe rupture. The globes are misshapen, there is hyperdensity in the vitreous because of blood, and the anterior chamber sizes are asymmetric.

3. **D.** <0. Dry pine is of very low density and fresh pine is denser; they measure −656 and −24 HU, respectively, in one study. This is well below 0.

4. **B.** Ehlers-Danlos syndrome. Marfan syndrome, Ehlers-Danlos syndrome, and homocystinuria are all associated with dislocation or subluxation of the lens.

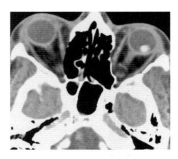

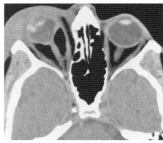

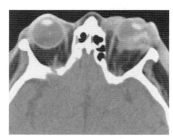

Comment

Computed Tomographic Imaging

On computed tomographic (CT) imaging, lens dislocation (Patient A, Figure 56-1) may be differentiated from other intraocular foreign bodies by confirming that the intraocular density has the configuration of a lens and, importantly, observing that the lens in that eye is not located in its normal position. Lens dislocation may be confirmed on physical examination. CT is the imaging modality of choice in the initial assessment of patients with orbital trauma because of its availability as well as the ease and rapidity with which the examination can be performed. In addition, CT readily establishes the presence of orbital foreign bodies, delineates orbital fractures, and assesses for retrobulbar complications of trauma.

In the Absence of Trauma

Subluxation or dislocation of the lens may be unrelated to trauma. It may be spontaneous or related to infection. There are also hereditary disorders that affect the connective (mesodermal) tissues that may be associated with lens dislocation; these disorders include Marfan syndrome, Ehlers-Danlos syndrome, and homocystinuria. In Marfan syndrome, lens subluxation or dislocation is superior and at the periphery of the globe (and usually bilateral), whereas in homocystinuria, subluxations are inferior ("down and out").

Details of Globe Rupture

Globe rupture indicates that the integrity of the outer membranes of the eye is disrupted. Globe rupture can occur when a blunt object impacts the orbit, causing anterior-posterior compression of the globe and raising intraocular pressure such that the sclera tears. Ruptures from blunt trauma usually occur at the sites where the sclera is thinnest, at the insertions of the extraocular muscles, at the limbus, and around the optic nerve. Sharp objects or those traveling at high velocity can perforate the globe directly. Globe rupture represents an ophthalmologic emergency and requires surgical intervention. Damage to the posterior segment of the eye is associated with a very high incidence of permanent loss of vision. Early recognition and ophthalmologic intervention are critical to maximizing functional outcome. On CT imaging, the presence of vitreous hemorrhage suggests an associated globe rupture. An enlarged anterior chamber and retraction of the lens indicate rupture of the posterior sclera. Other findings of globe rupture are a small, misshapen globe that contains blood or air (Patients B and C, Figures 56-2 and 56-3, respectively).

References

Maguire AM, Enger C, Eliott D, Zinreich SJ. Computerized tomography in the evaluation of penetrating ocular injuries. *Retina*. 1991;11: 405-411.

McGuckin JF Jr, Akhtar N, Ho VT, et al. CT and MR evaluation of a wooden foreign body in an in vitro model of the orbit. *AJNR Am J Neuroradiol*. 1996;17(1):129-133.

Weissman JL, Beatty RL, Hirsch WL, Curtin HD. Enlarged anterior chamber: CT finding of a ruptured globe. *Am J Neuroradiol*. 1995;16(suppl):936-938.

Cross-Reference

Neuroradiology: THE REQUISITES, 4th ed, pp 171, 317.

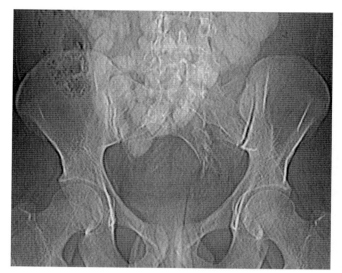

Figure 57-1

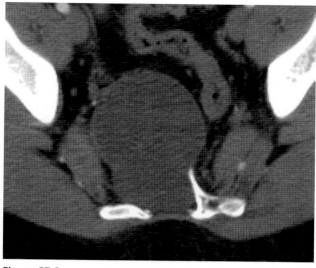

Figure 57-2

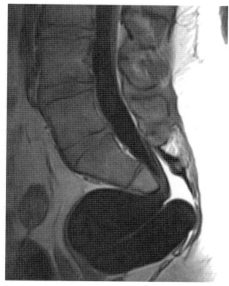

Figure 57-3

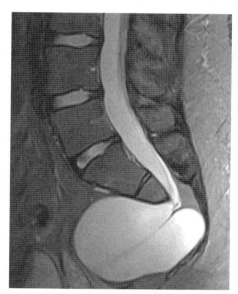

Figure 57-4

HISTORY: A 19-year-old man presents with a 4-month history of back pain and recent onset of urinary incontinence.

1. What should *least* likely be included in the differential diagnosis?
   A. Tarlov cyst
   B. Cystic schwannoma
   C. Chordoma
   D. Anterior sacral meningocele (ASM)

2. What sign has been associated with this lesion on plain films?
   A. Honda sign
   B. Scimitar sign
   C. Scottie dog sign
   D. Molar tooth sign

3. Which of the following is the *most dangerous* complication of ASM?
   A. Meningitis
   B. Constipation
   C. Urinary retention
   D. Leg weakness

4. Which of the following has *not* been associated with ASM?
   A. Currarino triad
   B. Marfan syndrome
   C. Chiari I malformation
   D. Spina bifida

CASE 57

Anterior Sacral Meningocele

1. **C.** Chordoma. The mass has no solid component as would a chordoma. All of the other diagnoses are cystic lesions that may remodel the surrounding bones.

2. **B.** Scimitar sign. Scimitar-shaped sacral deformity on radiography of the pelvis is pathognomonic for ASM. Honda sign has been associated with sacral insufficiency fracture, indicating horizontal involvement of the sacrum and vertical involvement of the sacral ala. Scottie dog sign has been associated with spondylolysis. Molar tooth sign has been associated with Joubert syndrome.

3. **A.** Meningitis. Spontaneous rupture of the sac can lead to severe bacterial meningitis, which is the most dangerous complication of ASM. Constipation is the most common symptom of ASM but is not the most dangerous complication. Urinary retention secondary to direct compression of the bladder by the herniated sac occurs but is not the most dangerous complication. A neurologic deficit such as leg weakness is rare.

4. **C.** Chiari I malformation. ASM may represent the presacral mass of the Currarino triad (anorectal, sacral, and presacral anomalies). ASM may be related to Marfan syndrome. ASM has been described in association with other spinal anomalies including spina bifida and tethered cord, and tumors such as lipomas. ASM is not associated with Chiari I.

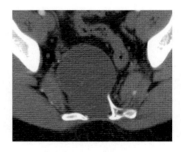

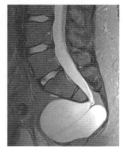

Comment

Demographics and Pathophysiology

ASM is a rare congenital malformation. The real incidence of the malformation is unknown, because it can remain asymptomatic for a long time. When symptomatic, ASMs are usually discovered before the third decade of life. ASM is usually classified among neurulation defects depending on the failure of the neural tube to close. The proposed pathogenetic mechanism is herniation of the arachnoid membrane through a primary dural defect, resulting in pulsatile stresses that erode the bone secondary to cerebrospinal fluid pressure oscillations. The sac of ASM is composed of two layers: outer dural and inner arachnoid membranes, which contain variable amounts of cerebrospinal fluid and occasionally neural roots or benign dysplastic tissues or tumors, or both. The sac may become progressively larger. Partial sacral agenesis is usually found. ASM usually occurs sporadically. Nevertheless, familial cases have been described, which may justify radiologic screening of the relatives of affected patients.

Clinical Findings

Clinical findings are mainly related to the mass effect exerted by the herniated sac on the pelvic structures. Constipation is the most common symptom of ASM, followed by urinary incontinence and dysmenorrhea. Sensory and motor neurologic deficits of the lower limbs and back are rare. The most frequent and dangerous complication of ASM is spontaneous rupture, which can lead to severe bacterial meningitis.

Imaging

On plain radiographs, the pathognomonic finding in ASM is the scimitar sign, a sickle-shaped smooth distortion of the sacrum simulating the shape of an arabic saber (Figure 57-1). A computed tomographic scan (Figure 57-2) can contribute further to the diagnostic work-up by showing the dysraphic sacrum. Magnetic resonance imaging (Figures 57-3 and 57-4) is the technique most frequently used for diagnosis and surgical planning because of its safety, its multiplanar imaging capability, and its effectiveness in discovering associated lesions such as intradural lipoma and tethering of the cord, as seen in this case.

Management

Surgical treatment is mandatory in nearly all cases because ASM does not undergo spontaneous regression and generally progresses in size, with a corresponding increase in the risk of complications. The goals of surgery are to obliterate the communication between ASM and the spinal subarachnoid space, to decompress the pelvis by sac excision, to remove associated tumors, and to untether the spinal cord when necessary.

References

Kovalcik PJ, Burke JB. Anterior sacral meningocele and the scimitar sign: report of a case. *Dis Colon Rectum*. 1988;31(10):806-807.

Massimi L, Calisti A, Koutzoglou M, et al. Giant anterior sacral meningocele and posterior sagittal approach. *Childs Nerv Syst*. 2003;19(10-11):722-728.

Cross-Reference

Neuroradiology: THE REQUISITES, 4th ed, p 299.

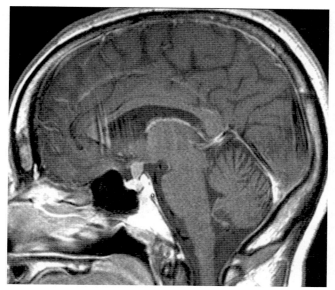

Figure 58-1 Patient A.

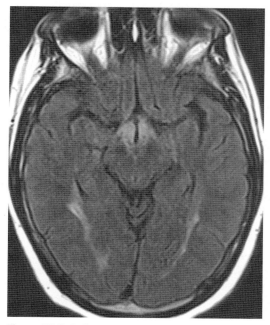

Figure 58-2 Patient B.

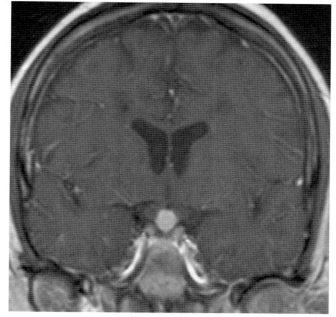

Figure 58-3 Patient B.

HISTORY: Withheld.

1. Which of the following should not be included in the differential diagnosis of these cases?
   A. Granulomatous disease
   B. Metastasis
   C. Germinoma
   D. Pituitary apoplexy

2. What structure is abnormal in Patient A (Figure 58-1), and what other structure is affected in Patient B (Figures 58-2 and 58-3)?
   A. Pituitary stalk and hypothalamus, respectively
   B. Pituitary stalk and pituitary gland, respectively
   C. Pituitary stalk and optic chiasm, respectively
   D. Hypothalamus and pituitary stalk, respectively

3. What is the most likely clinical presentation of infundibular masses?
   A. Ophthalmoplegia
   B. Diabetes mellitus
   C. Visual disturbances
   D. Diabetes insipidus

4. Which of the following is the most correct statement regarding the infundibulum?
   A. The supraoptic nucleus is within the infundibulum.
   B. The infundibulum contains a portal venous system.
   C. Rathke cysts most commonly arise in the infundibulum.
   D. In cases of microadenomas of the pituitary, the infundibulum deviates toward the lesion.

CASE 58

Lesions of the Pituitary Stalk and Hypothalamus: Sarcoidosis and Langerhans Cell Histiocytosis

1. **D.** Pituitary apoplexy. The differential diagnosis of infundibular lesions in adults includes granulomatous disease (sarcoid or tuberculosis), metastasis (especially lung and breast), and germinoma. Less commonly, lymphoma or a hypothalamic glioma can manifest in this way. Apoplexy is hemorrhage within the pituitary gland.

2. **A.** Pituitary stalk and hypothalamus, respectively. The abnormal structure is the pituitary stalk in Patient A; in Patient B, there is T2-FLAIR (fluid-attenuated inversion recovery) hyperintensity in the hypothalamus.

3. **C.** Visual disturbances. Visual disturbance is the most common presentation of infundibular masses, likely from compression of the optic chiasm.

4. **B.** The infundibulum contains a portal venous system. This is called the hypothalamo-hypophyseal portal system. The supraoptic nucleus is in the hypothalamus. Rathke cysts arise in the pituitary gland proper most frequently. The infundibulum commonly deviates away from the side of a pituitary mass.

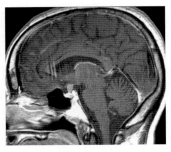

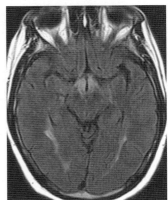

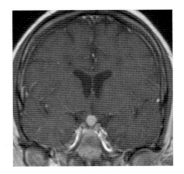

Comment

Patient A: Sarcoidosis

In Patient A, the midline sagittal enhanced T1-weighted magnetic resonance image shows abnormal thickening and enhancement along the pituitary stalk, which lacks normal tapering as it extends inferiorly toward the pituitary gland (Figure 58-1). This represents sarcoid, and it responded well to steroid treatment. This patient had a history of sarcoid with pulmonary involvement. Involvement of the central nervous system (CNS) by sarcoid occurs in approximately 5% to 15% of patients, with isolated involvement of the pituitary gland or stalk in less than 1% to 2% of all patients with sarcoid. When CNS sarcoid occurs with leptomeningeal involvement, the pituitary stalk is commonly involved.

Patient B: Langerhans Cell Histiocytosis

Patient B shows an enhancing mass in the hypothalamic region at the level of the upper pituitary stalk (Figures 58-2 and 58-3), and this represents Langerhans cell histiocytosis. The differential diagnosis of an infundibular mass in children includes germinoma, infection (meningitis or tuberculosis), and less commonly, lymphoma, leukemia, or glioma involving the hypothalamic region. In patients with Langerhans cell histiocytosis, the normal "bright spot" of the posterior pituitary gland in the sella may be absent on unenhanced T1-weighted images. Langerhans cell histiocytosis uncommonly affects the CNS. It is a disorder of the reticuloendothelial system. The most common cranial bone abnormality is a lytic, circumscribed, enhancing mass of the calvaria or skull base. In the cranium, it most commonly involves the temporal bone along the mastoid segment. It also can involve the frontal bone along the orbit.

Differential Diagnosis

The differential diagnosis of an infundibular lesion in adults includes granulomatous disease (sarcoid or tuberculosis) and metastasis (especially lung and breast). Less commonly, lymphoma or a hypothalamic glioma manifests in this way. Lymphocytic adenohypophysitis is a unique condition that almost always affects women. It is most common in the postpartum period or in the late stages (third trimester) of pregnancy. It is characterized by lymphocytic infiltration of the adenohypophysis and is usually self-limited.

Reference

Prayer D, Grois N, Prosch H, et al. MR imaging presentation of intracranial disease associated with Langerhans cell histiocytosis. *Am J Neuroradiol.* 2004;25:880-891.

Cross-Reference

Neuroradiology: THE REQUISITES, 4th ed, pp 202-204, 389.

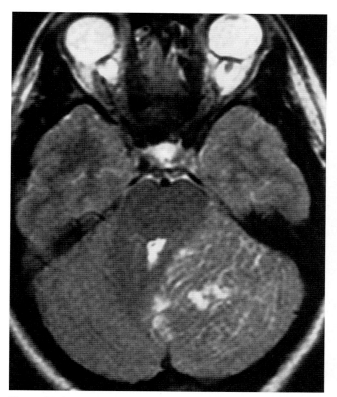

Figure 59-1

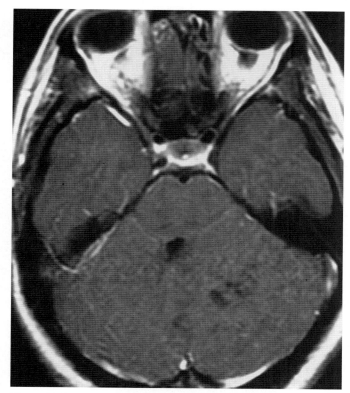

Figure 59-2

HISTORY: Nausea and vomiting.

1. What should *not* be included in the differential diagnosis of the case?
   A. Superior cerebellar artery infarct
   B. Dysplastic cerebellar gangliocytoma
   C. Tuberous sclerosis
   D. Glioblastoma

2. With what neurocutaneous syndrome are dysplastic gangliocytomas associated?
   A. Cowden syndrome
   B. Neurofibromatosis type 1
   C. Sturge-Weber syndrome
   D. Von Hippel–Lindau disease

3. In what location do primitive neuroectodermal tumors (PNETs) occur in adults most often?
   A. Fourth ventricle
   B. Supratentorial region
   C. Pons
   D. Lateral cerebellar hemisphere

4. Following intravenous gadolinium administration, what would you expect to see with this patient's mass?
   A. Solid enhancement
   B. Heterogeneous enhancement
   C. Nodular peripheral enhancement
   D. These lesions most likely do not enhance

CASE 59

Lhermitte-Duclos Disease (Dysplastic Gangliocytoma of the Cerebellum)

1. **D.** Glioblastoma. Differential considerations for Lhermitte-Duclos disease include superior cerebellar artery infarct, acute cerebritis, tuberous sclerosis, leptomeningeal metastatic disease, and granulomatous disease. This would be an atypical location and appearance for glioblastoma.

2. **A.** Cowden syndrome. Gangliocytomas are associated with Cowden syndrome.

3. **D.** Lateral cerebellar hemisphere. PNET occurs most commonly in the lateral cerebellum in adults.

4. **D.** These lesions most likely do not enhance. Enhanced images most often demonstrate no significant enhancement.

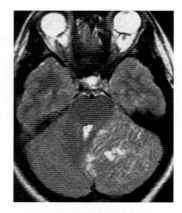

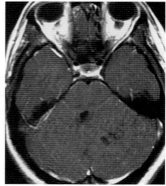

Comment

Lhermitte-Duclos disease is also known as dysplastic gangliocytoma of the cerebellum. Symptomatic patients typically have complaints related to mass effect in the second and third decades of life. Lhermitte-Duclos disease has been associated with Cowden disease (multiple hamartoma syndrome), an autosomal dominant disorder associated with an increased incidence of neoplasms in the pelvis, breast, colon, and thyroid. Intracranial meningiomas have also been noted with this syndrome.

Imaging

These lesions often occur in the cerebellar hemispheres and tend to be poorly demarcated, appearing on computed tomography as a mildly hypodense mass. Calcification has been reported. On magnetic resonance imaging, these lesions have a more characteristic appearance in which both gray and white matter of the cerebellar hemisphere are involved and are thickened and hyperintense on T2-weighted imaging, showing a somewhat characteristic laminated or "corduroy" appearance (Figure 59-1). They can exert mass effect. Hydrocephalus may be present. Dysplastic gangliocytomas do not demonstrate significant enhancement (Figure 59-2).

Controversy

Although this view is controversial, Lhermitte-Duclos disease is considered to represent a complex hamartomatous malformation, not a true neoplasm.

Pathology

On pathologic evaluation, these lesions usually appear as dysplasia with cellular disorganization of the normal laminar structure of the cerebellum and with hypertrophied granular cell neurons. Histologically there is hypermyelination of axons, and pleomorphic ganglion cells replace the granular and Purkinje cell layers.

References

Moonis G, Ibrahim M, Melhem ER. Diffusion-weighted MRI in Lhermitte-Duclos disease: report of two cases. *Neuroradiology*. 2004;46: 351-354.
Nagaraja S, Powell T, Griffiths PD, Wilkinson ID. MR imaging and spectroscopy in Lhermitte-Duclos disease. *Neuroradiology*. 2004;46:355-358.

Cross-Reference

Neuroradiology: THE REQUISITES, 4th ed, pp 67-69.

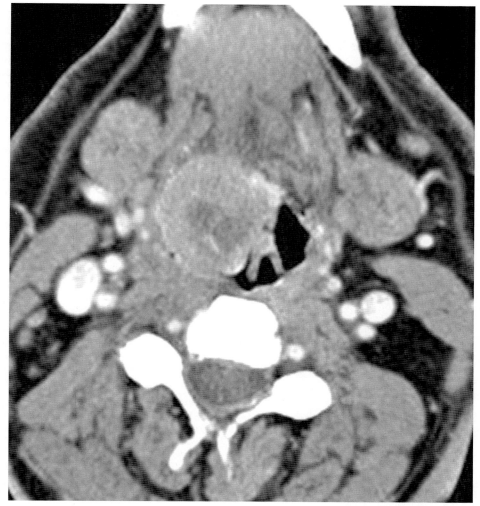

Figure 60-1

HISTORY: A patient has a 2-month history of globus sensation.

1. Which of the following is the single best diagnosis?
   A. Squamous cell carcinoma
   B. Mucus retention cyst
   C. Warthin tumor
   D. Synovial sarcoma

2. In which part of the head and neck is the vallecula located?
   A. Oral cavity
   B. Oropharynx
   C. Hypopharynx
   D. Submental space

3. What structure separates the two sides of the vallecula?
   A. The plica medialis
   B. The pharyngoepiglottic fold
   C. The plica anterialis
   D. The median glossoepiglottic fold

4. Based on the appearance of this cancer in Figure 60-1, what tumor stage is represented?
   A. T1
   B. T2
   C. T3
   D. T4

CASE 60

Squamous Cell Carcinoma of the Vallecula

1. **A.** Squamous cell carcinoma. This is the most common aerodigestive tract tumor. Minor salivary gland cancer may also occur here. Warthin tumor occurs only in and around the parotid gland. Synovial sarcoma is not known to be in this location; it can, however, occur in the hypopharynx.

2. **B.** Oropharynx. The vallecula is part of the oropharynx, along with the soft palate, base of tongue, tonsils, and posterior pharyngeal wall.

3. **D.** The median glossoepiglottic fold. This separates the two sides of the vallecula. The plica medialis does not exist here, and the pharyngoepiglottic fold is more lateral. There is no such structure as a plica anterialis.

4. **A.** T1. T1 staging is indicated in this figure; the cancer is less than 2 cm in greatest diameter. T2 staging implies a size of 2 to 4 cm.

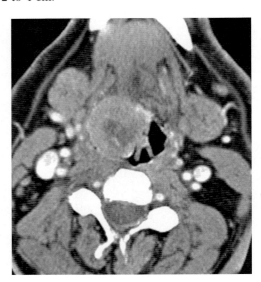

Comment

Treatment Considerations

The issues that are important in considering treatment options for oropharyngeal carcinomas include the following: (1) tumor stage; (2) whether the tumor crosses the midline, which would necessitate a total glossectomy; (3) whether the tumor has invaded mandibular or maxillary bone, which would necessitate flap reconstruction; (4) whether the tumor has invaded the pterygopalatine fossa, which could lead to perineural spread; (5) whether the internal carotid artery is encased, which would render the tumor unresectable; (6) whether the tumor has spread to muscles of mastication; (7) whether the tumor has invaded the skull base; and (8) nodal spread. All of these issues should be addressed with imaging.

Relevant Anatomy

The anatomic structures included in the oropharynx are the tongue base, soft palate, vallecula, tonsil, and posterolateral pharyngeal wall from the level of the hard palate to the pharyngoepiglottic fold. Below the pharyngoepiglottic fold are the larynx anteriorly and the hypopharynx posteriorly (Figure 60-1).

Imaging Findings

Advanced imaging techniques, such as those involving the apparent diffusion coefficient and perfusion parameters for primary tumors and nodal masses, can potentially differentiate those patients with advanced cancers who will respond to chemoradiation protocols from those who will not respond.

Reference

Kim S, Loevner LA, Quon H, et al. Prediction of response to chemoradiation therapy in squamous cell carcinomas of the head and neck using dynamic contrast-enhanced MR imaging. *AJNR Am J Neuroradiol.* 2010;31(2):262-268.

Cross-Reference

Neuroradiology: THE REQUISITES, 4th ed, pp 448, 461.

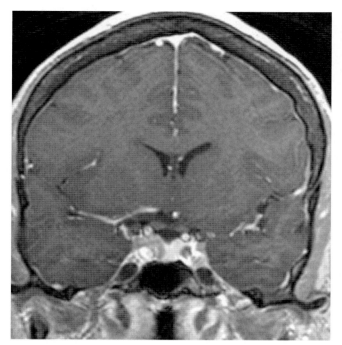

Figure 61-1

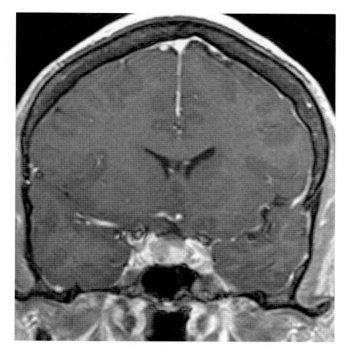

Figure 61-2

HISTORY: Withheld.

1. What is the single most likely diagnosis?
   A. Pituitary adenoma
   B. Lymphocytic hypophysitis
   C. Aneurysm
   D. Meningioma

2. What is the most common functional status of these tumors in autopsy series?
   A. Prolactin secreting
   B. Adrenocorticotropic hormone secreting
   C. Nonfunctional (no hormonal secretion)
   D. Growth hormone secreting

3. A patient with a known pituitary macroadenoma presents with acute onset of headache, nausea and vomiting, visual disturbance, cranial neuropathies, and a change in mental status. What is the likely secondary diagnosis related to the tumor?
   A. Encasement or occlusion of the internal carotid artery by pituitary macroadenoma
   B. Compression of cranial nerves by cavernous invasion
   C. Mass effect on the optic chiasm
   D. Pituitary apoplexy

4. What treatment is associated with an increased incidence of hemorrhage within an adenoma?
   A. Stereotactic radiosurgery
   B. Conventional radiation treatment
   C. Bromocriptine
   D. Transsphenoidal resection

CASE 61

Pituitary Microadenoma

1. **A.** Pituitary adenoma. Top differential considerations for a pituitary macroadenoma include pituitary hyperplasia, aneurysm, meningioma of the diaphragma sellae, metastasis, and lymphocytic hypophysitis.

2. **C.** Nonfunctional (no hormonal secretion). In autopsy series, approximately 50% of all pituitary adenomas are nonfunctional. Approximately 30% of all secreting tumors are prolactinomas. Clinically, functional tumors are more common, as many nonfunctional tumors are asymptomatic.

3. **D.** Pituitary apoplexy. Pituitary apoplexy is a clinical syndrome manifested by the acute onset of headache, nausea, vomiting, visual disturbance, cranial neuropathies, or a change in mental status. It is most commonly associated with hemorrhage within an adenoma, although it has been described with infarction. Most pituitary hemorrhages are asymptomatic.

4. **C.** Bromocriptine. Bromocriptine (a dopamine agonist) used to treat prolactinomas is associated with an increased incidence of hemorrhage within the adenoma.

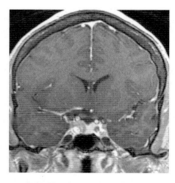

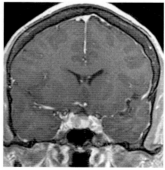

Comment

General and Imaging

Pituitary adenomas are slow-growing, benign epithelial neoplasms arising from the anterior lobe of the gland. They are typically demarcated with a "pseudocapsule" that separates them from the normal gland. Pituitary adenomas 10 mm or larger are referred to as macroadenomas, and those smaller than 10 mm in diameter are referred to as microadenomas. Many adenomas are incidental findings (asymptomatic). On imaging, they show hypoenhancement compared to the surrounding pituitary tissue initially (Figure 61-2) and hyperenhancement on delayed imaging, best seen on dynamic contrast-enhanced magnetic resonance imaging.

The clinical presentation of pituitary adenomas depends on their size, the presence of hormone secretion resulting in endocrine hyperfunction, and the presence of extension beyond the sella (leading to visual symptoms or cranial nerve palsies related to compression, Figure 61-1). In vivo, approximately 75% of pituitary adenomas are hormonally active; however, in autopsy series, nonsecreting adenomas are much more common. About 50% of all are nonsecreting. About 30% of those that secrete are prolactinomas.

Hormonally Active Tumors

The most common clinically significant secreting adenoma is the prolactinoma (which arises from the prolactin-secreting cells [lactotrophs]). In women, the most common clinical presentation is irregular menses, galactorrhea, and infertility. In men, impotence may be present. Hormonally active pituitary adenomas arising from somatotrophs, the growth hormone-secreting cells, cause acromegaly in adults and gigantism in children. In acromegaly, endochondral and periosteal bone formation is stimulated, as is proliferation of connective tissue. These changes result in bone overgrowth and increased soft tissue thickness, especially in the "acral" regions (feet, hands, mandible). There is enlargement of the mandible, thickening of the cranial vault, and frontal bossing (the result of enlargement of the frontal sinuses and prominence of the supraorbital ridges).

Reference

Indrajit IK, Chidambaranathan N, Sundar K, Ahmed I. Value of dynamic MRI imaging in pituitary adenomas. *Indian J Radiol Imaging.* 2001;11:185-190.

Cross-Reference

Neuroradiology: THE REQUISITES, 4th ed, pp 352-353.

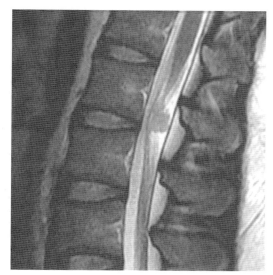

Figure 62-1

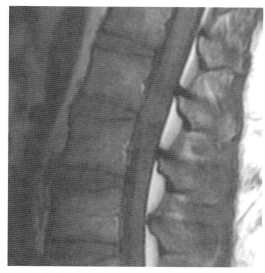

Figure 62-2

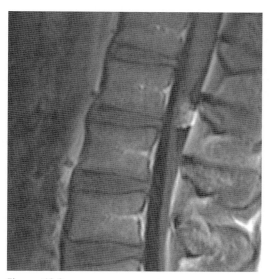

Figure 62-3

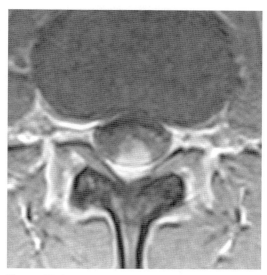

Figure 62-4

HISTORY: A 31-year-old man presents with a 2-year history of intermittent numbness and burning in the left anterior thigh.

1. Which of the following should *not* be included in the differential diagnosis?
   A. Myxopapillary ependymoma
   B. Paraganglioma
   C. Arachnoid cyst
   D. Schwannoma

2. What is the most common primary tumor involving the filum terminale?
   A. Hemangioblastoma
   B. Dermoid
   C. Ependymoma
   D. Astrocytoma

3. Which of the following statements regarding myxopapillary ependymoma subtype is true?
   A. Overall it accounts for approximately 70% of ependymomas.
   B. It arises almost exclusively from the filum terminale.
   C. It rarely manifests with subarachnoid hemorrhage.
   D. Calcifications are less common in this subtype than in other subtypes.

4. Which of the following best describes the imaging characteristics of myxopapillary ependymoma?
   A. Epidural mass showing hyperintense signal on T1-weighted images, hypointense signal on T2-weighted images, and no enhancement
   B. Well-circumscribed mass showing hypointense signal on T1-weighted and T2-weighted images and no enhancement
   C. Well-circumscribed enhancing mass showing isointense-to-hyperintense T1 signal, hyperintense T2 signal, and enhancement
   D. Well-circumscribed mass following cerebrospinal fluid signal on all pulse sequences

CASE 62

Myxopapillary Ependymoma

1. **C.** Arachnoid cyst. Arachnoid cysts typically have cerebrospinal fluid–like signal with no appreciable enhancement. Given the involvement of the filum terminale by this enhancing mass, myxopapillary ependymoma is the foremost consideration. Paragangliomas of the conus are rare, highly vascular tumors that demonstrate diffuse inhomogeneous avid enhancement. A schwannoma is a good possibility for an intradural extramedullary mass with inhomogeneous enhancement.

2. **C.** Ependymoma. A primary tumor involving the filum is most likely to be an ependymoma. Hemangioblastomas are more commonly intramedullary and in the cervicothoracic spine. Dermoids rarely occur in this location. Astrocytomas are intramedullary tumors.

3. **B.** It arises almost exclusively from the filum terminale. This statement is true; this subtype is rarely found elsewhere. The myxopapillary subtype accounts for only 30% of ependymomas. This subtype may manifest with subarachnoid hemorrhage. Calcifications are more common in this subtype.

4. **C.** Well-circumscribed enhancing mass showing isointense-to-hyperintense T1 signal, hyperintense T2 signal, and enhancement. These findings are typical for myxopapillary ependymomas, which are intradural in location and show hyperintense T2 signal. Since these lesions enhance, they do not follow cerebrospinal fluid signal on all pulse sequences.

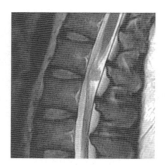

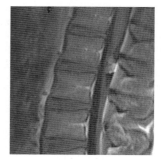

Comment

Demographics and Clinical Findings

Myxopapillary ependymomas of the filum terminale tend to occur in adults in the fourth decade of life. The most common clinical manifestation is low back pain, which may be accompanied by sciatic pain or other symptoms and signs of lumbosacral radiculopathy. There may be associated lower limb sensory disturbance or urinary sphincter disturbance.

Pathophysiology

Myxopapillary ependymomas are benign, slow-growing gliomas and are classified histologically as World Health Organization grade I. Myxopapillary ependymomas account for most ependymomas that arise in the lumbosacral area; involvement is usually limited to the conus medullaris and filum terminale. Uncommonly, these lesions may invade the nerve roots or sacrum. They are presumed to arise from ependymal cell rests normally present in the filum terminale.

Imaging

Magnetic resonance imaging (MRI) is the preferred imaging modality (Figures 62-1 through 62-4). Myxopapillary ependymomas are characteristically well-circumscribed, sausage-shaped tumors causing compression and displacement of the adjacent roots of the cauda equina (see Figure 62-4). These highly vascular tumors demonstrate mucinous changes not present in other histologic subtypes of ependymomas. The mucinous changes are presumed to be responsible for the increased frequency with which hyperintensity relative to cord signal is detected on precontrast T1-weighted images compared with the other subtypes. The hypervascularity of these tumors explains the features of intratumoral or subarachnoid hemorrhage (which can result in superficial siderosis) and the marked postcontrast enhancement sometimes observed on MRI. Generally, these tumors are hyperintense on T2-weighted images and isointense to hyperintense on T1-weighted images.

Management

The recognition of these tumors as a distinct entity is of considerable clinical importance because they are more amenable to radical surgical resection than most other variants of ependymoma. The goal of surgical resection, which is the primary mode of therapy, is to achieve complete resection while minimizing postoperative neurologic deficits. The extent of surgical resection is mainly related to tumor encapsulation and to involvement of the conus medullaris and cauda equina.

References

Bagley CA, Kothbauer KF, Wilson S, et al. Resection of myxopapillary ependymomas in children. *J Neurosurg*. 2007;106(4 suppl):261-267.

Wippold FJ II, Smirniotopoulos JG, Moran CJ, et al. MR imaging of myxopapillary ependymoma: findings and value to determine extent of tumor and its relation to intraspinal structures. *AJR Am J Roentgenol*. 1995;165(5):1263-1267.

Cross-Reference

Neuroradiology: THE REQUISITES, 4th ed, pp 573-574.

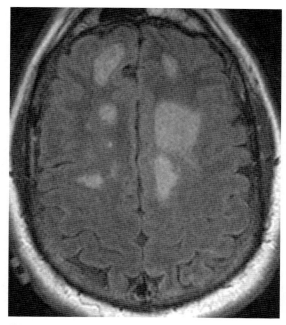

Figure 63-1

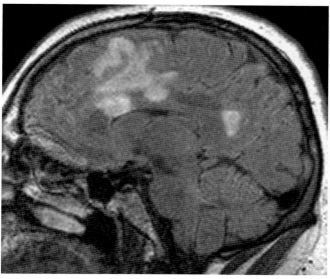

Figure 63-2

HISTORY: Weakness, numbness, tingling, and gait disturbance.

1. In a 29-year-old female, what would be the favored single diagnosis of the case?
   A. Multiple sclerosis
   B. Acute disseminated encephalomyelitis (ADEM)
   C. Lyme disease
   D. Vasculitis

2. What percentage of patients with this disease present in childhood and adolescence?
   A. 2% to 10%
   B. 15% to 25%
   C. 35% to 45%
   D. More than 75%

3. Which of the following is a correct statement regarding the revised McDonald diagnostic imaging criteria for this disease?
   A. Dissemination in space is considered when more than one lobe of the cerebrum is involved.
   B. Dissemination in time *cannot* be diagnosed on imaging if there is only one magnetic resonance image available.
   C. Dissemination in time can be diagnosed with the simultaneous presence of enhancing and non-enhancing lesions at any time.
   D. Dissemination in space can be diagnosed if there is a lesion in the pons and the cerebellum.

4. What finding may be present in the cerebrospinal fluid in patients with this disease?
   A. Elevated oligoclonal bands
   B. Reduced oligoclonal bands
   C. Reduced immunoglobulin G (IgG)
   D. Elevated aquaporin-4 antibodies (AQP4-Ab)

CASE 63

Multiple Sclerosis, Marburg Type

1. **A.** Multiple sclerosis (MS). Differential considerations include MS, ADEM, Lyme disease, vasculitis, and Susac syndrome.

2. **A.** 2% to 10%. The more precise range is approximately 3% to 5%.

3. **C.** Dissemination in time can be diagnosed with the simultaneous presence of enhancing and non-enhancing lesions at any time. This is a major revision in the imaging diagnosis of MS, where before a prior examination was necessary to show temporal changes. To identify dissemination in space, clinicians need hyperintense T2 lesions in at least two of the following four areas: juxtacortical, periventricular, infratentorial, and the spinal cord. (For further details, see Polman, Reingold, and Banwell, et al, 2011.)

4. **A.** Elevated oligoclonal bands. Elevated oligoclonal bands (≥90% of cases) and elevated IgG levels (approximately 75% of patients) are found in the cerebrospinal fluid in patients with this disease.

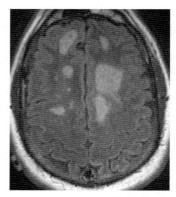

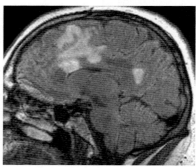

Comment

Although the etiology of MS is unknown, several causative factors have been implicated. These include autoimmune disease, infection (viral agent), and genetic factors. The prevalence of MS varies with geographic location.

Variants of Multiple Sclerosis

Variants of MS may be present on a clinical or imaging basis. A handful of rare borderline types of MS occur, including Marburg type (also known as acute, fulminant, or malignant MS), which is a form of acute MS usually seen in younger patients that may be preceded by fevers, is typically rapidly progressive, and can result in death. In such cases, there is extensive demyelination and there may be defined rings within or surrounding plaques of acute demyelination (Figures 63-1 and 63-2). Enhancement is typically seen in the region of these rings. Concentric sclerosis or Balo-type sclerosis is characterized histologically by alternating rings of demyelination and myelination (normal brain or areas of remyelination) and has a characteristic magnetic resonance imaging (MRI) appearance. Schilder disease is a rare progressive demyelinating disorder that usually begins in childhood. Symptoms can include dementia, aphasia, seizures, personality changes, tremors, imbalance, incontinence, muscle weakness, headache, and visual impairment.

"Tumefactive" MS on imaging may be mistaken for a neoplasm or occasionally an abscess, particularly in the absence of a clinical history. The age of the patient may be helpful (MS typically occurs in younger patients). In addition, on close questioning, patients often have neurologic symptoms that are spaced in both time and location. MRI might show white matter lesions separate from the mass, suggesting MS. Unlike neoplasms, tumefactive MS often has relatively little mass effect for the amount of signal abnormality present.

A Word on Neuromyelitis Optica

A demyelinating disease apart from MS that is usually limited to the optic nerves and spinal cord (either simultaneously or separately) is neuromyelitis optica, the main symptoms of which are loss of vision and spinal cord dysfunction. The visual impairment can consist of reduced visual fields, diminished light sensitivity, or loss of color vision. Spinal cord dysfunction includes muscle weakness, lack of coordination, reduced sensation, and incontinence. The brain is usually spared.

References

Cianfoni A, Niku S, Imbesi SG. Metabolite findings in tumefactive demyelinating lesions utilizing short echo time proton magnetic resonance spectroscopy. *Am J Neuroradiol.* 2007;28:272-277.

Polman CH, Reingold SC, Banwell B, et al. Diagnostic criteria for multiple sclerosis: 2010 revisions to the McDonald criteria. *Ann Neurol.* 2011;69(2):292-302.

Cross-Reference

Neuroradiology: THE REQUISITES, 4th ed, p 212.

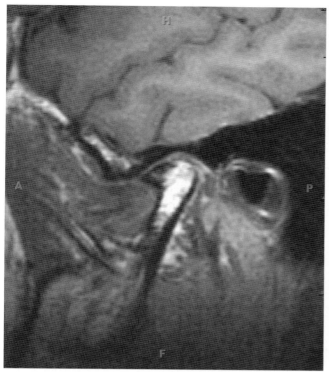

Figure 64-1

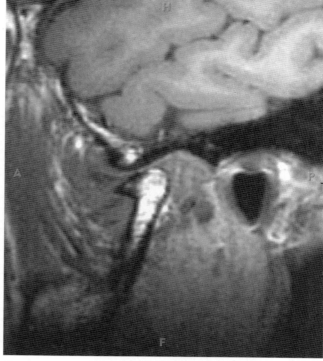

Figure 64-2

HISTORY: A 35-year-old woman complains about long-standing left-sided pain in the temporomandibular joint (TMJ).

1. Which of the following is the single best diagnosis?
   A. Anterior displacement with recapture
   B. Anterior displacement without recapture
   C. Normal
   D. Posterior meniscus displacement with recapture

2. To what does "sideways displacement of a meniscus" refer?
   A. Medial displacement
   B. Lateral displacement
   C. Medial or lateral displacement
   D. Anterior or posterior meniscus displacement

3. What percentage of the normal symptom-free population has meniscal abnormalities of the TMJ?
   A. Less than 10%
   B. 11% to 20%
   C. 21% to 40%
   D. 41% to 60%

4. What is the biggest technical challenge of evaluating the TMJ on magnetic resonance imaging (MRI)?
   A. Imaging the correct plane of the mandible
   B. Optimizing the contrast
   C. The timing of the enhancement
   D. Getting the patient to open the jaw sufficiently

CASE 64

Temporomandibular Joint Disease

1. **B.** Anterior displacement without recapture. The meniscus remains anterior in open- and closed-mouth views. Therefore, there is anterior displacement of the meniscus without recapture.

2. **C.** Medial or lateral displacement. "Sideways displacement of a meniscus" refers to either medial or lateral displacement. It does not refer to anterior or posterior displacement.

3. **C.** 21% to 40%. Approximately 30% of normal symptom-free people have meniscal abnormalities of the TMJ. These abnormalities usually reflect anterior displacement with recapture.

4. **D.** Getting the patient to open the jaw sufficiently. For patients with this condition, opening the jaw sometimes hurts, and the patient cannot keep it open for the duration of the examination. One must look at the degree of mandibular condyle displacement to determine whether the opening has been adequate.

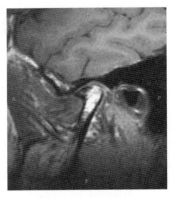

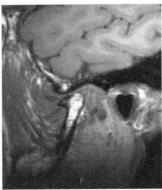

Comment

Difficulties with Imaging the Temporomandibular Joint

MRI of the TMJ is fraught with difficulty. Affected patients are often in discomfort. They move a lot. They do not want to open the mouth widely because it elicits discomfort. Once the mouth is open, it is hard to keep open for the sequence duration of 3 to 4 minutes, and so a bite block must often be used, but that can produce nonphysiologic artifact on images. The plane of section is difficult to achieve in sagittal and coronal views, especially because the right and left TMJs are oriented differently, and yet both are to be scanned at the same time. Furthermore, when the meniscus is anteriorly located, technicians must know to scan not through the joint alone but also in front of the joint to search for a sideways (medial-lateral) displacement of the meniscus (Figures 64-1 and 64-2).

Menisci Displacement

Most menisci become displaced anteriorly, anteromedially, or anterolaterally. They are rarely displaced only in a medial-to-lateral direction. They are not displaced posteriorly because the issue is laxity of the bilaminar zone, which allows the meniscus to slip anteriorly. When the meniscus pops back into place on opening of the jaw, it causes a clicking sound or feeling and, if it goes into the normal location on opening, the condition is termed *anterior displacement with recapture*. In the case described here, however, the meniscus remains anteriorly located, and thus the condition is termed *anterior displacement without recapture*. This is why the open- and closed-mouth views are imaged. The clicking may occur as the meniscus pops forward anteriorly on closing of the mouth as well.

Associations with Temporomandibular Joint Disease

TMJ disease occurs in young (premenopausal) women. Thus, most authorities believe it is hormonally mediated, potentially from the effect of estrogen on the connective tissue resulting in laxity of the bilaminar zone that attaches to the back of the meniscus.

References

Bag AK, Gaddikeri S, Singhal A, et al. Imaging of the temporomandibular joint: an update. *World J Radiol.* 2014;6(8):567-582.

Tomas X, Pomes J, Berenguer J, et al. MR imaging of temporomandibular joint dysfunction: a pictorial review. *Radiographics.* 2006; 26(3):765-781.

Cross-Reference

Neuroradiology: THE REQUISITES, 4th ed, pp 496-499.

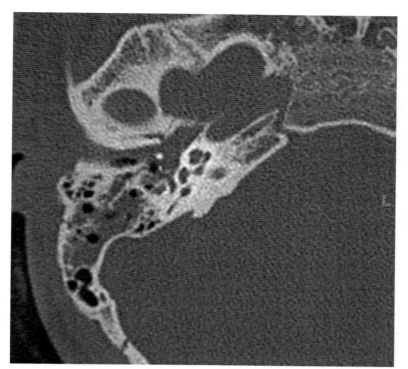

Figure 65-1

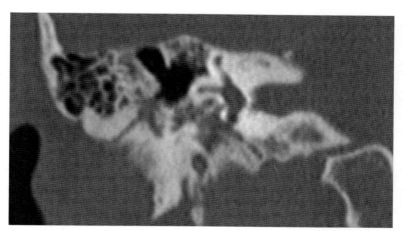

Figure 65-2

HISTORY: A 54-year-old man was involved in a high-speed collision that resulted in head trauma and hearing loss.

1. Which of the following is probably the cause of conductive hearing loss in this patient?
   A. Malleus fracture
   B. Incudomalleolar dislocation
   C. Middle ear hemotympanum
   D. Incudostapedial dislocation

2. Fractures along the plane of the petrous apex often extend into which of the following structures?
   A. The external auditory canal
   B. The jugular foramen
   C. The carotid canal
   D. The internal auditory canal

3. What is Battle sign?
   A. Bloodshot eyes
   B. "Shiners" under the eyelids
   C. Ecchymosis at the mastoid tip
   D. Blood in the external auditory canal

4. Which of the following is *not* a complication of temporal bone fracture?
   A. Meningitis
   B. Facial nerve palsy
   C. Perilymphatic fistula
   D. Cholesterol granuloma

CASE 65

Temporal Bone Fracture

1. **C.** Middle ear hemotympanum. Fluid of any kind in the middle ear can cause conductive hearing loss. Incudomalleolar and incudostapedial dislocation are common dislocations but not the most common cause of hearing loss. Malleus fracture and fracture through the cochlea are rare.

2. **C.** The carotid canal. Fractures in the plane of the petrous apex may extend along the carotid canal and then into the sphenoid sinus.

3. **C.** Ecchymosis at the mastoid tip. Ecchymosis at the mastoid tip may be associated with squamosal temporal bone fracture. Blood in the external auditory canal may be associated with any temporal bone fracture. "Shiners" under the eyelids are associated with orbital and skull base fractures.

4. **D.** Cholesterol granuloma. Cholesterol granuloma is not considered a complication of temporal bone fracture. Meningitis can occur with tegmen tympani disruption. Facial nerve palsy can result when the tympanic portion of the facial nerve is injured with oblique or horizontal temporal bone fractures. Perilymphatic fistula into the labyrinth can also be caused by temporal bone fractures.

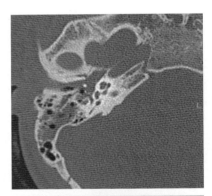

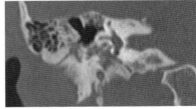

Comment

Classification of Temporal Bone Fractures

The classification of temporal bone fractures has undergone multiple revisions over time. Initially, the differentiation was between horizontal and vertical fractures according to the plane of the tegmen tympani. Physicians later realized that most fractures occurred in an oblique plane and that the classical vertical-versus-horizontal separation was relatively artificial. The current classification differentiates between fractures that involve the labyrinthine structures and those that do not. In describing temporal bone fractures, no matter what the classification, it is important to describe whether each of the following is present:

- Ossicular fracture
- Ossicular dislocation
- Facial nerve transection (canal intact?)
- Labyrinthine fracture
- Tegmen tympani disruption
- Carotid canal involvement
- Blood in the external auditory canal and/or middle ear

Facial Nerve Trauma

Facial nerve trauma occurs more commonly with classical horizontal (longitudinal) fractures and oblique fractures than with vertical (transverse) fractures (Figures 65-1 and 65-2). When facial nerve palsy occurs after trauma, decompression may be required; it should be performed between 2 weeks and 2 months after the injury. The classification of facial nerve injury is the House-Brackmann grading system (see table).

Grade	Characteristics
I. Normal	Normal facial function in all areas
II. Mild dysfunction	**Gross** Slight weakness noticeable on close inspection Possible presence of slight synkinesis At rest, normal symmetry and tone
	Motion Forehead: moderate-to-good function Eye: complete closure with minimal effort Mouth: slight asymmetry
III. Moderate dysfunction	**Gross** Obvious but not disfiguring difference between the two sides Noticeable but not severe synkinesis, contracture, or hemifacial spasm At rest, normal symmetry and tone
	Motion Forehead: slight-to-moderate movement Eye: complete closure with effort Mouth: slightly weak with maximum effort
IV. Moderately severe dysfunction	**Gross** Obvious weakness and/or disfiguring asymmetry At rest, normal symmetry and tone
	Motion Forehead: none Eye: incomplete closure Mouth: asymmetric with maximum effort
V. Severe dysfunction	**Gross** Only barely perceptible motion At rest, asymmetry
	Motion Forehead: none Eye: incomplete closure Mouth: slight movement
VI. Total paralysis	No movement

From House JW, Brackmann DE. Facial nerve grading system. *Otolaryngol Head Neck Surg.* 1985;93(2):146-147.

Reference

Ulug T, Arif Ulubil S. Management of facial paralysis in temporal bone fractures: a prospective study analyzing 11 operated fractures. *Am J Otolaryngol.* 2005;26(4):230-238.

Cross-Reference

Neuroradiology: THE REQUISITES, 4th ed, pp 407-409.

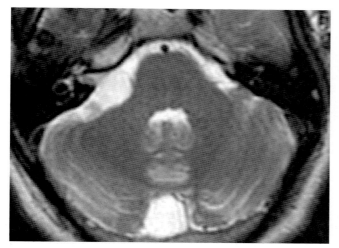

Figure 66-1

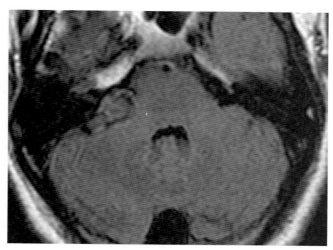

Figure 66-2

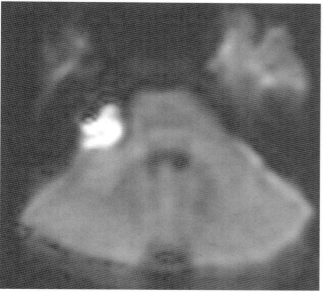

Figure 66-3

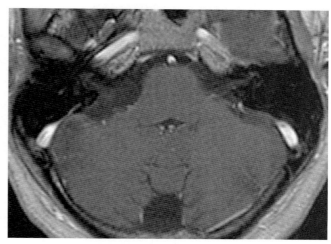

Figure 66-4

HISTORY: Ataxia.

1. Where is this lesion located?
   A. Prepontine cistern
   B. Cerebellopontine cistern
   C. Subdural space
   D. Epidural space

2. What is the single best diagnosis of the case?
   A. Arachnoid cyst
   B. Epidermoid
   C. Abscess
   D. Schwannoma

3. Which mass found in the lateral skull base is of the same histology as an epidermoid?
   A. Cholesterol granuloma
   B. Glomus tympanicum
   C. Mucocele
   D. Cholesteatoma

4. Which statement about K-space is correct?
   A. Each row represents one frequency encoding step.
   B. The central portion of K-space contains the higher spatial frequencies.
   C. The periphery of K-space contains the information about image contrast.
   D. Undersampling the high spatial frequencies can result in truncation artifact.

CASE 66

Epidermoid Cyst: Cerebellopontine Cistern

1. **B.** Cerebellopontine cistern. This is a classic location for an epidermoid cyst.

2. **B.** Epidermoid. The epidermoid cyst of the cerebellopontine angle shows restricted diffusion and does not completely suppress on fluid-attenuated inversion recovery (FLAIR).

3. **D.** Cholesteatoma. These lesions are lined by a single layer of stratified squamous epithelium, and they contain desquamated epithelium, keratin, and cholesterol crystals.

4. **D.** Undersampling the high spatial frequencies can result in truncation artifact. The periphery of K-space contains the higher frequencies related to detail. Increasing the matrix is a way to overcome the artifact.

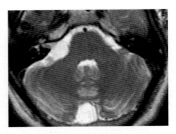

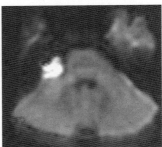

Comment

Epidermoid cysts are congenital lesions that result from incomplete separation of the neural and cutaneous ectoderm at the time of closure of the neural tube. These cysts are lined by a single layer of stratified squamous epithelium, and they contain desquamated epithelium, keratin, and cholesterol crystals. Many of these cysts are incidental findings, but when a patient is symptomatic, epidermoid cysts typically occur in the third or fourth decade of life. Men and women are equally affected. These cysts often do not cause symptoms, but in the cerebellopontine cistern, they can manifest with dizziness, trigeminal neuralgia, and facial nerve weakness.

Imaging

This case illustrates the typical appearance of an epidermoid cyst. There is a mass in the right cerebellopontine angle cistern that exerts mild mass effect on the adjacent brainstem (Figures 66-1 through 66-4). On unenhanced T1-weighted images (not shown), this mass is mildly hyperintense to cerebrospinal fluid (CSF), with fine internal architecture. On the T2-weighted image (see Figure 66-1), the lesion is isointense to CSF. Unlike arachnoid cysts, which are typically isointense to CSF on proton density and FLAIR images, epidermoid cysts are hyperintense relative to CSF on these pulse sequences (see Figure 66-2). This case illustrates hyperintensity on diffusion-weighted images, consistent with restricted diffusion, characteristic of these lesions (see Figure 66-3). After contrast, there is no enhancement, as in this case (see Figure 66-4). Other characteristic features of epidermoid cysts that distinguish them from arachnoid cysts (the major differential consideration here) are also present in this case, including the lobulated and scalloped borders of this lesion and its insinuating nature, which fills and conforms to the shape of the space that it occupies.

K-Space

K-space represents the collection of raw data from a magnetic resonance image. Each row represents one phase encoding step. The center of K-space contains the lower spatial frequencies related to image contrast. The periphery contains the higher frequencies related to detail. Undersampling the high spatial frequencies can result in truncation artifact.

References

Bushberg JT, Seibert JA, Leidholdt EM Jr, Boone JM. "K-space" data acquisition and image reconstruction. In: *The Essential Physics of Medical Imaging*. 3rd ed. Philadelphia: Lippincott Williams & Wilkins; 2011:444-446.

Kallmes DF, Provenzale JM, Cloft HJ, McClendon RE. Typical and atypical MR imaging features of intracranial epidermoid tumors. *AJR Am J Roentgenol*. 1997;169:883-887.

Tien RD, Felsberg GJ, Lirng JF. Variable bandwidth steady-state free-precession MR imaging: a technique for improving characterization of epidermoid tumor and arachnoid cyst. *AJR Am J Roentgenol*. 1995;164:689-692.

Cross-Reference

Neuroradiology: THE REQUISITES, 4th ed, pp 53-55.

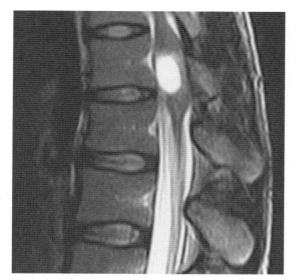

Figure 67-1

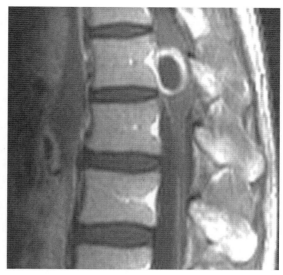

Figure 67-2

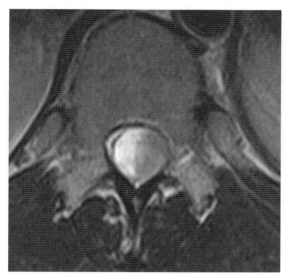

Figure 67-3

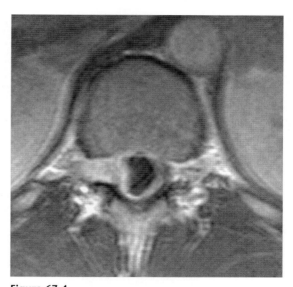

Figure 67-4

HISTORY: A 33-year-old man with a 6-month history of back pain, progressive weakness of the lower extremities, constipation, and bladder dysfunction presents to the emergency department with recent worsening of symptoms.

1. Which of the following should *not* be included in the differential diagnosis?
   A. Myxopapillary ependymoma
   B. Cystic meningioma
   C. Cystic schwannoma
   D. Congenital arachnoid cyst

2. Which term best describes this lesion's location?
   A. Intradural extramedullary
   B. Extradural
   C. Intramedullary
   D. Epidural

3. Which of the following cystic lesions should *not* be included in the differential diagnosis of the lesion shown?
   A. Enterogenous (neurenteric) cyst
   B. Epidermoid
   C. Tarlov cyst
   D. Arachnoid cyst

4. The depicted lesion is more frequently observed in patients with which of the following conditions?
   A. Neurofibromatosis type 1
   B. Neurofibromatosis type 2
   C. Von Hippel–Lindau disease
   D. Chiari I malformation

CASE 67

Cystic Schwannoma of Conus Medullaris Region

1. **D.** Congenital arachnoid cyst. Congenital arachnoid cysts typically are located in the dorsal thoracic epidural space. These lesions do not show enhancement. Myxopapillary ependymomas are intradural and found in the lumbar canal. They may show a cystic component. Meningiomas and schwannomas are the most common intradural tumors. Cystic meningiomas have been described. Cystic schwannoma is the most likely diagnosis considering the foraminal extension seen in this case.

2. **A.** Intradural extramedullary. The lesion displaces the conus medullaris. An intramedullary lesion of this size would be expected to cause cord edema.

3. **C.** Tarlov cyst. Tarlov cysts are extradural and typically located in the sacrum. A neurenteric cyst may manifest as an intradural rim-enhancing cystic lesion. Epidermoid follows cerebrospinal fluid signal on all pulse sequences and may appear as a cystic lesion. An infected arachnoid cyst may manifest as an intradural rim-enhancing cystic lesion.

4. **B.** Neurofibromatosis type 2. Patients with neurofibromatosis type 2 present with multiple schwannomas, meningiomas, and ependymomas. There is no increase in frequency of intraspinal schwannomas in patients with neurofibromatosis type 1. Von Hippel–Lindau disease is associated with the development of hemangioblastomas, and there is no increase in frequency of intraspinal schwannomas. In Chiari I malformation, there is tonsillar ectopia, and intraspinal schwannomas do not occur with increased frequency.

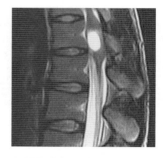

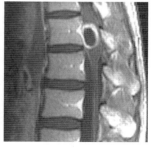

Comment

Demographics

Intraspinal schwannomas are most frequently seen in the lumbar region with a predilection for the thoracolumbar junction. Spinal schwannomas may be well circumscribed, intradural, or extradural, or combined intradural-extradural. The percentage of purely intradural nerve sheath tumors increases from 8% in the upper cervical region to 80% in the thoracolumbar region. This increase may be explained by the anatomic features of the spinal nerve roots, which have a longer intradural component at the caudal portion of the spinal axis.

Clinical Presentation

Back pain is the most common symptom of lumbar schwannomas. In schwannomas of the conus region, features of cauda equina and conus compression, including progressive pain, neurologic deficits, and bladder dysfunction, may be observed. These features help differentiate tumor from mechanical causes of back pain. A delayed presentation is common because these tumors are slow growing, and the affected patients are young and otherwise healthy.

Imaging

Magnetic resonance imaging is the preferred imaging modality (Figures 67-1 through 67-4). Peripheral contrast enhancement is a feature of intradural schwannomas that can help clinicians differentiate these lesions from neurofibromas, which tend to have more homogeneous, solid enhancement (see Figures 67-2 and 67-4). This pattern of peripheral enhancement has been observed when patients are scanned immediately after contrast agent injection. Delayed scans may or may not reveal this pattern. The hyperintense, nonenhancing regions within the tumor on T2-weighted images (see Figures 67-1 and 67-4) often correspond pathologically to areas of cyst formation and necrosis; however, these regions may also represent areas of diminished vascularity or increased compactness of the tumor. No correlation has been established between signal characteristics or enhancement patterns and the prevalence of Antoni type A or type B tissue within intradural schwannomas.

Management

Cystic schwannomas behave in a similar fashion to solid schwannomas and should be treated with surgical excision, which can be difficult because of the adhesion of the tumor capsule to the surrounding structures, fragile tumor capsules, and difficulty in identifying the arachnoidal planes. Complete excision without resultant neurologic deficits may be feasible, provided that there is no entrapment of nerve roots. Prognosis is usually excellent with the exception of the melanotic variant, malignant forms, and cases of neurofibromatosis.

References

Borges G, Bonilha L, Proa M Jr, et al. Imaging features and treatment of an intradural lumbar cystic schwannoma. *Arq Neuropsiquiatr.* 2005;63(3A):681-684.

Jaiswal A, Shetty AP, Rajasekaran S. Giant cystic intradural schwannoma in the lumbosacral region: a case report. *J Orthop Surg (Hong Kong).* 2008;16(1):102-106.

Cross-Reference

Neuroradiology: THE REQUISITES, 4th ed, p 505.

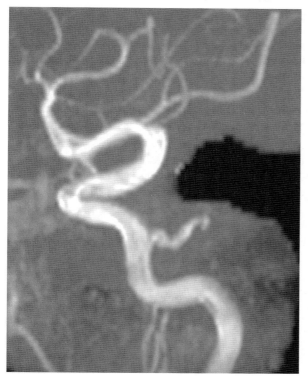

Figure 68-1

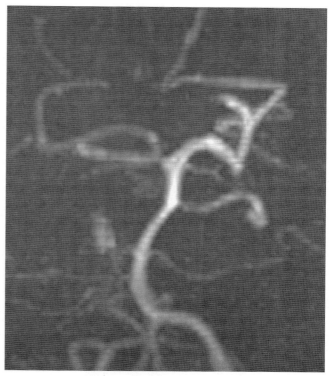

Figure 68-2

HISTORY: Trigeminal neuralgia.

1. What is the single best diagnosis of the case?
   A. Persistent trigeminal artery
   B. Persistent otic artery
   C. Persistent hypoglossal artery
   D. Fetal origin of the posterior cerebral artery

2. What is the most commonly recognized fetal-embryologic carotid-vertebrobasilar anastomosis, excluding posterior communicating arteries?
   A. Trigeminal artery
   B. Otic artery
   C. Hypoglossal artery
   D. Vertebrobasilar loops

3. What percentage of cerebral arteriograms reveal this finding?
   A. Less than 1%
   B. 5%
   C. 10%
   D. 50%

4. What other intracranial vascular abnormalities have been associated with this finding?
   A. Basilar fenestrations
   B. Developmental venous anomalies
   C. Cavernomas
   D. Aneurysms and arteriovenous malformations

CASE 68

Persistent Trigeminal Artery

1. **A.** Persistent trigeminal artery. This is a persistent trigeminal artery with communication between the precavernous internal carotid artery and the basilar artery.

2. **A.** Trigeminal artery. Otic artery is controversial and not found in lower order species. The hypoglossal artery is less common than the trigeminal artery. Vertebrobasilar loops are not an anterior-posterior communication.

3. **A.** Less than 1%. Approximately 0.1% to 0.5% of cerebral arteriograms reveal this finding.

4. **D.** Aneurysms and arteriovenous malformations have been associated with this finding.

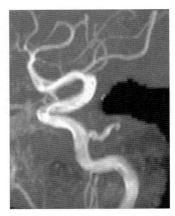

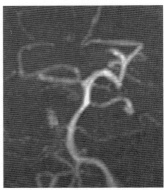

Comment

The trigeminal, otic, and hypoglossal arteries (named after the cranial nerves with which they course) are the three embryologic anastomoses between the anterior internal carotid artery and the posterior vertebrobasilar circulations. The persistent trigeminal artery is the most common embryonic carotid-vertebrobasilar anastomosis to persist into adulthood, reported in as many as 0.1% to 0.5% of cerebral arteriograms. Persistent trigeminal artery may be associated with hypoplasia or absence of the ipsilateral posterior communicating artery, or it can be associated with hypoplasia of both posterior communicating arteries. In addition, the proximal basilar artery and the distal vertebral arteries are often hypoplastic.

Imaging

A persistent trigeminal artery usually arises from the precavernous internal carotid artery (Figure 68-1); however, origin from the intracavernous internal carotid artery has been reported. In some cases, trigeminal arteries course through the sella turcica before joining the basilar artery (Figure 68-2); knowledge of this variant is critical in patients before transsphenoidal surgery.

Associations and Implications

Persistent trigeminal arteries are associated with a variety of intracranial vascular abnormalities, including aneurysms and arteriovenous malformations, as well as a spectrum of clinical syndromes, such as trigeminal neuralgia or other cranial neuropathies, and vertebrobasilar insufficiency. Aneurysms arising from the trigeminal artery itself have been reported. Correct identification and an understanding of this anatomic variation are important because interventional neuroradiologic and neurosurgical procedures (often performed to treat an associated vascular abnormality) may need to be modified appropriately.

References

Boyko OB, Curnes JT, Blatter DD, Parker DL. MRI of basilar artery hypoplasia associated with persistent primitive trigeminal artery. *Neuroradiology*. 1996;38:11-14.

Piotin M, Miralbes S, Cattin F, et al. MRI and MR angiography of persistent trigeminal artery. *Neuroradiology*. 1996;38:730-733.

Cross-Reference

Neuroradiology: THE REQUISITES, 4th ed, pp 29-30.

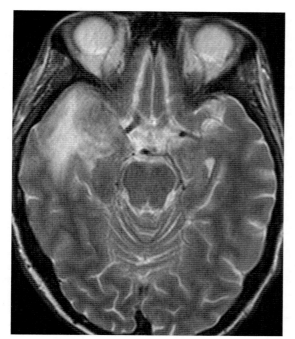

Figure 69-1

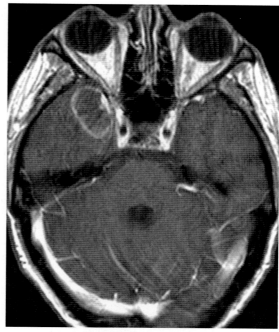

Figure 69-2

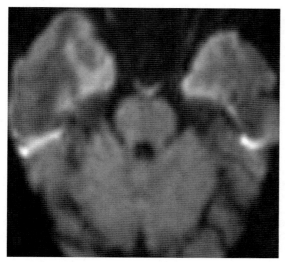

Figure 69-3

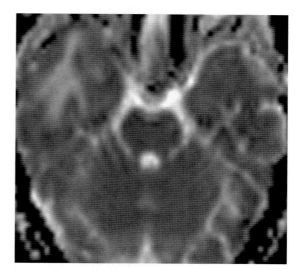

Figure 69-4

HISTORY: Headache in an immunocompromised patient.

1. In differentiating lymphoma from toxoplasmosis, which statement is most correct?
   A. Human immunodeficiency virus (HIV) lymphoma is more frequently multifocal, and toxoplasmosis is often solitary.
   B. Ring enhancement is more common with lymphoma.
   C. Hemorrhage is more often seen in untreated lymphoma than in toxoplasmosis.
   D. Lymphoma typically demonstrates increased cerebral blood volume (CBV) on perfusion, and toxoplasmosis has decreased CBV.

2. What animal is the primary host of this disease?
   A. Dog
   B. Rabbit
   C. Cat
   D. Ferret

3. In infants congenitally infected with toxoplasmosis, what is a typical neuroimaging finding?
   A. Mycotic-type aneurysm
   B. Parenchymal calcification
   C. Dysgenesis of the corpus callosum
   D. Cortical dysplasia

4. Which of the following lesions in an immunocompromised patient demonstrates increased uptake on thallium-201 scintigraphy?
   A. Glioblastoma
   B. Abscess
   C. Toxoplasmosis
   D. Lymphoma

CASE 69

Toxoplasmosis Infection in Acquired Immunodeficiency Syndrome

1. **D.** Lymphoma typically demonstrates increased CBV on perfusion, and toxoplasmosis has decreased CBV. Lymphoma is more frequently a solitary lesion. Ring enhancement can occur in both, but is more common in toxoplasmosis. Hemorrhage is less common in untreated lymphoma.

2. **C.** Cat. Although it is common in all warm-blooded animals, including humans, the primary host is the cat family (Felidae).

3. **B.** Parenchymal calcification. There are multiple calcifications in the basal ganglia and cortex as well as hydrocephalus. In severe cases, the infant can be microcephalic.

4. **D.** Lymphoma. Lymphoma shows increased uptake of thallium-201, which differentiates it from toxoplasmosis.

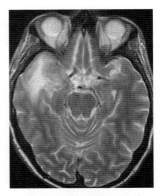

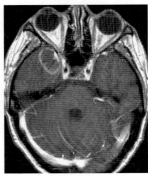

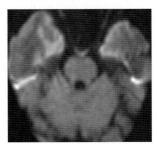

Comment

Central nervous system toxoplasmosis is caused by the intracellular protozoan *Toxoplasma gondii*. *Toxoplasma* encephalitis is most commonly seen in immunocompromised patients with impaired cellular immunity, especially in the setting of acquired immunodeficiency syndrome (AIDS). Other immunodeficient conditions associated with increased infection include prior organ transplantation, long-term steroid therapy or chemotherapy, and impaired immunity from an underlying malignancy.

Differentiating Toxoplasmosis from Lymphoma

In the setting of AIDS, radiologic differentiation between toxoplasmosis and lymphoma can be difficult. Both entities can have multiple lesions, and both can have solid or ring enhancement. Toxoplasmosis has a predilection for the basal ganglia and the corticomedullary junction. Lesions are often hyperintense on T2-weighted imaging (Figure 69-1) and show rim enhancement (Figure 69-2), but they vary widely in their signal characteristics. Lesions may be hemorrhagic. Findings favoring lymphoma are hyperdense masses on unenhanced computed tomography (CT), ependymal spread on enhanced magnetic resonance imaging (MRI; rare in toxoplasmosis), and a periventricular distribution.

Distinguishing these two disease processes is important because they are treated differently. Primary lymphoma responds to radiation therapy; however, the benefit of radiation therapy is diminished when treatment is delayed, as can happen in patients first treated empirically for toxoplasmosis. Thallium-201 SPECT (single-photon emission CT) can be effective (sensitive and specific) in distinguishing lymphoma (takes up thallium) from toxoplasmosis (normally does not take up thallium). Positron emission tomography has been shown to be useful in accurately differentiating hypometabolic toxoplasmosis lesions from metabolically active lymphoma.

Diffusion-weighted imaging with apparent diffusion coefficient (ADC) maps has been used to distinguish these two lesions. Toxoplasmosis lesions have demonstrated significantly greater diffusion than lymphoma, with increased diffusion relative to that in normal white matter. This is in contrast to the restricted diffusion seen within pyogenic abscesses (Figure 69-3). Increased diffusion in toxoplasmosis lesions has been postulated to reflect relatively decreased viscosity within the central cores of the lesions, perhaps because of an impaired cellular immune response related to the immunocompromised state of these patients. Although considerable overlap of ADC ratios between 1.0 and 1.6 has been reported, ADC ratios greater than 1.6 have been associated solely with toxoplasmosis. The core of the lesion in this case demonstrates increased diffusion relative to white matter (Figure 69-4): the ADC value was 1.3. Recent investigations with perfusion MRI have shown decreased regional blood volumes in toxoplasmosis lesions (attributed to the avascularity of abscesses) compared with increased blood volumes in lymphoma (attributed to increased vascularity in regions of metabolically active tumor).

References

Camacho DL, Smith JK, Castillo M. Differentiation of toxoplasmosis and lymphoma in AIDS patients by using apparent diffusion coefficients. *AJNR Am J Neuroradiol.* 2003;24:633-637.

Ernst TM, Chang L, Witt MD, et al. Cerebral toxoplasmosis and lymphoma in AIDS: perfusion MR imaging experience in 13 patients. *Radiology.* 1998;208:663-669.

Cross-Reference

Neuroradiology: THE REQUISITES, 4th ed, pp 199-200.

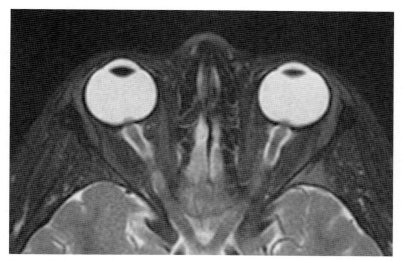

Figure 70-1

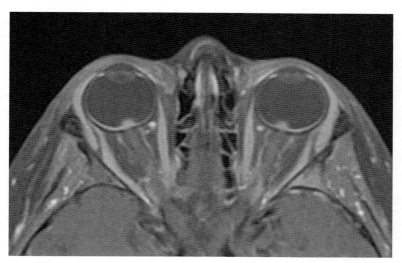

Figure 70-2

HISTORY: An obese patient presents with severe headache, vomiting, and blurred vision.

1. Which of the following should *not* be included in the differential diagnosis?
   A. Increased intracranial pressure (ICP)
   B. Idiopathic intracranial hypertension (IIH)
   C. Optic neuritis
   D. Pseudotumor cerebri

2. What is the major potential danger of papilledema?
   A. Retinal hemorrhage
   B. Choroidal detachment
   C. Cerebrospinal fluid (CSF) leakage
   D. Ischemic optic neuropathy

3. Which are the findings on magnetic resonance imaging (MRI) of papilledema?
   A. Enlarged optic nerve sheath complex, flattening of the optic nerve insertion on the globe, protrusion of the papilla into the globe, and tortuosity of the nerve
   B. Enlarged optic nerve sheath complex, optic nerve swelling, protrusion of the papilla into the globe, and tortuosity of the nerve
   C. Enlarged optic nerve sheath complex, optic nerve swelling, protrusion of the papilla into the globe, and increased optic nerve signal intensity
   D. Enlarged optic nerve sheath complex, proptosis, protrusion of the papilla into the globe, and tortuosity of the nerve

4. Which of the following is *not* a long-term effect of papilledema?
   A. Optic nerve atrophy
   B. Optic nerve ischemic injury
   C. Cataract formation
   D. Enlargement of the sheath

CASE 70

Papilledema

1. **C.** Optic neuritis. Increased ICP and IIH (also known as pseudotumor cerebri) cause papilledema. In optic neuritis, the optic nerve itself usually appears bright on T2-weighted images.

2. **D.** Ischemic optic neuropathy. Ischemic optic neuropathy can occur as a result of the pressure on the vasculature of the optic nerve. Choroidal detachment and CSF leakage are not associated with papilledema. Retinal hemorrhage is a rare phenomenon.

3. **A.** Enlarged optic nerve sheath complex, flattening of the optic nerve insertion on the globe, protrusion of the papilla into the globe, and tortuosity of the nerve. These all appear on MRI. The optic nerve might not swell or produce a bright signal, and proptosis is not a feature.

4. **C.** Cataract formation. Cataract formation is unrelated to papilledema. Optic nerve atrophy occurs as a chronic condition. Optic nerve ischemic injury can result from diminished vascular flow. The sheath is often enlarged in papilledema.

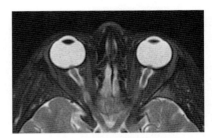

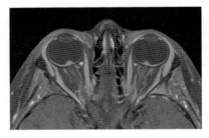

Comment

Imaging Findings

The patient demonstrates enlarged optic nerve sheath complexes, flattening of the optic nerve insertion on the globe, protrusion of the papilla into the globe (Figure 70-1), tortuosity of the nerve, and enhancement of the papilla (Figure 70-2). The finding of papilledema on MRI of the brain may indicate the presence of IIH, a disease that can, if untreated, lead to blindness. In addition to papilledema, affected patients often have partially or completely empty sella, flattening of the pituitary gland by CSF, and stenosis of the venous sinus. The sinus stenosis may be a source or result of the elevation in ICP caused by venous outflow obstruction and diminished CSF resorption. In some cases, ICP may be elevated as a result of a mass, hematoma, or obstruction of the CSF flow through the ventricles or arachnoid villi. In such cases, the presence of papilledema might suggest the acuity of such a process and the urgency of treatment.

Complications of Papilledema

Papilledema must be addressed because when pressure around the optic nerve sheath complex is elevated for a long time, blood flow can be reduced. This, in turn, can lead to ischemic injury of the nerve and to blindness. In IIH, CSF drainage via multiple taps and/or medications to reduce CSF production are usually necessary. If the condition is recurrent and difficult to treat, fenestration of optic nerve sheath may eliminate the risk. For mass lesions, neurosurgical intervention to remove the obstruction, craniectomy (in the most severe cases), or ventriculostomy for alternative CSF drainage and to reduce pressure may be required.

Tortuosity of the Optic Nerve

Tortuosity of the optic nerve occurs in relation to the fixation points of the distal and proximal nerves. Tortuosity may be in the horizontal or vertical plane and is a relatively nonspecific finding. The "smear sign" refers to partial volume averaging on an axial image of the nerve with fat as the nerve coils upward or downward in the vertical plane.

Incidence

As an indicator of increased ICP, papilledema seen on MRI is not specific. The findings are often delayed. IIH can occur without papilledema. Enhancement of the prelaminar optic nerve as a sign of elevated ICP and IIH is found in only 30% of cases.

Reference

Passi N, Degnan AJ, Levy LM. MR imaging of papilledema and visual pathways: effects of increased intracranial pressure and pathophysiologic mechanisms. *AJNR Am J Neuroradiol.* 2013;34(5):919-924.

Cross-Reference

Neuroradiology: THE REQUISITES, 4th ed, pp 324-326.

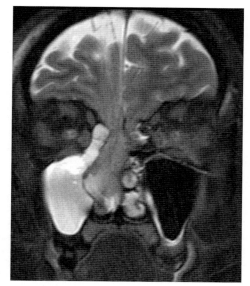

Figure 71-1

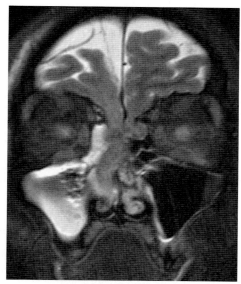

Figure 71-2

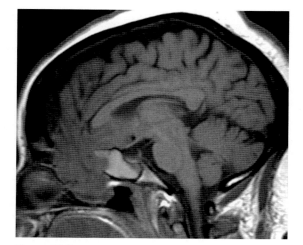

Figure 71-3

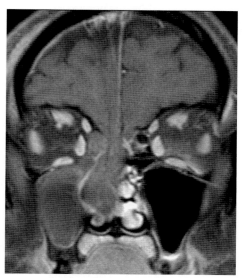

Figure 71-4

HISTORY: Incidental finding.

1. What is the single best diagnosis of the case?
   A. Encephalocele
   B. Meningocele
   C. Esthesioneuroblastoma
   D. Nasal glioma

2. What finding in this case suggests that this abnormality is developmental rather than acquired?
   A. Cortical dysplasia of the bifrontal lobes
   B. Herniation of brain parenchyma into the right nasal cavity
   C. Opacification of the right maxillary sinus
   D. Obstructive mucocele

3. What are the most common causes of acquired cephaloceles?
   A. Infection
   B. Inflammation
   C. Osseous dysplasias
   D. Trauma

4. Regarding iatrogenic cerebrospinal fluid (CSF) leaks resulting in CSF rhinorrhea, what is the most specific and sensitive examination that would help in identifying the leak and its location?
   A. Nuclear cisternography
   B. β2-Transferrin assay
   C. Computed tomography (CT) cisternography
   D. Magnetic resonance imaging (MRI) of brain

CASE 71

Encephalocele, Developmental

1. **A.** Encephalocele or meningoencephalocele, depending on the classification system used. All herniations of intracranial contents into extracranial spaces are cephaloceles as a generic term. This lesion has meninges, brain, and CSF within the herniated tissue, so it is appropriately called a meningoencephalocele. Meningocele implies that there is no brain tissue present.

2. **A.** Cortical dysplasia of the bifrontal lobes. Because there are other congenital defects, this is likely also to be congenital. Midline herniations also suggest a congenital etiology.

3. **D.** Trauma. This includes surgery.

4. **C.** CT cisternography. The higher spatial resolution of CT compared with standard MRI and the identification of the CSF leaking into the nasal cavity give this examination higher overall accuracy than the other answer options. Evaluation of β2-transferrin is very sensitive but not specific for location of leak, although it has supplanted the use of nuclear cisternography.

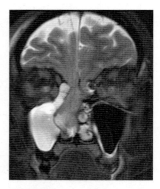

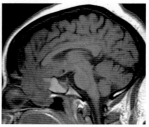

Comment

This case illustrates a large congenital basal encephalocele associated with bilateral frontal lobe cortical dysplasia (Figures 71-1 through 71-4). Cephalocele refers to herniation of the meninges, CSF, or brain through an osseous defect in the cranium. Meningoencephaloceles are more common than meningoceles. Congenital encephaloceles are due to an abnormality in the process of invagination of the neural plate. During embryogenesis, the dura around the brain contacts the dermis in the facial or nasion region as the neural plate regresses. When there is failure of dermal regression, a cephalocele, dermoid cyst, sinus tract, or nasal glioma can develop. Dermoid sinus tracts can have an intracranial connection in up to 25% of cases, and they may be complicated by infection (osteomyelitis, meningitis, and abscesses). Vietnamese and southeastern Asian women have a higher incidence of congenital nasofrontal and sphenoethmoidal meningoencephaloceles. Nasofrontal and sphenoethmoidal meningoencephaloceles are often clinically occult, and the differential diagnosis is broad when this entity is seen through the nasoscope on clinical examination. Anterior basal encephaloceles have an association with other developmental anomalies, as in this case, including migrational abnormalities, agenesis of the corpus callosum, and cleft lip and palate.

In the setting of trauma or surgery, most meningoencephaloceles involve the nasal cavity and paranasal sinuses or the temporal bone. Patients can present with rhinorrhea.

A combination of imaging modalities, including nuclear scintigraphy, CT, and MRI, can be used to assess CSF leaks and cephaloceles. It is important to determine whether the CSF leak is due to a dural laceration or an encephalocele. Radionucleotide cisternography has fallen out of favor because it has been shown to have low specificity in localizing leaks. The noninvasive nature, avoidance of radiation exposure, and cost-effectiveness as well as the specificity of β2-transferrin analysis is often sufficient and may be preferred to radionuclide cisternography. Once a leak is established, CT without contrast may be performed for anatomic localization by identifying an osseous defect. If the aforementioned evaluation fails to localize the leak, iodinated contrast CT cisternography may be necessary. If an encephalocele is suspected, MRI is most useful in establishing this diagnosis by showing direct continuity of the tissue in the sinonasal cavity with the intracranial brain.

References

Allbery SM, Chaljub G, Cho NL, et al. MR imaging of nasal masses. *Radiographics*. 1995;15:1311-1327.

Hudgins PA, Browning DG, Gallups J, et al. Endoscopic paranasal sinus surgery: radiographic evaluation of severe complications. *AJNR Am J Neuroradiol*. 1992;13:1161-1167.

Labruzzo SV, Aygun N, Zinreich SJ. Imaging of the paranasal sinuses: mitigation, identification, and workup of functional endoscopic surgery complications. *Otolaryngol Clin North Am*. 2015;48(5):805-815.

Cross-Reference

Neuroradiology: THE REQUISITES, 4th ed, p 285.

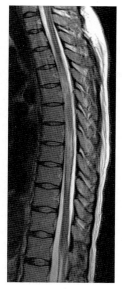

Figure 72-1

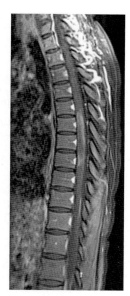

Figure 72-2

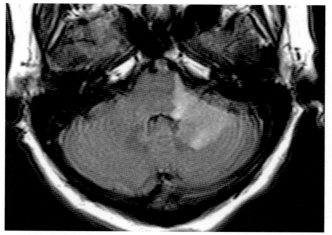

Figure 72-3

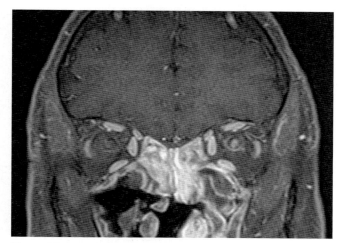

Figure 72-4

HISTORY: A 52-year-old woman presents with shooting pain and numbness in the legs followed by loss of vision in her left eye.

1. What should *not* be included in the differential diagnosis?
   A. Neuromyelitis optica (NMO)
   B. Sarcoid
   C. Acute disseminated encephalomyelitis
   D. Multiple sclerosis (MS)

2. Which of the following statements regarding NMO is true?
   A. The symptoms in NMO are less profound than in MS.
   B. Most patients are NMO–immunoglobulin G (IgG) seropositive.
   C. NMO is monophasic in most cases.
   D. Brain lesions found on magnetic resonance imaging (MRI) exclude the diagnosis of NMO.

3. Which of the following findings is more characteristic of MS or other inflammatory lesions than it is of NMO?
   A. Spinal cord lesion at a single level
   B. Severe cord atrophy
   C. Cord necrosis
   D. Hypointense spinal cord lesions on T1-weighted imaging

4. Which of the following brain lesions is more characteristic of MS than it is of NMO?
   A. Lesions in the dorsal medulla
   B. Hypothalamic lesions
   C. Lesions involving the posterior limb of the internal capsule (PLIC)
   D. Ovoid periventricular or corpus callosum signal abnormality oriented perpendicular to the longitudinal axis of the lateral ventricles

CASE 72

Neuromyelitis Optica

1. **C.** Acute disseminated encephalitis. This would not explain the optic nerve findings. NMO is the most likely diagnosis. Sarcoid and MS may produce these findings.

2. **B.** Most patients are NMO-IgG seropositive. Symptoms are typically *more* profound in NMO than in MS. Most NMO patients have a relapsing course. The presence of brain lesions does not exclude NMO.

3. **A.** Spinal cord lesion at a single level. NMO lesions are characteristically longitudinally extensive, which is a major imaging criterion. Severe spinal cord atrophy can be seen in many diseases, including MS and NMO. Spinal cord necrosis supports a diagnosis of NMO. Hypointensity on T1-weighted imaging also supports a diagnosis of NMO.

4. **D.** Ovoid periventricular or corpus callosum signal abnormality oriented perpendicular to the longitudinal axis of the lateral ventricles. This is more typical for MS than for NMO. Cortical spinal tract lesions are characteristic of NMO. Dorsal medullary, hypothalamic, cerebral peduncle, and PLIC lesions are seen in NMO.

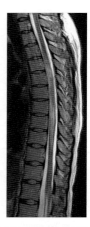

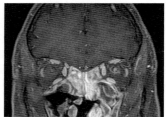

Comment

Clinical Features

NMO is an idiopathic inflammatory disorder of the central nervous system that preferentially affects the optic nerves and spinal cord. A monophasic course of acute transverse myelitis simultaneously associated with optic neuritis is classic; however, more than 90% of patients experience a relapsing course. Optic neuritis can be separated from transverse myelitis by months or years, and episodes tend to relapse, resulting in significant disability.

Pathophysiology and Diagnostic Criteria

More recent clinical, pathologic, immunologic, and imaging studies have suggested that NMO is distinct from MS. The identification of a disease-specific autoantibody, NMO-IgG, in the serum of patients with NMO facilitated the diagnosis of NMO and was incorporated into new diagnostic criteria. The autoantibody targets aquaporin-4 (AQP4), the most abundant water channel in the central nervous system, localized on astrocytic end-feet. The autoantibody, found in most patients with NMO, binds to AQP4 and, in conjunction with complement, causes lysis of astrocytes. NMO has occasionally been associated with other autoimmune diseases, such as Sjögren syndrome, systemic lupus erythematosus, rheumatoid arthritis, and mixed connective tissue disorders.

There are three major criteria for diagnosis of NMO. These include optic neuritis (Figure 72-4), transverse myelitis with spinal cord lesion extending over three spinal segments (Figures 72-1 and 72-2), and the absence of other neurologic disease. There are minor criteria, which include positive NMO-IgG in the serum or cerebrospinal fluid; normal brain MRI or nonspecific brain T2 signal; lesions in the dorsal medulla, hypothalamus, or brainstem (Figure 72-3); and linear periventricular white matter signal abnormalities. All three major and at least one minor criteria must be met for a positive diagnosis.

Imaging

MRI typically shows a longitudinally extensive lesion that extends over three or more vertebral segments with sensitivity of 98% and specificity of 83%. MRI of the orbit often reveals gadolinium enhancement of the optic nerve during an acute attack of optic neuritis. Patients with NMO are frequently found to have symptomatic or asymptomatic brain lesions. Brain lesions characteristically occur in the hypothalamus and periventricular areas, which correspond to brain regions with high levels of AQP4 expression.

Management

The optimal treatment for NMO has not yet been established. High-dose corticosteroids have been used for treatment of acute attacks. Therapeutic plasmapheresis should be considered in patients who fail to improve with high-dose corticosteroid therapy. Another treatment option is immunosuppressants.

References

Cabrera-Gomez JA, Kister I. Conventional brain MRI in neuromyelitis optica. *Eur J Neurol.* 2012;19(6):812-819.

Kim W, Kim SH, Kim HJ. New insights into neuromyelitis optica. *J Clin Neurol.* 2011;7(3):115-127.

Cross-Reference

Neuroradiology: THE REQUISITES, 4th ed, pp 215-216.

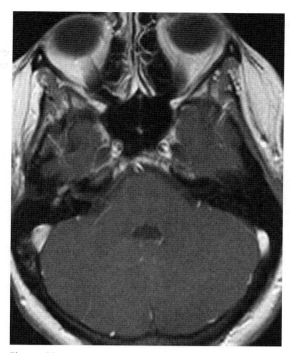

Figure 73-1

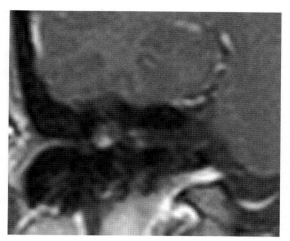

Figure 73-2

HISTORY: Upper respiratory infection.

1. In this patient with upper respiratory tract infection, what is the most likely clinical diagnosis?
   A. Ramsay Hunt syndrome
   B. Lyme disease
   C. Metastatic disease
   D. Bell palsy

2. What portion of the facial nerve normally enhances?
   A. Cisternal
   B. Intracanalicular
   C. Anterior genu
   D. Foraminal

3. What structure separates the internal auditory canal into superior and inferior components?
   A. Tegmen tympani
   B. Scutum
   C. Bill bar
   D. Crista falciformis

4. What cranial nerve runs in the anteroinferior portion of the internal auditory canal?
   A. Facial nerve
   B. Superior division of the vestibular nerve
   C. Inferior division of the vestibular nerve
   D. Cochlear division of the vestibulocochlear nerve

CASE 73

Facial Nerve Inflammation (Viral)

1. **D.** Bell palsy. Statistically, the most common cause of pathology involving cranial nerves VII and VIII is infection. Clinically this often presents as hemifacial paresis that resolves within 6 to 8 weeks.

2. **C.** Anterior genu. The portions within the temporal bone (descending mastoid tympanic and geniculate ganglia) normally enhance because they have a rich circumneural venous plexus. The labyrinthine portion, the portion within the internal auditory canal, and the cisternal portions do not normally enhance. The presence of enhancement implies pathology.

3. **D.** Crista falciformis. This separates the apex of the internal auditory canal into superior and inferior segments, with the cochlear nerve in the anterior inferior quadrant, the facial nerve in the anterior superior quadrant, and the superior and inferior divisions of the vestibular nerve posteriorly. The Bill bar separates the anterior and posterior portions.

4. **D.** Cochlear division of the vestibulocochlear nerve. See answer to Question 3.

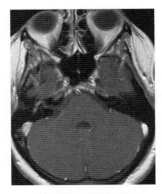

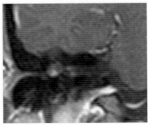

Comment

Images

This case shows enlargement and thickening of the right facial nerve (cranial nerve VII) along the tympanic portion (Figure 73-1), as well as enhancement of the facial nerve in the fundus of the internal auditory canal (Figure 73-2). Enhancement of the right cochlear nerve below the facial nerve in the antero-inferior internal auditory canal is also seen.

Infection/Inflammation

The patient presented with Bell palsy. Statistically speaking, inflammatory processes (i.e., viral) are most likely. Other infectious causes associated with cranial nerve VII involvement, in addition to viral causes, include Lyme disease. In immunocompromised patients, especially those with human immunodeficiency virus (HIV) infection, cytomegalovirus can affect the nerves in the internal auditory canal. Other inflammatory processes such as sarcoidosis can also affect the cranial nerves.

Neoplasms

Neoplasms that can involve cranial nerve VII include schwannoma (unlikely in this case because multiple cranial nerves are involved and this patient's clinical presentation was acute). Subarachnoid seeding of tumor can involve the internal auditory canals and can be seen in lymphoma and carcinomatosis (lung, breast, or seeding of primary brain tumors). Perineural spread of malignancies along the facial nerve is often associated with destructive changes in the temporal bone. Perineural spread of temporal bone squamous cell carcinoma, primary parotid malignancies, and skin cancers of the ear and cheek are probably the most common.

Management

Often, imaging is not necessary in the work-up of Bell palsy. However, when Bell palsy is bilateral, is recurrent, or does not show significant improvement in 6 to 8 weeks, imaging is indicated to assess for causes other than viral disease.

Reference

Gebarski SS, Telian SA, Niparko JK. Enhancement along the normal facial nerve in the facial canal: MR imaging and anatomic correlation. *Radiology.* 1992;183:391-394.

Cross-Reference

Neuroradiology: THE REQUISITES, 4th ed, pp 26-27, 395-396.

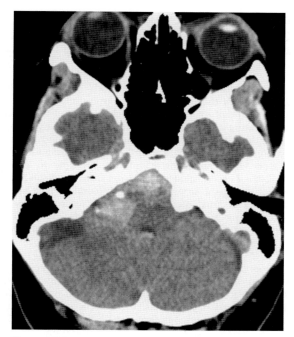

Figure 74-1

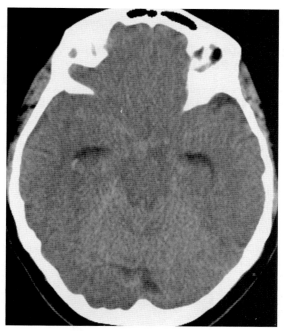

Figure 74-2

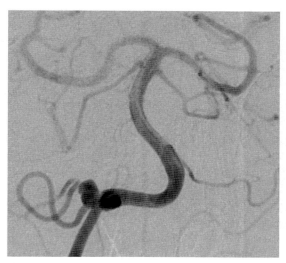

Figure 74-3

HISTORY: Severe headache.

1. What is the single best diagnosis in this case?
   A. Rupture of a right posterior inferior cerebellar artery (PICA) aneurysm
   B. Traumatic intradural right vertebral artery dissection
   C. Perimesencephalic hemorrhage
   D. Epidermoid

2. What statement regarding radiation intensity from an x-ray tube is correct?
   A. It decreases with the square root of the distance from the source.
   B. It decreases linearly with the distance from the source.
   C. It remains constant regardless of distance.
   D. It decreases with the square of the distance from the source.

3. During acquisition of the examination in Figure 74-3, digital subtraction angiography (DSA), what step should have been taken to decrease the radiation dose to the patient?
   A. Use air gaps to increase magnification.
   B. Utilize continuous fluoroscopy rather than pulsed fluoroscopy.
   C. Position the image receptor as close as possible to the patient.
   D. Use open collimation to increase incident photons on the detector.

4. What is the most common site of origin for aneurysms in the posterior circulation?
   A. PICA
   B. Anterior inferior cerebellar artery
   C. Superior cerebellar artery
   D. Tip of the basilar artery

CASE 74

Right Posterior Inferior Cerebellar Artery Aneurysm Rupture

1. **A.** Rupture of a right PICA aneurysm. There is subarachnoid blood, greatest in the right side of the posterior fossa. The DSA image shows a saccular outpouching at the right PICA.

2. **D.** It decreases with the square of the distance from the source. Radiation from a point source decreases with square of the distance. For example, a twofold increase in distance results in a fourth of the radiation intensity.

3. **C.** Position the image receptor as close as possible to the patient. This maximizes the incident radiation on the receptor, therefore requiring fewer photons to make the image. All the other answer options would increase radiation dose.

4. **D.** Tip of the basilar artery. This is the most common location for posterior fossa circulation aneurysm.

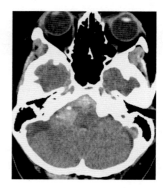

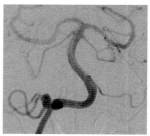

Comment

Aneurysm rupture manifests with subarachnoid hemorrhage (Figures 74-1 and 74-2) and hydrocephalus (see Figure 74-2).

Anterior Circulation

The majority of intracranial aneurysms arise from the supraclinoid segment of the internal carotid artery and its branches. More than 80% of saccular aneurysms arise from the anterior communicating artery, the distal internal carotid artery at the origin of the posterior communicating artery, the bifurcation of the supraclinoid internal carotid artery, and the middle cerebral artery. Intracranial aneurysms are multiple in approximately 20% of cases. Aneurysms arising from the distal internal carotid artery at the origin of the ophthalmic artery account for 5% of intracranial aneurysms and have interesting associations, including a preponderance in women, multiplicity in 10% to 20% of cases, and bilateralism in up to 20% of cases.

Posterior Circulation

Aneurysms arising from the posterior circulation are not uncommon; however, they occur much less commonly than do their anterior circulation counterparts. Most originate from the tip of the basilar artery. Basilar tip aneurysms can become quite large, and not uncommonly, the origins of one or both posterior cerebral arteries may be incorporated into the aneurysm. The next most common site for aneurysms in the posterior circulation is the origin of the PICA, as in this case (Figure 74-3). In rare cases, aneurysms arise from the superior cerebellar artery or the anteroinferior cerebellar artery.

Acquired Aneurysms

Aneurysms arising from distal arterial branches are usually acquired rather than congenital. They are often secondary to infection of the arterial wall (mycotic) or to trauma (aneurysms arising from the posterior circulation may be related to compression along the tentorium), and occasionally they are related to neoplasms.

Reference

Jayaraman MV, Mayo-Smith WW, Tung GA, et al. Detection of intracranial aneurysms: multi-detector row CT angiography compared with DSA. *Radiology*. 2004;230:510-518.

Cross-Reference

Neuroradiology: THE REQUISITES, 4th ed, pp 141-145.

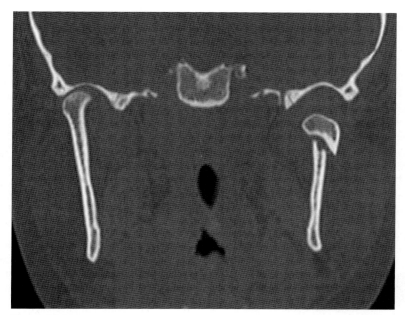

Figure 75-1

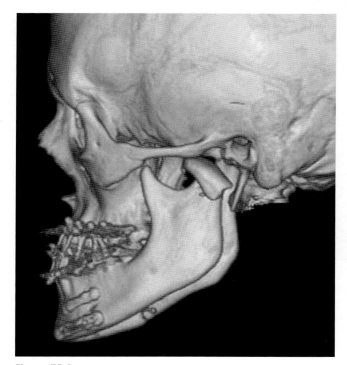

Figure 75-2

HISTORY: A patient presents with jaw pain after having been in an altercation.

1. Which of the following is the single best diagnosis?
   A. Osteosarcoma
   B. Meniscus dislocation
   C. Traumatic fracture
   D. Pathologic fracture

2. What is the main danger of a mandibular neck fracture?
   A. Rotatory subluxation
   B. Avascular necrosis
   C. Persistent dislocation
   D. Pseudarthrosis

3. What part of the mandible is fractured most commonly?
   A. Body
   B. Angle
   C. Neck
   D. Condyle

4. Which of the following is considered an open fracture?
   A. Fractures that affect the alveolus and teeth
   B. Condylar fracture
   C. Ascending ramus fracture
   D. Neck of mandible fracture

CASE 75

Condylar Fracture

1. **C.** Traumatic fracture. The left mandibular neck fracture is evident on the coronal two-dimensional image.

2. **B.** Avascular necrosis. Of all mandibular fractures, the rate of avascular necrosis is highest with fractures of the mandibular neck.

3. **A.** Body. The body fractures more commonly than the angle, which is fractured more commonly than the condyle. The neck is not frequently the site of fracture.

4. **A.** Fractures that affect the alveolus and teeth. By definition, a fracture affecting the alveolus and teeth is analogous to a fracture that protrudes through the skin and increases the risk of infection, and is therefore considered "open."

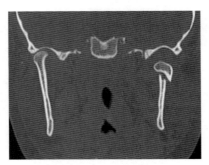

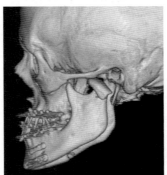

Comment

Location of Fractures

The mandible, orbital walls, and nasal bones are most commonly fractured in facial trauma. Although one should suspect multiple fractures with any mandibular fracture, nearly 30% of mandibular fractures are isolated, particularly those caused by direct blows. Mandibular condylar fractures and parasymphyseal fracture are more commonly multiple than fractures of other portions of the mandible. The left side is affected more commonly than the right, possibly because of a right-handed blow (men have mandibular fractures three to four times more often than do women) and because passengers tend to flinch to the right during a motor vehicle accident. The locations of fractures vary with the cause: parasymphyseal fractures tend to occur with motor vehicle accidents, body fractures with gunshot wounds, and angle fractures with assaults.

Displacement of Mandibular Fractures

Displacement of mandibular fractures is dependent on the pull of the muscles of mastication (Figures 75-1 and 75-2). The masseter and temporalis muscles exert upward pull on the angle of the mandible, which distract fractures vertically, whereas the medial and lateral pterygoid muscles distract fractures medially.

Complications

In addition to occurring with fractures, avascular necrosis of the mandible can occur with bisphosphonate therapy, steroid therapy, osteoporosis, and sickle cell disease. Other complications, such as technical failure and infections, increase with open fractures, delays in surgical reduction, and intravenous drug use.

Reference

Anyanechi CE, Saheeb BD. Mandibular sites prone to fracture: analysis of 174 cases in a Nigerian tertiary hospital. *Ghana Med J.* 2011;45(3):111-114.

Cross-Reference

Neuroradiology: THE REQUISITES, 4th ed, p 600.

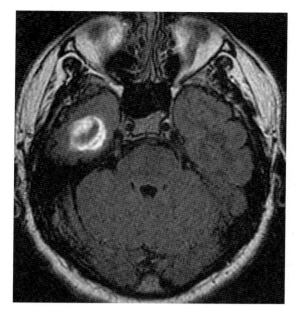

Figure 76-1

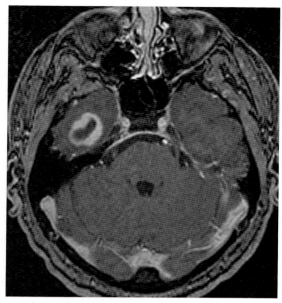

Figure 76-2

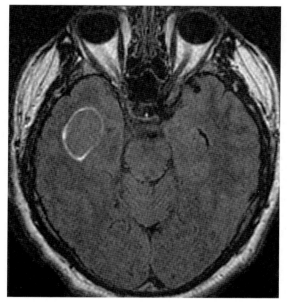

Figure 76-3

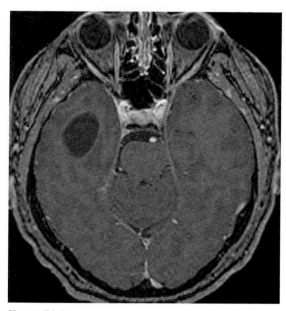

Figure 76-4

HISTORY: Seizures.

1. If this patient is 17 years old, what is the single best diagnosis?
   A. Lung cancer metastasis
   B. Oligodendroglioma
   C. Cavernous malformation
   D. Ganglioglioma

2. Gangliogliomas typically arise in which portion of the cerebrum?
   A. Frontal lobe
   B. Parietal lobe
   C. Temporal lobe
   D. Occipital lobe

3. What is the World Health Organization (WHO) grading of a gangliocytoma?
   A. I
   B. II
   C. III
   D. IV

4. Which of the following temporal lobe masses is most commonly associated with seizures?
   A. Ganglioglioma
   B. Astrocytoma
   C. Dysembryoplastic neuroepithelial tumor
   D. Oligodendroglioma

CASE 76

Ganglioglioma

1. **D.** Ganglioglioma. Not only would lung cancer be rare in a 17-year-old, but a large solitary metastasis without surrounding vasogenic edema would be very atypical. Oligodendrogliomas can occur in the temporal lobe with a cystic component, similar to this case. This mass would be rare in a 17-year-old and is most commonly seen in patients in the 30- to 60-year age range. A good differential in this case, given the patient's age, would consist of astrocytoma, ganglioglioma, dysembryoplastic neuroepithelial tumor, and pleomorphic xanthoastrocytoma.

2. **C.** Temporal lobe. Most gangliogliomas (85%) are located in the temporal lobe, followed by the frontal lobe.

3. **A.** I. These are WHO grade I, low-grade, slow-growing tumors.

4. **A.** Ganglioglioma. From among the answer options, this tumor has the highest association with seizures.

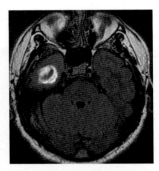

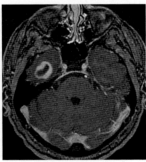

Comment

Imaging

Gangliogliomas and ganglioneuromas are slow-growing, low-grade tumors that most commonly affect children and young adults. In children and young adults, the main differential considerations for ganglioglioma on imaging studies include low-grade astrocytoma, juvenile pilocytic astrocytoma, dysembryoplastic neuroepithelial tumor, and pleomorphic xanthoastrocytoma.

Gangliogliomas typically occur in the cerebrum, most commonly arising in the temporal lobe (Figures 76-1 through 76-4), followed by the frontal lobe, parietal lobe, occipital lobe, and region of the hypothalamus and third ventricle. They may also be infratentorial, arising within the cerebellum or brainstem. Gangliogliomas are typically circumscribed tumors that occur superficially in the brain parenchyma, with little or no surrounding edema (see Figures 76-1 and 76-3). They are usually cystic (purely cystic or cystic with solid components) (see Figures 76-1 through 76-4), although solid tumors without cyst formation may occur. Calcification is frequently present, and these neoplasms can demonstrate variable contrast enhancement, ranging from mild to marked. However, contrast enhancement need not be present.

Pathology

Because gangliogliomas are composed of both glial (usually astrocytes) and neural elements, they can undergo malignant degeneration. When neuronal elements make up the majority of the mass, the neoplasm is referred to as a ganglioneuroma. Gangliocytomas are composed of mature ganglion cells. They rarely have glial elements and therefore have no potential for malignant change.

References

Koeller KK, Henry JM. From the archives of the AFIP: superficial gliomas: radiologic-pathologic correlation. *Radiographics.* 2001;21: 1533-1556.

Provenzale JM, Ali U, Barboriak DP, et al. Comparison of patient age with MR imaging features of gangliogliomas. *AJR Am J Roentgenol.* 2000;174:859-862.

Cross-Reference

Neuroradiology: THE REQUISITES, 4th ed, pp 266-268.

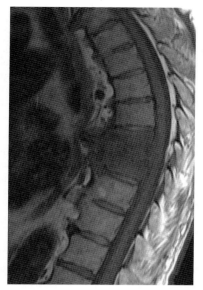

Figure 77-1

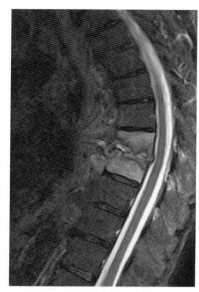

Figure 77-2

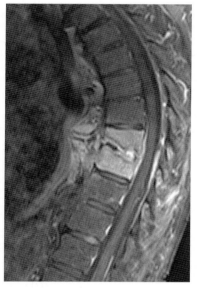

Figure 77-3

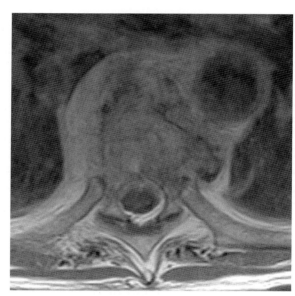

Figure 77-4

HISTORY: A 78-year-old man presents with a 3-month history of back pain.

1. What is the single best diagnosis?
   A. Primary spinal tumor
   B. Discitis osteomyelitis
   C. Metastatic disease
   D. Degenerative disc disease

2. Regarding the differences in tuberculous versus pyogenic spondylitis, which statement is correct?
   A. Tuberculous abscesses tend to have thicker and more irregular walls than pyogenic abscesses.
   B. Tuberculous spondylitis is less often associated with paraspinal abscess.
   C. Subligamentous spread to three or more vertebral levels is more frequently observed in tuberculous spondylitis.
   D. Thoracic spine involvement is less common in tuberculous spondylitis.

3. In what percentage of patients are findings considered "typical" of discitis osteomyelitis observed?
   A. 5%
   B. 35%
   C. 75%
   D. 95%

4. Which of the following organisms most commonly causes discitis osteomyelitis?
   A. *Mycobacterium tuberculosis*
   B. *Staphylococcus aureus*
   C. Gram-negative organisms
   D. *Escherichia coli*

157

CASE 77

Thoracic Discitis Osteomyelitis

1. **B.** Discitis osteomyelitis. The findings in this case are typical of this entity. Primary spinal tumors infrequently cross the disc space. There is a paraspinal abscess, which should not be found with degenerative changes alone or metastasis.

2. **C.** Subligamentous spread to three or more vertebral levels is more frequently observed in tuberculous spondylitis. Tuberculosis-related paraspinal abscesses tend to have thin smooth walls. There is a higher incidence of abscess with tuberculosis versus pyogenic infection. Thoracic spinal involvement is more frequent in tuberculosis infection than in pyogenic infection.

3. **D.** 95%. In 1996, Dagirmanjian and colleagues reported that "typical" findings were observed in approximately 95% of patients.

4. **B.** *Staphylococcus aureus. S. aureus* is the most commonly found organism at time of fine-needle aspiration or biopsy. Although less common, gram-negative organisms are often found in intravenous drug users, and *E. coli* is often associated with urinary tract infections and urosepsis.

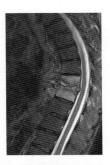

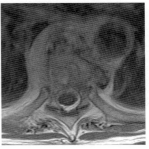

Comment

Background

Vertebral osteomyelitis occurs primarily in adults, with most affected patients older than 50 years. The lumbar region is most commonly affected, followed by the cervical spine and thoracic spine. Adult discitis osteomyelitis has a slow, insidious onset, which may result in a delayed diagnosis. Pain with localized tenderness is the initial presenting symptom.

Histopathology

Discitis and vertebral osteomyelitis are almost always present together and share much of the same pathophysiology. In most cases, the infection does not originate in the vertebra or disc space but rather spreads to the involved intervertebral disc hematogenously from a systemic infection (urinary tract infections, pneumonia, and soft tissue infections are the most common sources).

Imaging

In this case, magnetic resonance imaging (MRI) shows the findings that are considered "typical" of discitis osteomyelitis: decreased vertebral body signal on T1-weighted images (Figure 77-1), loss of endplate definition on T1-weighted images, increased disc signal intensity on T2-weighted images (Figure 77-2), and contrast enhancement of the disc and adjacent vertebral bodies (Figure 77-3). Dagirmanjian et al. reported that each of these findings was observed with a frequency of approximately 95%. In comparison, increased vertebral body signal on T2-weighted images was observed in only 56% of spinal levels affected by discitis osteomyelitis. The absence of this finding should not dissuade the clinician from making an MRI diagnosis of discitis osteomyelitis when the typical findings are present (as in this case). The variation in signal intensity of the involved vertebral bodies on T2-weighted images has been attributed, in part, to variability in the ratio of sclerotic bone (as seen on standard radiographs) to edematous marrow.

The contrast enhancement pattern of the involved disc can be highly variable. It may be thick and patchy, linear and continuous, or a mixture. The intensity of vertebral body enhancement is variable. Enhancement of epidural and paraspinal associated soft tissue masses provides additional evidence of infection (Figure 77-4). Homogeneous enhancement favors phlegmon, and ring enhancement favors mature abscess.

Management

Elevated erythrocyte sedimentation rate and C-reactive protein are the most consistent laboratory abnormalities seen in cases of discitis, whereas leukocytosis is frequently absent. Blood cultures are positive in 50% to 70% of patients and should be obtained for any patient suspected of having discitis osteomyelitis. Treatment includes antibiotics and immobilization to allow the vertebral bodies to fuse in an anatomically aligned position. Indications for surgery include neurologic deficit and spinal deformity.

References

Dagirmanjian A, Schils J, McHenry M, et al. MR imaging of vertebral osteomyelitis revisited. *AJR Am J Roentgenol.* 1996;167(6): 1539-1543.

Jung NY, Jee WH, Ha KY, Park CK, Byun JY. Discrimination of tuberculous spondylitis from pyogenic spondylitis on MRI. *AJR Am J Roentgenol.* 2004;182(6):1405-1410.

Cross-Reference

Neuroradiology: THE REQUISITES, 4th ed, pp 559-560.

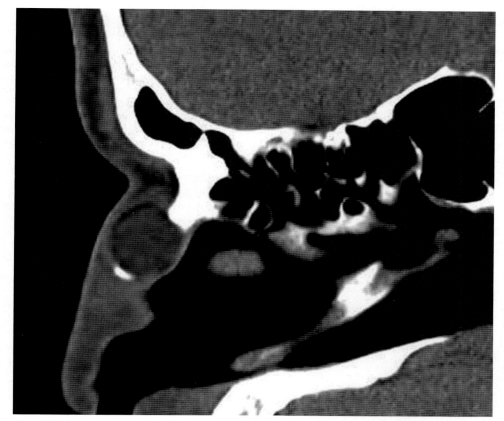

Figure 78-1

HISTORY: An adolescent is not happy with the cosmetic appearance of her nose.

1. Which of the following is the single best diagnosis?
   A. Aneurysmal bone cyst
   B. Nasal glioma
   C. Dermoid
   D. Encephalocele

2. What is the name of the passageway of a dermal sinus tract from the sinonasal cavity to the intracranial compartment?
   A. Anterior neuropore
   B. Foramen cecum
   C. Frontalis ponticulus
   D. Cribriform plate

3. What percentage of nasal dermoids have an intracranial connection?
   A. 0% to 20%
   B. 21% to 40%
   C. 41% to 60%
   D. More than 60%

4. What percentage of patients with nasal dermoids present with an infection?
   A. 0% to 20%
   B. 21% to 40%
   C. 41% to 60%
   D. More than 60%

CASE 78

Nasal Dermoid

1. **C.** Dermoid. The location and density indicate a dermoid. The location is a less likely site for a lipoma, although lipomas contain fat; encephaloceles do not contain fat. The density is not characteristic of nasal glioma. Aneurysmal bone cysts are multiseptated with fluid levels.

2. **B.** Foramen cecum. The foramen cecum is the passageway from the sinonasal cavity to the intracranial compartment. The anterior neuropore is an embryologic channel and not located through the nose. There is no such thing as "frontalis ponticulus."

3. **A.** 0% to 20%. Twelve percent to 18% of nasal dermoids have an intracranial connection.

4. **B.** 21% to 40%. Thirty percent of patients with nasal dermoids present with an infection.

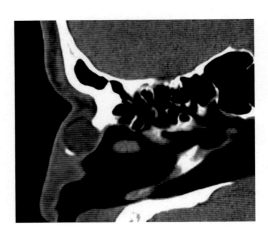

Comment

Imaging Findings

Nasal dermoids typically manifest as a soft tissue mass and/or a tract leading from the nasal bridge or glabella in the midline (Figure 78-1). However, infection may occur, and in some cases, a cheesy off-white material may be expressed from the lesion through the sinus tract. In rare cases, patients may present with an intracranial infection because the pathogens can travel from the dermoid via the dermal sinus tract, through the foramen cecum, to the meninges, which may then result in meningitis.

Incidence of Nasal Dermoids

Boys are affected more commonly than girls, and the average age at discovery is approximately 3 years. Nasal dermoids are the most common midline congenital masses of the face and represent approximately 10% of all head and neck dermoids. Most nasal dermoids are superficial, but 16% affect the nasal cartilage, 12% the cribriform plate, and 10% the nasal bone (like this one).

Reference

Rahbar R, Shah P, Mulliken JB, et al. The presentation and management of nasal dermoid: a 30-year experience. *Arch Otolaryngol Head Neck Surg.* 2003;129(4):464-471.

Cross-Reference

Neuroradiology: THE REQUISITES, 4th ed, pp 55, 415-417.

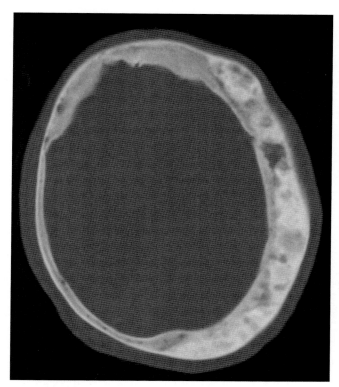

Figure 79-1

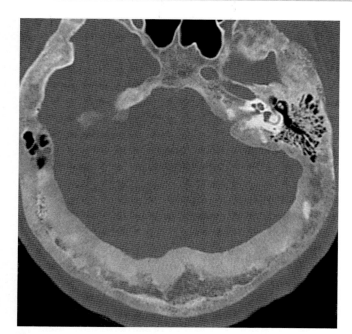

Figure 79-2

HISTORY: Enlarging head size.

1. Of the choices provided, what is the single best diagnosis?
   A. Eosinophilic granuloma
   B. Multiple myeloma
   C. Hyperostosis internus frontalis
   D. Paget disease

2. What is the name of the osteolytic phase of this disease in the calvarium?
   A. Calcinosis circumscripta
   B. Melanosis circumscripta
   C. Osteitis deformans
   D. Osteoporosis circumscripta

3. Which characteristic is helpful in distinguishing fibrous dysplasia from this disease?
   A. Polyostosis
   B. Paranasal sinus involvement
   C. If the lesion crosses the suture lines
   D. If there is diploic widening

4. Which systemic condition can result from this disease?
   A. Anemia
   B. Rheumatoid arthritis
   C. Diabetes
   D. Kidney stones

CASE 79

Paget Disease: Osteitis Deformans

1. **D.** Paget disease. The differential diagnosis of Paget disease of the skull includes other sclerotic bone lesions, hyperostosis frontalis, fibrous dysplasia, and metastatic disease. The extensive skull base involvement virtually eliminates hyperostosis. Eosinophilic granuloma manifests as an erosive, lytic lesion, often with a beveled edge, and is associated with a soft tissue mass, whereas in this case there is mixed lysis and sclerosis and thickening of the skull. Multiple myeloma manifests with multiple lytic lesions, with no definite thickening of the skull.

2. **D.** Osteoporosis circumscripta. Calcinosis circumscripta is deposition of calcium deposits in the skin and subcutaneous soft tissues. Melanosis circumscripta is a melanoma in situ of the skin. Osteitis deformans is another name for Paget disease, and it does not specifically refer to the osteolytic phase.

3. **B.** Paranasal sinus involvement. Fibrous dysplasia is more likely to involve the sinuses than is Paget disease. Both fibrous dysplasia and Paget can be polyostotic. Both can cross the suture lines. Both can cause diploic widening.

4. **D.** Kidney stones. Heart disease and kidney stones can result from Paget disease, not anemia, rheumatoid arthritis, or diabetes mellitus.

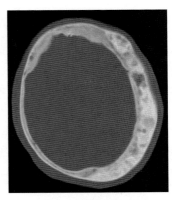

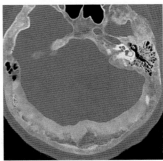

Comment

In Paget disease, there is malfunction in the normal process of bone remodeling. When an area of bone is destroyed, the new bone replacing it is soft and porous. Bone affected with Paget disease also has increased vascularity. The cause of Paget disease is unknown; however, a viral cause is favored. Paget disease is more common in men than in women, and it usually occurs after the age of 40 years. It is often an incidental finding detected on radiographs obtained for other reasons. Patients may be symptomatic, depending on the distribution of disease. Involvement of the calvarium (Figure 79-1) can manifest with enlarging head size. Involvement of the skull base, resulting in platybasia, can lead to neurologic symptoms (weakness and paralysis) (Figure 79-2). Conductive hearing loss can result if there is involvement of the ossicles. Compression of the eighth cranial nerve as a result of bone overgrowth can cause sensorineural hearing loss. There is usually relative sparing of the otic capsule (see Figure 79-2).

Stages of Disease

Paget disease has multiple stages, including an initial osteolytic phase characterized by osteoclastic activity with resorption of normal bone. This phase is followed by excessive and sporadic new bone formation as a result of osteoblastic activity. Eventually, Paget disease enters its inactive stage.

Neoplastic Involvement

Neoplastic involvement within pagetoid bone is not uncommon and includes sarcomatous degeneration, giant cell tumors, superimposed hematologic neoplasms (myeloma, lymphoma), and metastatic disease. Giant cell tumors are typically confined to the skull and less often to the facial bones. It is speculated that the increased blood flow within pagetoid bone can make it more susceptible to deposition of metastases. Clinically, the development of neoplastic disease in pagetoid bone should be suspected if there is increased pain or an associated soft tissue mass.

Differential Diagnosis

The differential diagnosis of Paget disease of the skull includes other sclerotic bone lesions, hyperostosis frontalis, fibrous dysplasia, and metastatic disease. In older adults, metastatic disease (prostate cancer in men and breast cancer in women) can have the cotton-wool appearance of Paget disease.

References

Richards PS, Bargiota A, Corrall RJ. Paget's disease causing an Arnold-Chiari type 1 malformation: radiographic findings. *AJR Am J Roentgenol.* 2001;176:816-817.

Tehranzadeh J, Fung Y, Donohue M, et al. Computed tomography of Paget's disease of the skull versus fibrous dysplasia. *Skeletal Radiol.* 1998;27:664-672.

Cross-Reference

Neuroradiology: THE REQUISITES, 4th ed, pp 403, 584.

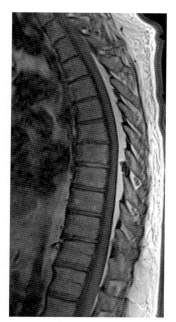

Figure 80-1

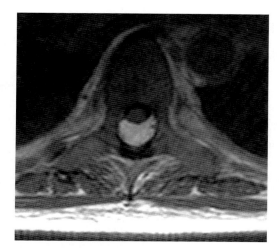

Figure 80-2

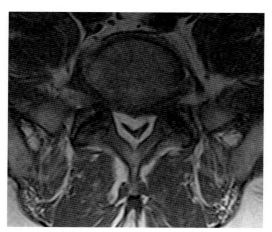

Figure 80-3

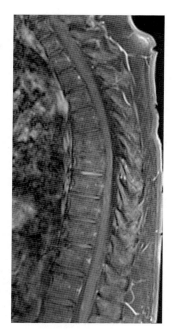

Figure 80-4

HISTORY: A 66-year-old man presents with back pain and lower extremity numbness.

1. What is the single best diagnosis?
   A. Lipoma
   B. Meningioma
   C. Angiolipoma
   D. Spinal epidural lipomatosis

2. What finding on axial images has been described as pathognomonic of this abnormality when it involves the lumbar spine?
   A. "Y" sign
   B. "Shiny corner" sign
   C. "Empty sac" sign
   D. "Dural tail" sign

3. Which of the following statements regarding this entity is true?
   A. Involvement of the cervical spine is rare.
   B. The idiopathic form of this entity typically favors the thoracic spine.
   C. Males are affected more than females.
   D. Neurologic deficits occur more frequently with involvement of the thoracic spine compared to the lumbar spine.

4. Which of the following is *not* a cause of this entity?
   A. Cushing syndrome
   B. Exogenous steroid use
   C. Idiopathic origin
   D. Addison syndrome

CASE 80

Spinal Epidural Lipomatosis

1. **D.** Spinal epidural lipomatosis (SEL). There is no evidence of a capsule or masslike appearance to indicate a focal lipoma. Meningiomas are typically intradural and do not have the signal intensity of fat. Angiolipomas are typically hyperintense on T1-weighted images; however, they are often inhomogeneous and show enhancement.

2. **A.** "Y" sign. This finding is also known as the Mercedes-Benz sign. The "shiny corner" sign is described in ankylosing spondylitis. The "empty sac" sign is described in arachnoiditis. The "dural tail" sign is described in meningiomas.

3. **C.** Males are affected more than females. A strong male predominance exists. The distal lumbar spine and the midthoracic and distal thoracic spine are the most commonly involved sites. Secondary SEL typically favors the thoracic spine, whereas idiopathic SEL favors the lumbar spine. Lumbar SEL is typically associated with radiculopathy.

4. **D.** Addison syndrome. Adrenal cortex insufficiency results in weight loss and decreased body fat. Cushing syndrome and exogenous steroid use are known causes. Some cases have no predisposing factors.

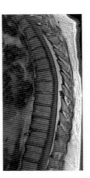

Comment

Background

SEL is a rare disorder defined as a pathologic overgrowth of normal extradural fat. It is most often associated with the administration of exogenous steroids and conditions of endocrine dysfunction, such as Cushing disease and hypothyroidism. Obesity is the second most common association. Cervical spine involvement is extremely rare. Several authors assert that the term *idiopathic* should be used solely to characterize cases of SEL that develop in nonobese patients, who were not receiving corticosteroid therapy, and who do not have any other underlying SEL-related disease.

Pathophysiology

The presence of excessive adipose tissue in the confines of the spinal canal may result in direct compression of the neural elements as well as venous structures. Venous engorgement may contribute to myelopathy and/or radiculopathy. Back pain and weakness are the most frequent presenting complaints.

Imaging

Magnetic resonance imaging (MRI) is the diagnostic test of choice. The normal range for epidural fat thickness in the sagittal plane is 3 to 6 mm, whereas a thickness of 7 to 15 mm has been reported for patients with symptomatic SEL (Figures 80-1 and 80-2). The thecal sac may be completely effaced, revealing the typical Mercedes-Benz sign on axial images (Figure 80-3). The most commonly involved levels in the thoracic and lumbar spine are T6-T8 and L4-L5. Epidural lipomatosis should be differentiated from other extradural mass lesions such as lipoma and angiolipoma. Lipomatosis consists of unencapsulated, diffuse fatty tissue derived from preexisting epidural fat by hypertrophy, whereas lipomas or angiolipomas are typically well-encapsulated, circumscribed masses. Angiolipoma may also show enhancement, which was not seen in this case (Figure 80-4).

Management

Surgical decompression is the treatment of choice when patients present with abnormal neurologic signs. Weight reduction may be beneficial in patients who present with mild symptoms.

References

Al-Khawaja D, Seex K, Eslick GD. Spinal epidural lipomatosis—a brief review. *J Clin Neurosci.* 2008;15(12):1323-1326.

Lee SB, Park HK, Chang JC, et al. Idiopathic thoracic epidural lipomatosis with chest pain. *J Korean Neurosurg Soc.* 2011;50(2): 130-133.

Cross-Reference

Neuroradiology: THE REQUISITES, 4th ed, pp 587-588.

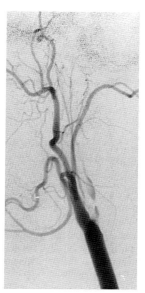

Figure 81-1   Patient A.

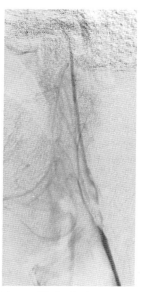

Figure 81-2   Patient A.

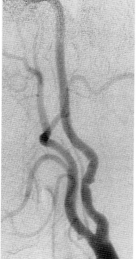

Figure 81-3   Patient A.

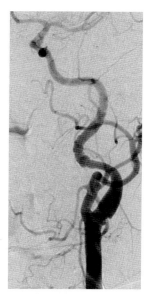

Figure 81-4   Patient B.

HISTORY: Stroke.

1. What acute abnormality is present in the left internal carotid artery of Patient A?
   A. Aneurysm
   B. Atherosclerosis
   C. Dissection
   D. Pseudoaneurysm

2. What common underlying pathology do both patient A and B have that predisposed them to stroke?
   A. Atrial fibrillation
   B. Common carotid artery stenosis
   C. Takayasu arteritis
   D. Fibromuscular dysplasia

3. What is the most common location for an intracranial arterial dissection?
   A. Cavernous internal carotid artery
   B. Distal vertebral artery
   C. Basilar artery
   D. Supraclinoid internal carotid artery

4. Which of the following statements is correct regarding collimators in radiography/fluoroscopy?
   A. Collimators change the effective focal spot size.
   B. Collimators reduce scatter radiation.
   C. Collimators decrease exposure time.
   D. Collimators reduce lower energy photons.

CASE 81

Fibromuscular Dysplasia

1. **C.** Dissection. The left common carotid artery injection (Figure 81-1) shows marked narrowing with an irregularity to the proximal left internal carotid artery and poor filling of the distal vessel, consistent with a dissection. The delayed angiographic image (Figure 81-2) following the same injection shows prolonged anterograde flow.

2. **D.** Fibromuscular dysplasia. Alternating dilated and narrowed segments of the internal carotid arteries are demonstrated in both patients, although more evident in Patient B. This is the most common appearance of fibromuscular dysplasia.

3. **D.** Supraclinoid internal carotid artery. This is the most common location for intracranial dissection.

4. **B.** Collimators reduce scatter radiation. Collimators may reduce scatter by decreasing the volume of tissue through which the radiation passes. They do not affect the focal spot size. They can increase exposure time by decreasing incident photons on the detector. Collimators do not reduce low energy photons, but filters do.

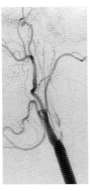
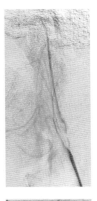
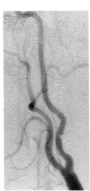
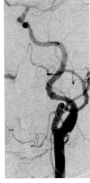

Comment

Angiography

Digital subtraction angiography (DSA) demonstrates findings consistent with an extracranial dissection of the proximal left internal carotid artery (Figure 81-1). There is marked narrowing and irregularity of the proximal internal carotid artery, with poor distal filling and very slow antegrade flow seen on the delayed image (Figure 81-2).

In these cases, injection of the right common carotid arteries demonstrates normal appearances of the common carotid artery. Distal to the carotid bifurcation, however, there is irregularity, with regions of narrowing alternating with dilation, producing a "string of beads" appearance that is commonly described in fibromuscular dysplasia (Figures 81-3 and 81-4).

Causes of Extracranial Dissection

An extracranial dissection can result from major or minor trauma, including chiropractic manipulation. Alternatively, extracranial dissection can result from an underlying vascular abnormality or dysplasia.

Types of Fibromuscular Dysplasia

There are many subtypes (medial, intimal, and adventitial) of fibromuscular dysplasia in which one or all of the layers of the arterial wall may be involved; however, involvement of the media with hyperplasia or dysplasia is most common, seen in up to 90% of cases. Thinning of the media is associated with abnormalities in the internal elastic lamina, resulting in the dilations seen in this condition. The cervical internal carotid artery is most commonly affected, and the proximal 2 cm of this vessel is usually spared because of architectural differences in this part of the vessel's wall. The extracranial vertebral artery and external carotid arteries may be involved; however, intracranial fibromuscular dysplasia is relatively uncommon. The incidence of intracranial aneurysms is increased in patients with this condition.

Reference

Manninen HI, Koivisto T, Saari T, et al. Dissecting aneurysms of all four cervicocranial arteries in fibromuscular dysplasia: treatment with self-expanding endovascular stents, coil embolization, and surgical ligation. *AJNR Am J Neuroradiol.* 1997;18:1216-1220.

Cross-Reference

Neuroradiology: THE REQUISITES, 4th ed, p 118.

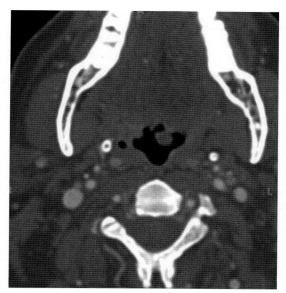

Figure 82-1

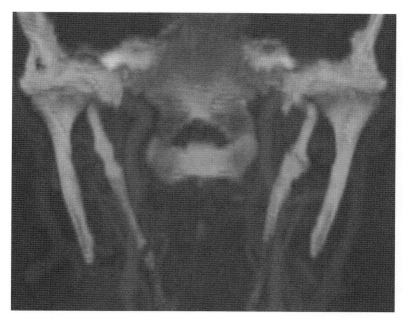

Figure 82-2

HISTORY: An elderly man presents with right ear pain during eating.

1. Which of the following is the single best diagnosis?
   A. Osteochondroma of the styloid process
   B. Fracture of the styloid process
   C. Myositis ossificans
   D. Eagle syndrome

2. What is the other name for the poststyloid parapharyngeal space?
   A. The retropharyngeal space
   B. The carotid space
   C. The deep lobe of the parotid gland
   D. The longus space

3. What structure does the stylomastoid foramen mark?
   A. The exit of the facial nerve from the skull base
   B. The otic ganglion
   C. Cranial nerve V_3
   D. Cranial nerve V_2

4. What are the two nerves that run along the styloglossus-stylohyoid musculature?
   A. Cranial nerves V_3 (lingual branch) and XII
   B. Cranial nerves IX and XII
   C. Cranial nerves V_2 (buccal branch) and X
   D. Chorda tympani and cranial nerve X

CASE 82

Eagle Syndrome

1. **D.** Eagle syndrome. Eagle syndrome is a condition involving elongation and calcification of the styloid process, which cause pain on swallowing.

2. **B.** The carotid space. The carotid space is the other name for the poststyloid parapharyngeal space because it is posterior to the styloid musculature. The deep lobe of the parotid gland is anterior to the styloid musculature and therefore not "poststyloid."

3. **A.** The exit of the facial nerve from the skull base. The facial nerve exits from the skull base and leaves the temporal bone via the stylomastoid foramen. The otic ganglion is nearby, but the stylomastoid foramen is not its marker. Cranial nerve V_3 leaves via the foramen ovale, and cranial nerve V_2 leaves via the foramen rotundum.

4. **A.** Cranial nerves V_3 (lingual branch) and XII. Cranial nerves V_3 (lingual branch) and XII run along the sublingual space. Cranial nerves IX, X, and V_2 (buccal branch) are not located in this space, nor is the chorda tympani.

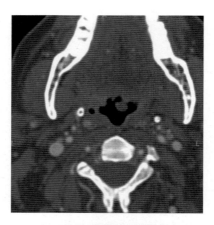

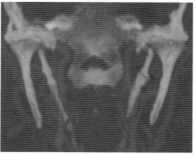

Comment

Characteristics of Eagle Syndrome

Eagle syndrome is an unusual entity, and some authorities do not believe that it causes pain on swallowing. It results from prominence with calcification of the stylohyoid ligament in such a way that the styloid process becomes elongated. The elongated styloid process often indents the pharyngeal mucosa when symptomatic (Figures 82-1 and 82-2). Compression of cranial nerve IX (most commonly) or XII and/or the sympathetic nervous plexus along the carotid artery may yield unusual complaints. The syndrome is named for Watt W. Eagle, a Duke University otolaryngologist who published a report of about 200 affected patients in 1937.

Incidence of Eagle Syndrome

The styloid process is elongated in 4% of the population; the length is usually described as more than 3 to 4 cm. However, fewer than 10% of patients with this elongation have symptoms. Treatment is resection of a portion of the elongated styloid process via an intraoral or extraoral approach. Some physicians inject local anesthetic in the ligament beforehand to ensure that this is the source of the otalgia, dysphagia, and/or headaches.

Reference

Costantinides F, Vidoni G, Bodin C, Di Lenarda R. Eagle's syndrome: signs and symptoms. *Cranio.* 2013;31(1):56-60.

Cross-Reference

Neuroradiology: THE REQUISITES, 4th ed, pp 502-504.

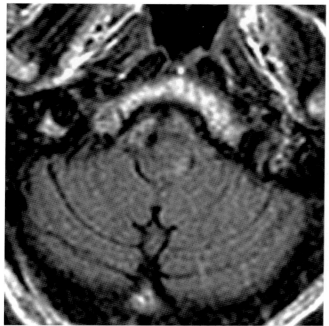

Figure 83-1

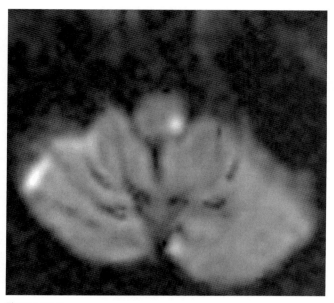

Figure 83-2

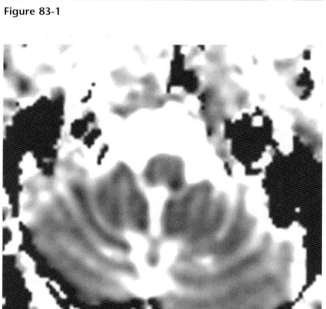

Figure 83-3

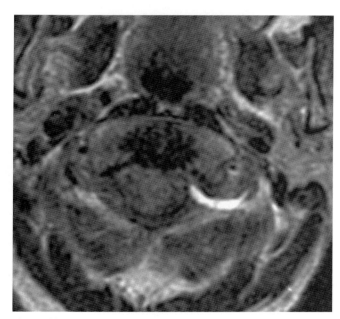

Figure 83-4

HISTORY: Acute sensory deficits.

1. What is the single best diagnosis of the case?
   A. Infarct
   B. Osmotic demyelination syndrome
   C. Brainstem glioma
   D. Human immunodeficiency virus (HIV) encephalitis

2. What part(s) of the brainstem does the posterior inferior cerebellar artery (PICA) supply?
   A. Central medulla
   B. Lateral medulla
   C. Lateral and posterior medulla
   D. Lateral and anterior medulla

3. What part(s) of the brainstem does the superior cerebellar artery (SCA) supply?
   A. Central pons
   B. Lateral pons
   C. Lateral and posterior pons
   D. Lateral and anterior pons

4. What is the most common cause of ischemia in the posterior circulation in an older patient?
   A. Dissection
   B. Thromboembolic disease
   C. Vasospasm
   D. Vasculitis

CASE 83

Lateral Medullary (Wallenberg) Syndrome

1. **A.** Infarct. Considering the clinical history of acute sensory deficits and the imaging, especially the restricted diffusion (Figures 83-2 [B1000] and 83-3 [ADC]) ipsilateral to the hyperintensity in the left vertebral artery (Figure 83-4), infarct is the favored diagnosis. Osmotic demyelination syndrome typically occurs in the pons, and thus this would be an unlikely etiology for this case. HIV encephalitis manifests with atrophy and bilateral diffuse white matter abnormalities. Although gliomas can involve the brainstem, it would be unlikely to have an isolated lesion in the medulla.

2. **C.** Lateral and posterior medulla. The PICA supplies the lateral and posterior aspects of the medulla.

3. **C.** Lateral and posterior pons. The SCA supplies the lateral and posterior aspects of the pons.

4. **B.** Thromboembolic disease. The most common cause is thromboembolic disease from accelerated atheromatous disease or emboli from a cardiac source.

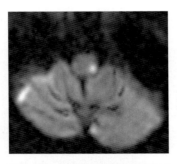

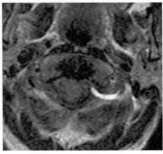

Comment

Clinical Presentation

Infarcts of the lateral medulla (PICA territory) can result in lateral medullary (Wallenberg) syndrome. This is characterized by loss of pain and temperature of the body on the contralateral side (lateral spinothalamic tract) and face on the ipsilateral side (descending trigeminothalamic tract), ataxia, ipsilateral swallowing and taste disorders, hoarseness, vertigo and nystagmus, and ipsilateral Horner syndrome.

Causes

In older patients, the most common cause of posterior circulation ischemia is thromboembolic disease resulting from accelerated atheromatous disease or embolic disease from a cardiac source. However, because the vasculature (including the vertebral arteries) becomes more tortuous as a patient ages, in the older adult population in the setting of embolic disease from a systemic source, it is less common to have embolic disease isolated to the posterior fossa (usually patients also have embolic disease to the anterior circulation). Isolated posterior fossa embolic disease is more common in young patients. In young patients with posterior fossa ischemia, in addition to embolic disease, the diagnosis of a dissection should also be considered.

Imaging

This can be evaluated with magnetic resonance imaging (MRI) and magnetic resonance angiography (MRA) or with computed tomography angiography (CTA). MRI should include unenhanced axial T1-weighted images through the distal vertebral arteries with fat suppression, when possible, to look for clot in the vessel wall, which is hyperintense owing to methemoglobin. In addition, the dissected vessel may be enlarged as a result of mural hematoma, and occlusion (absence of signal void) or luminal narrowing (reduced size of the signal void) may be seen. In this case, the patient's ischemic disease was related to thrombosis of the distal left vertebral artery as a result of dissection (Figure 83-4). There is subtle T2-FLAIR hyperintensity correlating to the recent infarct (Figure 83-1).

Reference

Min WK, Kim YS, Kim JY, et al. Atherothrombotic cerebellar infarction: vascular lesion-MRI correlation of 31 cases. *Stroke.* 1999;30:2376-2381.

Cross-Reference

Neuroradiology: THE REQUISITES, 4th ed, pp 33, 89-90.

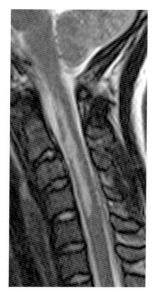

Figure 84-1

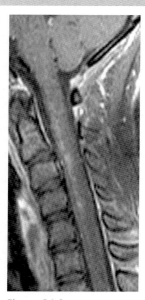

Figure 84-2

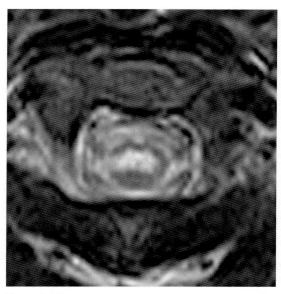

Figure 84-3

HISTORY: A 14-year-old girl develops acute paralysis and respiratory failure following upper respiratory infection.

1. Considering the imaging and clinical history, what is the single most likely diagnosis?
   A. Acute disseminated encephalomyelitis (ADEM)
   B. Systemic lupus erythematosus (SLE)
   C. Neuromyelitis optica (NMO)
   D. Astrocytoma

2. Which of the following statements is true?
   A. Diagnosis of acute transverse myelitis (ATM) is made on spinal cord biopsy.
   B. ATM is clinically characterized by the development of motor sensory and autonomic dysfunction.
   C. Angiography is the imaging modality of choice in evaluation of ATM.
   D. ATM is more frequent in adults than children.

3. Which of the following statements regarding ADEM is true?
   A. Antibodies to myelin oligodendrocyte glycoprotein are found in children with ADEM.
   B. Adults are more often affected than children.
   C. Two thirds of patients have relapses.
   D. Cerebrospinal fluid analysis typically reveals oligoclonal bands.

4. Regarding spinal cord lesions in multiple sclerosis (MS) and ADEM, which of the following statements is correct?
   A. Spinal cord lesions extending over a longer segment are more likely characteristic of MS than ADEM.
   B. Spinal cord lesions showing ringlike enhancement can occur in both.
   C. Spinal cord lesions with well-defined margins are characteristic of ADEM.
   D. Spinal cord lesions affecting the cervical cord present with equal incidence in both MS and ADEM.

CASE 84

Acute Disseminated Encephalomyelitis

1. **A.** Acute disseminated encephalomyelitis (ADEM). ADEM affects children and adolescents. Patients typically present with extensive lesions involving the spinal cord. SLE may produce the findings present in this case. Longitudinally extensive lesions involving the spinal cord have been associated with NMO. Astrocytoma should be included in the differential diagnosis of an enhancing intramedullary lesion; however, the lack of cord expansion and the history provided make it unlikely.

2. **B.** ATM is clinically characterized by the development of motor sensory and autonomic dysfunction. ATM is characterized clinically by acute or subacute development of symptoms and signs of neurologic dysfunction in motor, sensory, and autonomic nerve tracts of the spinal cord. Spinal cord biopsy is not a practical option in the routine evaluation of these patients. Enhanced spinal magnetic resonance imaging (MRI) and a lumbar puncture are mandatory in the evaluation of suspected ATM. Children are affected more often than adults.

3. **A.** Antibodies to myelin oligodendrocyte glycoprotein are found in children with ADEM. Antibodies to myelin oligodendrocyte glycoprotein are present in 35% of pediatric patients with ADEM. ADEM most commonly affects young children and adolescents. Although ADEM is classically considered to be a monophasic disorder, one third of patients experience relapses. Oligoclonal bands are typically absent or rare in ADEM.

4. **B.** Spinal cord lesions showing ringlike enhancement can occur in both. Both ADEM and MS may show a ring-enhancing lesion. Large lesions, or longitudinally extensive lesions involving the spinal cord, have been associated with ADEM, in contrast to spinal lesions in MS, which tend to be small (one to two spinal segments in length). In contrast to lesions in MS, lesions in ADEM have poorly defined margins. ADEM more commonly affects the thoracic spine, whereas MS more commonly affects the cervical spine.

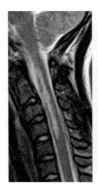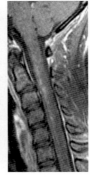

Comment

Background

ADEM is a monophasic demyelinating disease of the central nervous system that occurs in most cases following a viral illness, vaccination, or nonspecific respiratory infection. ADEM most commonly affects young children and adolescents. It typically affects the gray matter and white matter of the brain and spinal cord (30%). Symptoms include fever, headache, ataxia, and seizures. Symptoms may progress for 2 weeks. The prognosis is favorable, with complete recovery within 6 months. Although ADEM is classically considered to be a monophasic disorder, one third of patients experience relapses. ADEM relapses occurring within 3 months of the inciting ADEM episode are considered part of the same acute event. At least 18% of all children ultimately diagnosed with MS experience a first demyelinating event clinically indistinguishable from typical ADEM.

Pathophysiology

The pathogenesis of ADEM is unclear; however, it is thought to be an immune-mediated disorder resulting from an autoimmune reaction to myelin. In the acute stages, ADEM is characterized histologically by perivenous edema, demyelination, and infiltration with macrophages and lymphocytes, with relative axonal sparing, whereas the late course of the disease is characterized by perivascular gliosis.

Imaging

Although the MRI features of ADEM and MS cannot be reliably distinguished, large lesions, or longitudinally extensive lesions involving the spinal cord (Figures 84-1 and 84-2), have been associated with ADEM and with neuromyelitis optica, in contrast to spinal lesions in MS, which tend to be small (one to two spinal segments in length). Lesions may involve the gray matter or white matter (Figure 84-3) and may or may not enhance (see Figure 84-2).

Management

Cerebrospinal fluid analysis typically reveals lymphocytes and mildly increased protein. Treatment includes early use of high-dose intravenous steroids. Severe cases may be treated with a combination of intravenous corticosteroids and intravenous immunoglobulin, immunosuppressants, or plasmapheresis. The prognosis is favorable, with complete recovery within 6 months.

References

Callen DJ, Shroff MM, Branson HM, et al. Role of MRI in the differentiation of ADEM from MS in children. *Neurology.* 2009;72(11): 968-973.

Pröbstel AK, Dornmair K, Bittner R, et al. Antibodies to MOG are transient in childhood acute disseminated encephalomyelitis. *Neurology.* 2011;77(6):580-588.

Rossi A. Imaging of acute disseminated encephalomyelitis. *Neuroimaging Clin N Am.* 2008;18(1):149-161, ix.

Cross-Reference

Neuroradiology: THE REQUISITES, 4th ed, pp 216-217.

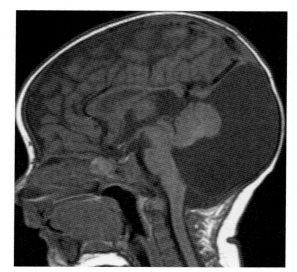

Figure 85-1

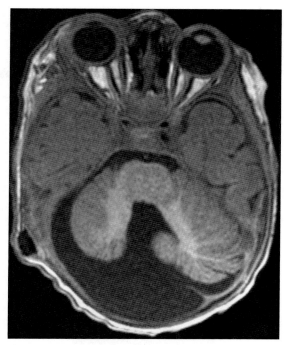

Figure 85-2

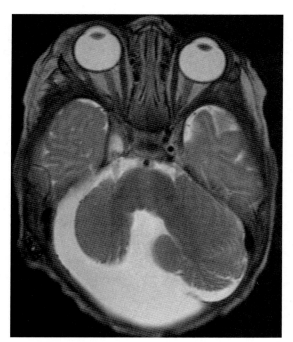

Figure 85-3

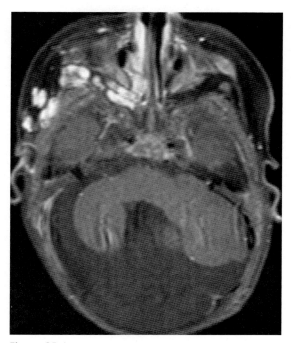

Figure 85-4

HISTORY: Macrocephaly.

1. What is the single best diagnosis?
   A. Joubert syndrome
   B. Dandy-Walker
   C. Postoperative changes
   D. Rhombencephalosynapsis

2. What is believed to be the cause of this entity?
   A. Genetic
   B. Neoplastic
   C. In utero insult
   D. Postpartum injury

3. What is the most common presentation of this entity?
   A. Macrocephaly
   B. Paresthesia
   C. Ataxia
   D. Developmental delay

4. What percentage of this entity is associated with hydrocephalus?
   A. 0%
   B. 25%
   C. 50%
   D. 75%

CASE 85

Dandy-Walker Malformation

1. **B.** Dandy-Walker. There is a large posterior fossa cyst with dysplasia of the vermis. This is part of the Dandy-Walker complex. There is no molar tooth deformity, as seen in Joubert syndrome; no fusion of the cerebellum; and no evidence of surgery in the calvarium.

2. **C.** In utero insult. An in utero insult is believed to be the cause of the malformation, with severity dependent on when in development it occurs.

3. **A.** Macrocephaly. This is the most common presenting sign or symptom.

4. **D.** 75%. Dandy-Walker is associated with hydrocephalus 75% of the time.

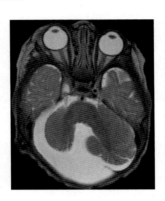

Comment

The Dandy-Walker complex (which includes Dandy-Walker malformation and its variants) is a congenital anomaly believed to be related to an in utero insult to the fourth ventricle leading to complete or partial outflow obstruction of cerebrospinal fluid. As a result, there is cystlike dilation of the fourth ventricle, which protrudes up between the cerebellar hemispheres to prevent their fusion, and there is incomplete formation of all or part of the inferior vermis. The spectrum of Dandy-Walker variant depends on the time in utero at which the insult occurs, as well as the severity of the insult (the degree of fourth ventricular outflow obstruction).

Associations

Dandy-Walker malformations are associated with hydrocephalus in approximately 75% of cases, which usually develops in the postnatal period. Dandy-Walker malformations may be associated with atresia of the foramen of Magendie and, possibly, the foramen of Luschka; however, atresia of the ventricular outlet foramina is not an essential feature of the condition. In addition, 70% of patients have associated supratentorial anomalies, including dysgenesis of the corpus callosum, migrational anomalies, and encephaloceles.

Imaging

This case demonstrates characteristic magnetic resonance (MR) findings of a Dandy-Walker malformation, including a large retrocerebellar cyst; enlargement of the posterior fossa with osseous remodeling; abnormally high position of the straight sinus, torcular Herophili, and tentorium; and torcular-lambdoid inversion (Figures 85-1 through 85-4). The radiologic hallmark of Dandy-Walker malformation is communication of the retrocerebellar cyst with the fourth ventricle, which is readily appreciated on the sagittal MR image (see Figure 85-1).

Differential Diagnosis

A mega cisterna magna consists of an enlarged posterior fossa secondary to an enlarged cisterna magna but with a normal cerebellar vermis and fourth ventricle. Retrocerebellar arachnoid cysts of developmental origin are clinically important. They displace the fourth ventricle and cerebellum anteriorly and show significant mass effect. Differentiation of posterior fossa arachnoid cyst from Dandy-Walker malformation is essential because surgical therapy differs between the two entities.

Reference

Glenn OA, Barkovich J. Magnetic resonance imaging of the fetal brain and spine: an increasingly important tool in prenatal diagnosis: part 2. *Am J Neuroradiol.* 2006;27:1807-1814.

Cross-Reference

Neuroradiology: THE REQUISITES, 4th ed, pp 280-281.

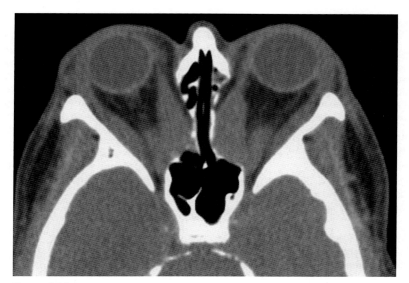

Figure 86-1

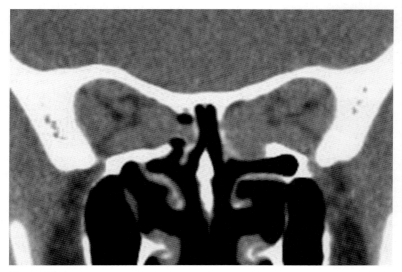

Figure 86-2

HISTORY: Agitation and tachycardia.

1. What is the single best diagnosis of the case?
   A. Fibrous dysplasia
   B. Sinusitis and myositis
   C. Silent sinus syndrome
   D. Thyroid orbitopathy

2. Which of the extraocular muscles is typically spared in thyroid orbitopathy?
   A. Superior rectus
   B. Inferior rectus
   C. Medial rectus
   D. Lateral rectus

3. Which symptom usually necessitates surgery for thyroid eye disease?
   A. Exposure keratitis
   B. Diplopia
   C. Optic neuropathy
   D. Poor cosmesis

4. What is the current recommended surgery for thyroid orbitopathy?
   A. Steroids
   B. Eyelid split and reconstruction
   C. Orbital floor decompression
   D. Endoscopic medial orbital wall decompression

CASE 86

Thyroid Eye Disease

1. **D.** Thyroid orbitopathy. Extraocular muscle enlargement and prior medial wall decompression bilaterally are compatible with thyroid eye disease. The history is supportive of the diagnosis of the patient with hyperthyroidism.

2. **D.** Lateral rectus. The lateral rectus and superior oblique are typically spared. The inferior and medial rectus muscles are most often affected.

3. **A.** Exposure keratitis. Although optic neuropathy often necessitates surgery, most patients who are operated on are so treated for exposure keratitis prior to developing neuropathy.

4. **D.** Endoscopic medial orbital wall decompression. As demonstrated in this case, the recommended surgery is endoscopic medial orbital wall decompression.

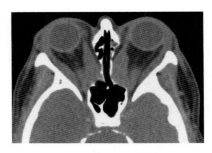

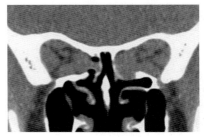

Comment

The terms *thyroid orbitopathy*, *thyroid eye disease*, *Graves ophthalmopathy*, *Graves orbitopathy*, *thyroid ophthalmopathy*, *dysthyroid eye disease*, and *Basedow disease* refer to the pathologic process in the eye that is associated with thyroid dysfunction. The acute phase is characterized by inflammation and edema of the extraocular muscles with lymphocytic infiltration. There is often injection of the fat as well. Thyroid ophthalmopathy is more common in women by a ratio of 4:1 and is often asymptomatic; however, when present, it may be seen in euthyroid or hyperthyroid states. The most common cause of unilateral or bilateral exophthalmos in adults is thyroid ophthalmopathy. The incidence of bilateral disease may be as high as 90% of cases.

The muscular enlargement (Figures 86-1 and 86-2) causes proptosis with associated eyelid retraction. The eyelid retraction leads to exposure of the cornea and the irritation and abrasions that can occur on the surface of the eye. The eyes are dry and painful. In addition, affected patients may have diplopia.

Most patients evaluated with computed tomography or magnetic resonance imaging (MRI) carry a known diagnosis of thyroid ophthalmopathy, and the role of imaging is to assess for the presence of optic nerve compression in the orbital apex by enlarged muscles. When vision is compromised in patients who do not respond to medical therapy, orbital decompression by removal of the osseous walls around the orbital apex may be necessary.

Imaging Findings

In the worst-case scenario, the optic nerve is compressed by the large muscles at the orbital apex. In Figures 86-1 and 86-2, fat remains visible around the optic nerve, but this patient has already been treated with orbital decompression (infracturing) of the medial walls to provide the space for the medial rectus muscle to come off of the optic nerves. The enlarged muscles paradoxically may lead to restriction of eye motion. On imaging, the effects typically seen are first on the inferior rectus and medial rectus muscles, most commonly followed by superior rectus, lateral rectus, and superior oblique muscles. Affected patients have proptosis, edema of the retrobulbar fat, displacement of the lacrimal glands out of the orbit, swelling of the eyelids, and proliferation of the orbital fat (both intraconal and extraconal). The muscular tendons are spared, whereas the bellies of the muscles are markedly expanded. On MRI, the muscles appear edematous and enhance avidly.

References

Aydin K, Guven K, Sencer S, et al. A new MRI method for the quantitative evaluation of extraocular muscle size in thyroid ophthalmopathy. *Neuroradiology*. 2003;45:184-187.

Kirsch E, Hammer B, von Arx G. Graves' orbitopathy: current imaging procedures. *Swiss Med Wkly*. 2009;139(43–44):618-623.

Cross-Reference

Neuroradiology: THE REQUISITES, 4th ed, pp 334-335.

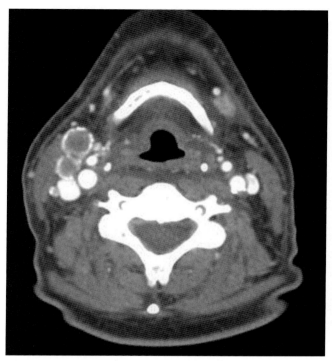

Figure 87-1

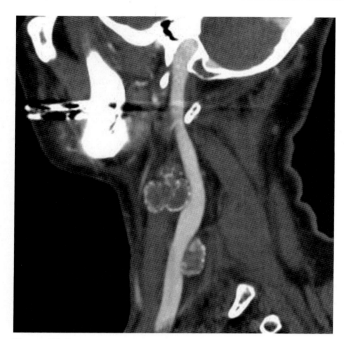

Figure 87-2

HISTORY: An adult presents with long-standing bilateral neck discomfort.

1. Which of the following is the best differential diagnosis?
   A. Calcified nodes from tuberculosis, irradiated lymphoma, or thyroid cancer
   B. Calcified nodes from thyroid cancer or embolization material in hypervascular nodal metastasis
   C. Extracranial meningiomas or schwannomas in a patient with neurofibromatosis type 2 (NF2)
   D. Hemangioma with peripheral enhancement or phleboliths in vascular malformations

2. Which of the following is *not* a manifestation of thyroid cancer adenopathy?
   A. Calcified nodes
   B. Highly enhancing nodes
   C. Cystic nodes
   D. Hemorrhagic nodes

3. How soon after radiation therapy do lymphoma nodes calcify?
   A. Within 3 months
   B. 3 to 6 months
   C. 6 to 9 months
   D. More than 9 months

4. What is the level of adenopathy of nodes that are between the hyoid bone and cricoid cartilage but completely behind the jugular vein?
   A. IIA
   B. IIB
   C. III
   D. IIIB

177

CASE 87

Calcified Nodes

1. **A.** Calcified nodes from tuberculosis, irradiated lymphoma, or thyroid cancer. Tuberculosis, irradiated lymphoma, Thorotrast use, and thyroid cancer are all potential causes of calcified nodes. Thorotrast was used as a contrast agent in the 1930s and 1940s. Embolization materials are usually higher density than calcification and would not appear like this. Schwannomas would not appear like this, and meningiomas rarely occur extracranially. These are not phleboliths.

2. **D.** Hemorrhagic nodes. Hemorrhagic lymph nodes are very uncommon. Thyroid cancer nodes may calcify, may enhance avidly, or may be cystic.

3. **D.** More than 9 months. Lymphoma nodes typically calcify 12 months after radiation therapy.

4. **C.** III. Level III adenopathy consists of lymph nodes that reside between the hyoid bone and cricoid cartilage. Unlike levels I, II, and V nodes, levels III, IV, VI, and VII nodes are not further subdivided into A and B levels.

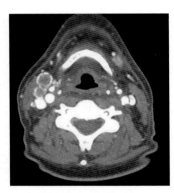

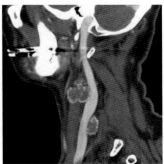

Comment

Calcified Lymph Node Associations

Calcification of lymph nodes may be secondary to a number of disorders, including treated granulomatous infections (e.g., tuberculosis, fungal infections), treated lymphoma, thyroid cancer, silicosis, sarcoidosis, and some mucinous adenocarcinomas. Much of the literature is based on plain radiographs; the onset of calcification in treated lymphoma after radiotherapy is quoted as being 12 months. High-resolution computed tomography may reveal it earlier.

Imaging Findings

Thyroid cancer is unusual in that the nodes associated with it may be calcified, cystic, or hypervascular and may even appear bright on T1-weighted magnetic resonance imaging, presumably because of high colloid content. The other primary tumor that may cause lymph nodes to appear bright on T1-weighted images is melanoma. Thyroid cancer also is unique in that it may lead to retropharyngeal nodes, and many nodes never meet the 1-cm size criterion (Figures 87-1 and 87-2).

Nodal Nomenclature

Nodal nomenclature for squamous cell carcinomas in the aerodigestive system is based on location: level IA nodes are submental; level IB nodes are submandibular; level IIA nodes are in the jugular chain above the hyoid bone and *not* completely behind the jugular vein; level IIB nodes are in the jugular chain above the hyoid and completely behind the jugular vein; level III nodes are in the jugular chain between the hyoid bone and the cricoid cartilage; level IV nodes are in the jugular chain below the cricoid cartilage and down to the clavicle; level VA nodes are completely behind the sternocleidomastoid muscle and above the cricoid cartilage; level VB nodes are completely behind the sternocleidomastoid muscle and below the cricoid cartilage; level VI nodes are anterior visceral; and level VII nodes are anterior mediastinal.

Reference

Gawne-Cain ML, Hansell DM. The pattern and distribution of calcified mediastinal lymph nodes in sarcoidosis and tuberculosis: a CT study. *Clin Radiol.* 1996;51(4):263-267.

Cross-Reference

Neuroradiology: THE REQUISITES, 4th ed, pp 446, 513.

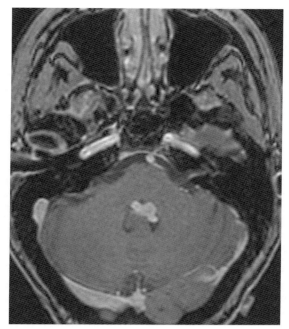

Figure 88-1 Patient A.

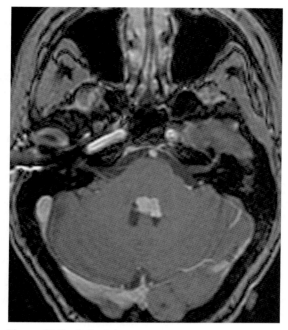

Figure 88-2 Patient A.

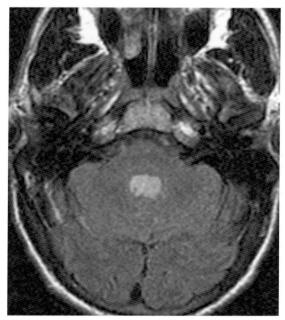

Figure 88-3 Patient B.

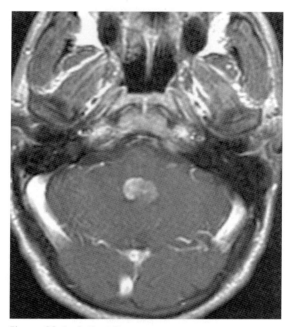

Figure 88-4 Patient B.

HISTORY: Nausea and vomiting.

1. What single answer should first be *excluded* from the differential diagnosis of these cases?
   A. Hemangioblastoma
   B. Meningioma
   C. Ependymoma
   D. Choroid plexus papilloma

2. Which of the following is the most common location for ependymomas?
   A. Lateral ventricles
   B. Filum terminale
   C. Posterior fossa
   D. Spinal cord

3. Where do choroid plexus papillomas most commonly occur in adults?
   A. Atria of the lateral ventricles
   B. Temporal horns of the lateral ventricles
   C. Third ventricle
   D. Fourth ventricle

4. Which infectious agent has been implicated in the evolution of both choroid plexus papillomas and ependymomas?
   A. JC virus
   B. Simian virus 40
   C. Human papillomavirus (HPV)
   D. Epstein-Barr virus

CASE 88

Fourth Ventricular Neoplasms: Choroid Plexus Papilloma and Ependymoma

1. **A.** Hemangioblastoma. A mass within the fourth ventricle could represent an ependymoma, a meningioma, a choroid plexus papilloma, a metastasis, or occasionally a hemangioma. A hemangioblastoma within the posterior fossa usually occurs as a mass within the cerebellum, it can contain a cyst, and it can also contain vascular flow voids.

2. **C.** Posterior fossa. The most common location for an ependymoma is the posterior fossa.

3. **D.** Fourth ventricle. The most common location for choroid plexus papillomas in an adult is the fourth ventricle. The most common location for choroid plexus papillomas in children is the atria of the lateral ventricles.

4. **B.** Simian virus 40. The JC virus is associated with progressive multifocal leukoencephalopathy (PML). HPV is associated with squamous cell carcinoma. Epstein-Barr virus has been associated with nasopharyngeal carcinoma, Burkitt lymphoma, and Hodgkin disease.

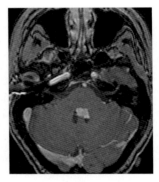

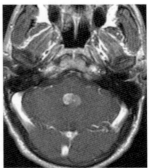

Comment

Case A

Choroid plexus papillomas (Patient A) are epithelial tumors arising from the surface of the choroid plexus. They occur most commonly in the lateral ventricles (45%). They may also arise within the fourth ventricle (40%) (Patient A, Figures 88-1 and 88-2) and the third ventricle (10%). In adults, the majority of choroid plexus papillomas occur in the fourth ventricle, whereas in children, 80% arise in the atria or trigone of the lateral ventricles. Choroid plexus papillomas can cause hydrocephalus as a result of overproduction of cerebrospinal fluid or obstructive hydrocephalus related to adhesions from proteinaceous or hemorrhagic material blocking the subarachnoid cisterns or ventricular outlets. In addition, large tumors cause focal expansion of the ventricle they fill; they can also cause trapping. These tumors are composed of vascularized connective tissue and frond-like papillae lined by a single layer of epithelial cells.

Case B

Intracranial ependymomas occur above or below the tentorium. The tumor arises in rests of ependymal cells lining the ventricles that extend into adjacent white matter. Infratentorial ependymomas occur in approximately two thirds of cases, and 75% of these posterior fossa tumors are located in the fourth ventricle (Patient B, Figures 88-3 and 88-4). Approximately 15% arise in the cerebellopontine angle, and the remaining small percentage arises within the cerebellar hemisphere. Approximately 50% of infratentorial ependymomas extend into the cerebellopontine angle cisterns and foramen magnum via the recesses of the fourth ventricle (foramina of Magendie and Luschka). Of infratentorial ependymomas, 12% occur with subarachnoid seeding, especially those demonstrating anaplastic histology.

Imaging of Both Tumors

Calcification, hemorrhage, and cysts are often present in both choroid plexus papillomas and ependymomas. Calcification is readily identified on computed tomography, as are large regions of cyst formation. On magnetic resonance imaging, hypointensity can correspond to calcium, vessels, or blood products. Tumors that are very cystic will be hyperintense on T2-weighted images, whereas those with large areas of old blood products may be hypointense. Both neoplasms can enhance avidly (Patient A, Figures 88-1 and 88-2) or heterogeneously (Patient B, Figure 88-4), depending on the degree of cyst formation, calcification, and hemorrhage. When contained in the fourth ventricle, choroid plexus papillomas and ependymomas may be identical in appearance, as in these cases (Patients A and B). Choroid plexus papillomas tend to demonstrate an intense blush on catheter-directed angiography, and enlarged choroidal arteries may be seen providing blood flow to the tumor.

Reference

Koeller KK, Sandberg GD. From the archives of the AFIP: cerebral intraventricular neoplasms. Radiologic-pathologic correlation. *Radiographics*. 2002;22:1473-1505.

Cross-Reference

Neuroradiology: THE REQUISITES, 4th ed, pp 49-52.

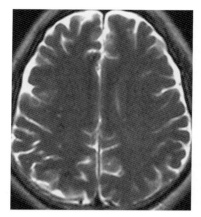

Figure 89-1 Patient A.

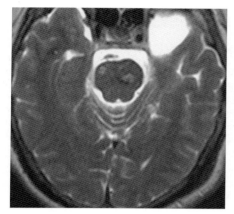

Figure 89-2 Patient A.

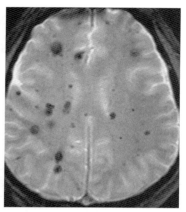

Figure 89-3 Patient A.

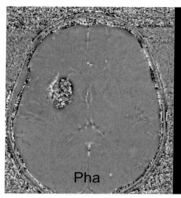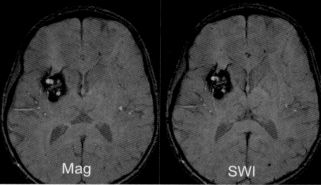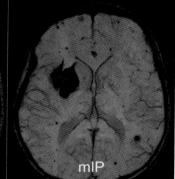

Pha   Mag   SWI   mIP

Figure 89-4 Patient B.

HISTORY: Withheld.

1. Choose the single best statement describing the T2-weighted images (Figures 89-1 and 89-2).
   A. There are subdural hematomas.
   B. There is acute parenchymal microhemorrhage.
   C. Crescentic and ring-like hypointensity in the right frontal lobe, right temporal lobe, and pons is due to hemosiderin related to cavernous malformations.
   D. Calcification and hemosiderin are easily differentiated on T2-weighted imaging.

2. The higher sensitivity to susceptibility effects of gradient echo imaging compared to conventional T2-weighted imaging are the result of what feature of the pulse sequence?
   A. Absence of a 180-degree rephasing pulse
   B. Short time to echo
   C. Flip angle
   D. Decreased cross-talk

3. Regarding the susceptibility-weighted imaging (SWI) series, Figure 89-4, Patient B, which statement is correct?
   A. The minimum intensity projection (mIP) image consists of projecting the voxel with the lowest signal intensity value on every view throughout the slab of data onto a two-dimensional image.
   B. There is more blooming on magnitude (Mag) than on the processed SWI.
   C. The mIP images are formed by multiplying the Mag and SWI data.
   D. The mIP images decrease conspicuity of microhemorrhage and vessel contiguity.

4. In SWI, what predominately contributes to increased sensitivity compared to T2* gradient echo (T2*GRE) imaging?
   A. Higher magnetic field strengths
   B. Increased time for acquisitions
   C. Utilization of magnitude and phase information to produce images
   D. There is no change in sensitivity between SWI and T2*GRE sequences

CASE 89

Multiple Cavernous Malformations

1. **C.** Crescentic and ring-like hypointensity in the right frontal lobe, right temporal lobe, and pons is due to hemosiderin related to cavernous malformations. These lesions are more evident on GRE and SWI. There are no definite acute hematomas or pathologic subdural collections. Both calcification and hemosiderin are hypointense on T2 and cannot easily be discriminated.

2. **A.** Absence of a 180-degree rephasing pulse. Gradient echo imaging is more sensitive to magnetic field inhomogeneities and susceptibility because of the lack of a 180-degree rephasing pulse. The other answer options are not determining factors of increased susceptibility.

3. **A.** The minimum intensity projection (mIP) image consists of projecting the voxel with the lowest signal intensity value on every view throughout the slab of data onto a two-dimensional image. There is less blooming on Mag images because they are higher resolution. SWI images are formed by multiplying phase and magnitude (Pha and Mag, Figure 89-4) data. A clinical utility of mIP images is to increase conspicuity of hemorrhage and vessel contiguity.

4. **C.** Utilization of magnitude and phase information to produce images. SWI is more sensitive than GRE when controlling for main field strength. The time of acquisition does not change sensitivity between the two techniques.

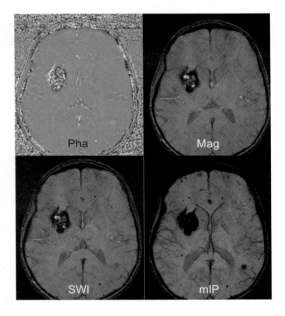

Comment

Cavernous malformations have a characteristic appearance on magnetic resonance imaging. Specifically, these lesions have central high signal intensity on unenhanced T1-weighted and T2-weighted imaging and are surrounded by a rim of hemosiderin that is hypointense on T2-weighted imaging (Figures 89-1 and 89-2) and blooms on gradient echo imaging (Figure 89-3).

In approximately 25% of cases, these lesions are multiple, and there is a familial pattern in a small percentage. Many patients with multiple cavernomas have lesions too numerous to count. As in this case, many of the lesions may be quite small and identifiable only on GRE or SWI. Although cavernomas are believed to be congenital lesions, de novo development is common in patients with a familial pattern, after radiation therapy, and in association with developmental venous anomalies.

T2*GRE

Gradient echo imaging has increased sensitivity to magnetic susceptibility because of the lack of a 180-degree rephasing pulse. Blood products (hemosiderin), calcium, iron, and other ions are more readily seen on this sequence as areas of marked hypointensity. T1 or T2 weighting of a gradient echo scan may be determined by selection of the flip angle and the time to echo. A small flip angle and a long time to echo result in more T2 weighting. Similarly, a smaller flip angle and a longer time to echo result in greater sensitivity to susceptibility effects (see Figures 89-1 through 89-3).

Susceptibility-Weighted Imaging

Although T2*GRE imaging can detect small venous structures and small areas of hemorrhage, the incorporation of phase information is what increases sensitivity (approximately four-fold) on SWI. SWI is a fully velocity-compensated high-resolution three-dimensional gradient echo sequence that uses magnitude and filtered-phase information to increase sensitivity, and in some cases specificity, in characterizing pathology. SWI of the whole brain takes approximately 4 minutes at 3T and since it is a three-dimensional acquisition, can be reformatted into virtually any plane. It is now standard on most platforms and most protocols for the evaluation of neurologic and degenerative disorders, including traumatic brain injury, hemorrhagic disorders, vascular malformations, cerebral infarct, and neoplasms (Figure 89-4).

The mIP reformations are formed by projecting the voxel with the lowest signal intensity value on every view throughout the slab of data onto a two-dimensional image. Typically, four 2-mm slices are incorporated into a slab of data measuring 8 mm.

References

Mori T, Fujimoto M, Sakae K, et al. Familial presumed cerebral cavernous angiomas diagnosed by MRI: three generations. *Neuroradiology.* 1996;38:641-645.

Rigamonti D, Hadley MN, Drayer BP, et al. Cerebral cavernous malformations: incidence and familial occurrence. *N Engl J Med.* 1988;319:343-347.

Cross-Reference

Neuroradiology: THE REQUISITES, 4th ed, pp 145-146.

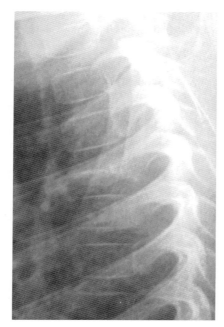

Figure 90-1

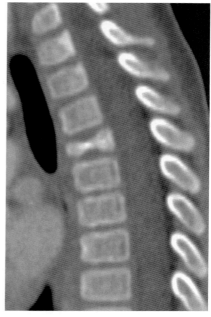

Figure 90-2

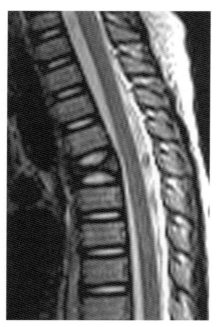

Figure 90-3

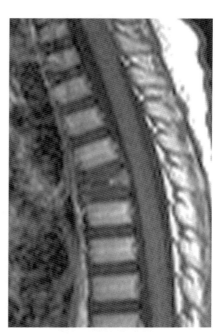

Figure 90-4

HISTORY: A 2-year-old girl presents with weakness and decreased appetite.

1. What should *not* be included in the differential diagnosis?
   A. Ewing sarcoma
   B. Langerhans cell histiocytosis
   C. Osteomyelitis
   D. Giant cell tumor

2. What is the most common skeletal site of involvement in patients with this disorder?
   A. Spine
   B. Skull
   C. Pelvis
   D. Ribs

3. What would be the most likely treatment in this case?
   A. Surgery
   B. Radiotherapy
   C. Conservative treatment
   D. Vertebroplasty

4. Which of the following is *not* a cause of vertebra plana in adults?
   A. Trauma
   B. Osteopoikilosis
   C. Metastatic disease
   D. Multiple myeloma

CASE 90

Langerhans Cell Histiocytosis with Vertebra Plana

1. **D.** Giant cell tumor. Giant cell tumor is usually seen in patients older than age 20. Ewing sarcoma, Langerhans cell histiocytosis, osteomyelitis, lymphoma, and trauma should be included in the differential diagnosis of vertebra plana in a child.

2. **B.** Skull. The skull is the most common site, although it can occur almost anywhere.

3. **C.** Conservative treatment. Most lesions spontaneously regress and are treated conservatively. Surgery is rarely indicated and is reserved for patients with spinal instability or neurologic deficit. Radiotherapy is suggested only when immobilization fails to relieve the symptoms and the lesion continues to progress. Efficacy of vertebroplasty in children is not proven.

4. **B.** Osteopoikilosis. Osteopoikilosis is a benign hereditary condition characterized by the presence of numerous bone islands in the skeleton. It is not a cause of vertebra plana. Trauma, metastatic disease, and multiple myeloma may all cause vertebra plana.

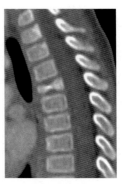

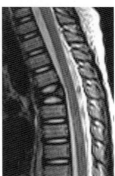

Comment

Background

Vertebra plana represents marked flattening of a vertebral body with preserved intervertebral disc space and lack of kyphosis. Langerhans cell histiocytosis is the most common cause of vertebra plana in children. Other causes of vertebra plana include multiple myeloma, metastatic disease, Ewing sarcoma, lymphoma, leukemia, Gaucher disease, aneurysmal bone cyst,

trauma, and infection. Langerhans cell histiocytosis is predominantly a disease of childhood, with more than 50% of cases diagnosed between ages 1 and 15 years. Boys are affected slightly more often than girls. The disease may be focal or systemic. The most frequent site of skeletal lesions is in the skull. Other sites include the pelvis, spine, mandible, ribs, and tubular bones. In the spine, Langerhans cell histiocytosis mainly involves the vertebral bodies, with a predilection for the thoracic spine followed by the lumbar and cervical spine. Involvement of posterior elements is less common. Involvement of the vertebral body may result in anterior wedging or, more commonly, near collapse with marked flattening of a vertebral body, a characteristic "vertebra plana" appearance.

Histopathology

Langerhans cell histiocytosis refers to a set of clinicopathologic entities (previously referred to as histiocytosis X) that result from abnormal clonal proliferation of Langerhans cells. Eosinophilic granuloma is the unifocal clinical variant.

Imaging

When a clinical diagnosis of Langerhans cell histiocytosis is suspected, further evaluation by radiographic skeletal survey or bone scintigraphy should be performed to detect other bony lesions; however, lesions may be missed on both bone scan and radiographs. Rib, spine, and pelvic lesions are more easily missed on radiographs (Figure 90-1). On computed tomography (CT) scan, Langerhans cell histiocytosis initially manifests as a lytic area with poorly defined margins. The body of the vertebra is usually involved, with bony destruction leading to a pathologic fracture with a resultant characteristic vertebra plana deformity. Involvement of the posterior elements is less common. Sagittal reformatted CT images help in identifying the vertebra plana and its surrounding anatomy. Preservation of the disc space above and below the vertebral body collapse (Figure 90-2) helps in differentiating the lesion from vertebral osteomyelitis. Magnetic resonance imaging on initial presentation usually shows a lesion that is hyperintense on T2-weighted images and hypointense on T1-weighted images and shows enhancement after contrast agent administration (relative to unaffected vertebrae). Later, the involved vertebral body becomes isointense on T1-weighted images; becomes isointense to hypointense on T2-weighted images (Figure 90-3); shows no enhancement (Figure 90-4); and appears as a thin plane of collapsed bone separating the two adjacent, intact intervertebral discs. The adjacent discs are similar in stature and intensity to normal nonadjacent discs (see Figures 90-3 and 90-4). The posterior portion of the vertebra plana may be displaced into the canal, resulting in an epidural mass. Some authors have suggested that the variations in signal intensity in the collapsed vertebral body over time are manifestations of a healing stage.

Management

Partial or almost complete height reconstitution is the usual healing pattern observed in vertebra plana lesions. Neurologic deficits usually resolve as osseous healing progresses. Because most lesions spontaneously regress, vertebra plana is often treated conservatively. Surgery is rarely indicated for spinal lesions in these patients unless there are symptoms secondary to compression of the spinal cord by the collapsed vertebra.

Reference

Azouz EM, Saigal G, Rodriguez MM, et al. Langerhans' cell histiocytosis: pathology, imaging and treatment of skeletal involvement. *Pediatr Radiol.* 2005;35(2):103-115.

Cross-Reference

Neuroradiology: THE REQUISITES, 4th ed, p 584.

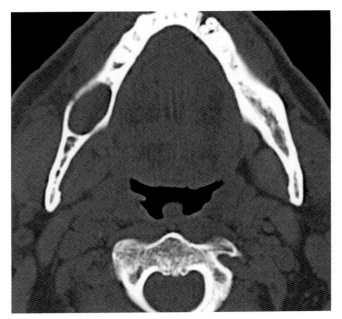

Figure 91-1

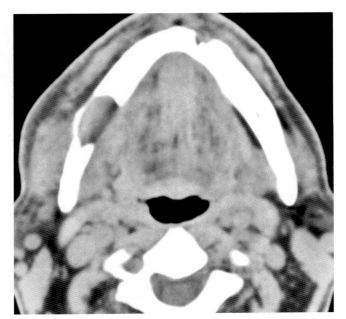

Figure 91-2

HISTORY: A 30-year-old patient is experiencing right-sided jaw pain.

1. Which of the following is the most likely cause of the bone lesion in this patient in view of the history provided?
   A. Keratocystic odontogenic tumor (KOT)
   B. Metastasis
   C. Osteonecrosis from bisphosphonate administration
   D. Radicular cyst

2. The long axis of which lesion is usually parallel to the long axis of the mandible?
   A. Nasopalatine cyst
   B. Dentigerous cyst
   C. Radicular cyst
   D. KOT

3. What syndrome is associated with KOTs?
   A. Gardner
   B. Gradenigo
   C. Gorham
   D. Gorlin

4. Which of the following cysts is more commonly multilocular than unilocular?
   A. Unicameral bone cyst
   B. Dentigerous cyst
   C. Nasopalatine cyst
   D. Aneurysmal bone cyst

CASE 91

Keratocystic Odontogenic Tumor

1. **A.** Keratocystic odontogenic tumor (KOT). Aside from KOT, a unicameral bone cyst may also be a consideration for a lesion such as the one presented.

2. **D.** KOT. The long axis of a KOT is parallel to the long axis of the mandible. The dentigerous cyst and radicular cyst are more vertically oriented to the mandible. The nasopalatine cyst occurs in the maxilla, not in the mandible.

3. **D.** Gorlin. Gorlin syndrome is associated with KOTs. Gardner syndrome is associated with osteomas; Gradenigo syndrome, with petrous apicitis; and Gorham syndrome, with vanishing bone or osteolysis.

4. **D.** Aneurysmal bone cyst. Unicameral bone, dentigerous, nasopalatine, and radicular cysts are more commonly unilocular than multilocular. Aneurysmal bone cysts are often multilocular.

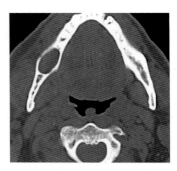

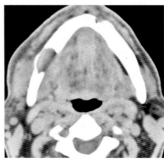

Comment

Classification of Keratocystic Odontogenic Tumors

Because of their neoplastic nature—their aggressive behavior, high mitotic activity histologically, and associated mutation of the protein patched homolog 1 *(PTCH1)* gene—the World Health Organization designated odontogenic keratocysts as KOTs (i.e., neoplasms). Thus these lesions are considered tumors rather than cysts, and KOTs now represent nearly one third of all primary odontogenic tumors, surpassing odontomas and ameloblastomas in frequency. Of all other odontogenic cysts, 50% are radicular cysts, 30% are dentigerous cysts, and 15% are residual cysts (radicular cysts after a tooth has been removed).

Orientation of Keratocystic Odontogenic Tumors

KOTs are sometimes distinguished from other odontogenic cysts because they are usually oriented in the long axis, not the short axis, of the mandible or maxilla (Figures 91-1 and 91-2). It is usually not associated with a carious tooth (radicular/periapical cyst) and may or may not be associated with an undescended unerupted tooth (dentigerous cyst). KOTs are three times more common in the mandible than in the maxilla and usually occur in the premolar-molar regions.

Imaging Findings

On imaging, KOTs have smooth, expanded, scalloped margins. Most KOTs are multilocular, but the presence of a unilocular lesion, as in this case, should not exclude the diagnosis of KOT. On unenhanced computed tomography, they often appear hyperdense because of keratin content. Their solid portions do not enhance, and the lesions can therefore be distinguished from benign ameloblastomas.

Components of Gorlin Syndrome

Patients with Gorlin syndrome (also known as *basal cell nevus syndrome* and *nevoid basal cell carcinoma syndrome*) may have (1) basal cell carcinomas of the skin (90% of cases), (2) falcine and dural calcification, (3) KOTs (75% of cases), (4) bifid or fused ribs, (5) palmar and plantar pits, and (6) first-degree relatives with the disorder. In comparison with the general population, such patients have a higher rate of medulloblastomas. The origin of the disease has been isolated to an autosomal dominant genetic defect of chromosome 9 that leads to mutations of the *PTCH1* gene.

Reference

Avelar RL, Antunes AA, Carvalho RW, Bezerra PG, Oliveira Neto PJ, Andrade ES. Odontogenic cysts: a clinicopathological study of 507 cases. *J Oral Sci.* 2009;51(4):581-586.

Cross-Reference

Neuroradiology: THE REQUISITES, 4th ed, pp 449-450.

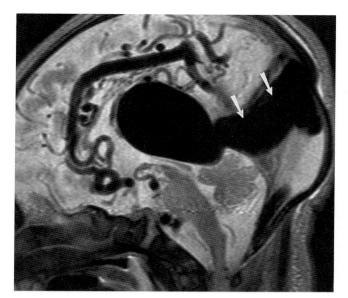

Figure 92-1

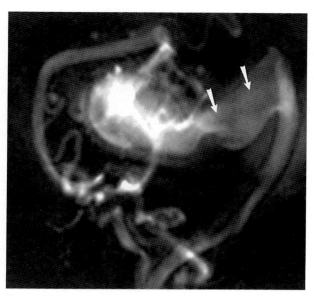

Figure 92-2

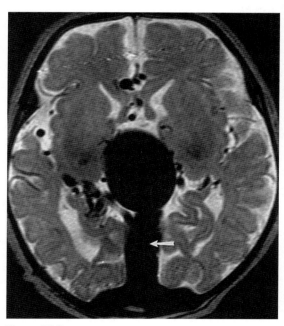

Figure 92-3

HISTORY: Child with large head.

1. What is the correct diagnosis?
   A. Vein of Galen malformation
   B. Hematoma
   C. Calcified mass
   D. Meningioma

2. Which of the following is *not* a classical clinical presentation for this entity?
   A. High-output congestive heart failure
   B. Hydrocephalus
   C. Macrocephaly
   D. Seizure

3. What are the two major types of high flow vascular malformations associated with this entity?
   A. Arteriovenous malformation (AVM) and direct arteriovenous fistula (AVF)
   B. Cavernous malformation and AVM
   C. Venolymphatic malformation and AVF
   D. Cavernous malformation and venolymphatic malformation

4. What anatomic structure or variant is denoted by the *arrows* in Figures 92-1 through 92-3?
   A. Falcine sinus
   B. Superior sagittal sinus
   C. Inferior sagittal sinus
   D. Suboccipital sinus

CASE 92

Vein of Galen Malformation

1. **A.** Vein of Galen malformation. A large flow void is consistent with a vein of Galen AVM rather than a hematoma, meningioma, or calcified mass.

2. **D.** Seizure. Classical presentation includes high-output congestive heart failure resulting from the large left-right shunt, hydrocephalus, and macrocephaly resulting from increased intracranial pressure.

3. **A.** AVM and direct AVF. The two major types of vascular malformations are true AVMs and direct AVFs (between choroidal arteries and the vein of Galen). Cavernous malformations and venolymphatic malformations are low-flow lesions not associated with vein of Galen malformations.

4. **A.** Falcine sinus. In the setting of a persistent median prosencephalic vein, the straight sinus may not develop because the median prosencephalic vein provides diencephalic venous drainage. Instead, a falcine sinus is frequently noted, as in this case *(arrows)*.

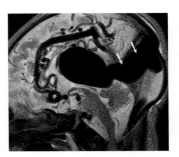

Comment

Computed Tomography

The computed tomographic appearance of a vein of Galen aneurysm in an infant is characteristic. On unenhanced images, the vein of Galen appears as a hyperdense, demarcated mass at the level of the posterior third ventricle and diencephalon. After intravenous contrast agent administration, there is marked homogeneous enhancement of the malformation.

Magnetic Resonance Imaging

Magnetic resonance imaging (MRI) not only confirms the presence of flow within this abnormality (Figures 92-1 and 92-2) but also better delineates the arterial and the venous anatomy. In combination with magnetic resonance angiography (MRA) (Figure 92-3), MRI may show large choroidal AVFs or the presence of a parenchymal AVM. In this case, a vein of Galen aneurysm is associated with a large AVM confirmed by MRA.

Fetal Ultrasound

Because many women undergo obstetric ultrasound as part of prenatal care, many of these malformations are detected in utero with color-flow Doppler sonography.

Causes

Early in embryologic development, the deep brain structures and diencephalon are drained by the median prosencephalic vein. As the internal cerebral veins begin to develop, this vein slowly regresses. A caudal remnant of the median prosencephalic vein becomes the normal vein of Galen. In patients with vein of Galen aneurysms related to either a parenchymal AVM or a direct AVF between the choroidal vessels, a persistent median prosencephalic vein may occur. Because this vein provides diencephalic venous drainage, the straight sinus may not form. Instead, a falcine sinus is frequently noted, as in this case *(arrows)*. Vein of Galen malformations resulting from direct AVFs are frequently associated with venous obstruction and venous hypertension. High-output heart failure in newborns and hydrocephalus secondary to obstruction of the aqueduct of Sylvius by the enlarged vein of Galen with macrocephaly are common clinical scenarios in infants.

Treatment

Treatment of these malformations is catheter angiography and possibly venography with embolization of the shunt, utilizing glue, coils, and potentially other occlusion devices. Several embolization procedures may be necessary to completely obliterate the vascular shunts and communications. This treatment is often performed over several months before the child is a toddler.

Reference

Hassan T, Timofeev EV, Ezura M, et al. Hemodynamic analysis of an adult vein of Galen aneurysm malformation by use of 3D image-based computational fluid dynamics. *AJNR Am J Neuroradiol.* 2003;24:1075-1082.

Cross-Reference

Neuroradiology: THE REQUISITES, 4th ed, p 147.

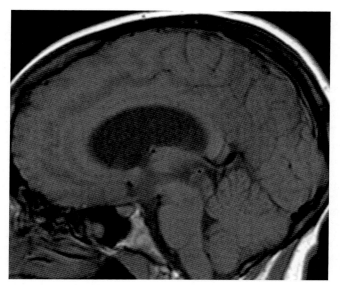

Figure 93-1

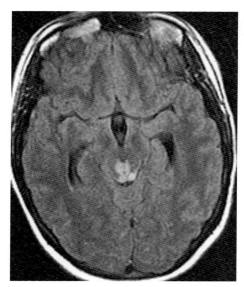

Figure 93-2

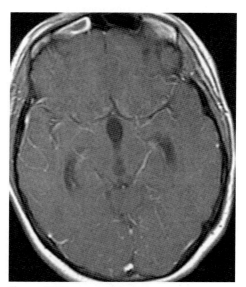

Figure 93-3

HISTORY: 17-year-old with headache and diplopia.

1. What is the single best diagnosis?
   A. Tectal glioma
   B. Glioblastoma
   C. Pineoblastoma
   D. Congenital aqueductal stenosis

2. What secondary imaging finding is associated with this lesion?
   A. Hydrocephalus
   B. Herniation
   C. Hemorrhage
   D. Infarct

3. What is the most likely additional sign or symptom that this patient may have?
   A. Auditory hallucinations
   B. Decreased light perception
   C. Upward gaze palsy
   D. Gelastic seizures

4. What congenital anomaly is usually associated with "beaking" of the tectum?
   A. Chiari I malformation
   B. Chiari II malformation
   C. Chiari III malformation
   D. Dysgenesis of the corpus callosum

CASE 93

Glioma of the Tectum (Quadrigeminal Plate)

1. **A.** Tectal glioma. There is no enhancement or edema to suggest a high-grade neoplasm. Subtle cystic appearance and no enhancement in this location suggest a low-grade glioma. Lymphoma should also be considered, although this usually enhances and may show restricted diffusion secondary to hypercellularity.

2. **A.** Hydrocephalus. There is obstructive hydrocephalus resulting from compression of the aqueduct of Sylvius. There is no evidence of parenchymal herniation, blood, or infarct. One may consider artery of Percheron infarct, but the age of the patient, symptoms, and characteristics of hydrocephalus make this less common.

3. **C.** Upward gaze palsy. This lesion affects the superior colliculus and may result in Parinaud syndrome. Auditory hallucinations are not frequently reported with these tumors. Gelastic seizures are a classic presentation of hypothalamic hamartomas or other tumors. Light perception should not be affected.

4. **B.** Chiari II malformation. This is associated with "beaking" of the tectum.

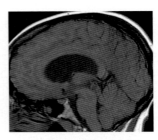

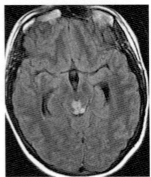

Comment

Imaging and Differential Diagnosis

These images show a mildly expansile mass lesion of the tectal plate that is predominantly cystic (Figures 93-1 and 93-2). There is no significant pathologic enhancement after contrast agent administration (Figure 93-3). There is resultant compression of the aqueduct of Sylvius, as is typically seen in patients with tectal gliomas. In many patients, the clinical presentation is that of obstructive hydrocephalus. Gliomas arising from the tectum are usually low-grade astrocytomas. They may be solid or cystic masses and have a wide spectrum of enhancement characteristics, ranging from none to prominent. Because most of these are low-grade neoplasms, the absence of enhancement is not surprising.

Anatomy Review

The midbrain is separated into the tegmentum and the tectum, which are portions of the midbrain anterior and posterior to the aqueduct of Sylvius. The tectum (roof) consists of the quadrigeminal plate, which contains the paired superior and inferior colliculi. The tectum is affected more frequently by extrinsic rather than intrinsic lesions. It is often compressed (particularly the superior colliculi), along with the aqueduct of Sylvius, by pineal region masses, such as meningiomas in adults; germ cell tumors (e.g., germinoma, embryonal carcinoma, choriocarcinoma, teratoma); tumors of pineal origin (e.g., pineoblastoma, pineocytoma); and aneurysms of the vein of Galen, which may result in Parinaud syndrome. In this case, an *asterisk* denotes the normal pineal gland (see Figure 93-1).

Occasionally, the tectum may be affected by demyelinating disease, vascular abnormalities, or trauma. In addition, the tectum may be abnormal in congenital malformations, most notably Chiari II malformation, in which there may be a spectrum of abnormalities ranging from collicular fusion to tectal "beaking."

References

Sherman JL, Citrin CM, Barkovich AJ, et al. MR imaging of the mesencephalic tectum: normal and pathologic variations. *AJNR Am J Neuroradiol.* 1987;8:59-64.
Sun B, Wang CC, Wang J. MRI characteristics of midbrain tumours. *Neuroradiology.* 1999;41:158-162.

Cross-Reference

Neuroradiology: THE REQUISITES, 4th ed, pp 3, 59-60.

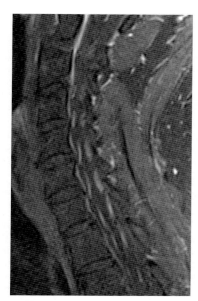

Figure 94-1

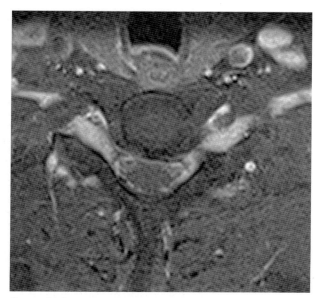

Figure 94-2

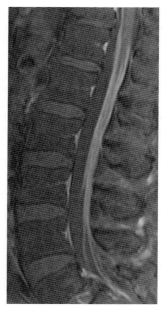

Figure 94-3

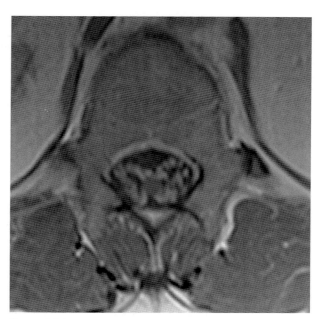

Figure 94-4

HISTORY: A 50-year-old patient presents with progressive numbness and weakness in the upper and lower extremities for the past 4 months.

1. Which of the following should be excluded from the differential diagnosis based on the imaging and clinical history?
   A. Guillain-Barré syndrome (GBS)
   B. Chronic inflammatory demyelinating polyradiculoneuropathy (CIDP)
   C. Sarcoidosis
   D. Acute disseminated encephalomyelitis (ADEM)

2. Which of the following features *correctly* differentiates CIDP from GBS?
   A. Illness usually develops and progresses over months, rather than acutely, in GBS.
   B. GBS tends to relapse more frequently than CIDP.
   C. Motor involvement is often absent in CIDP.
   D. Intrathecal nerve root enlargement and enhancement are more common in CIDP than GBS.

3. Which of the following statements regarding enhancement of the nerve roots is true?
   A. Nerve root enhancement is often seen in patients with Charcot-Marie-Tooth disease.
   B. Radiculopathy secondary to focal disc herniation may be associated with nerve root enhancement.
   C. Nerve root enhancement in the neural foramina is a concerning finding requiring further investigation.
   D. Leptomeningeal carcinomatosis may cause enhancement but *not* enlargement of the nerve roots.

4. Which of the following disease-associated radiculoneuropathies is often present without nerve root enhancement?
   A. Radiation-induced polyradiculopathy
   B. Lymphoma
   C. Cytomegalovirus (CMV) polyradiculitis
   D. Diabetic amyotrophy

CASE 94

Chronic Inflammatory Demyelinating Polyradiculoneuropathy

1. **D.** Acute disseminated encephalomyelitis. ADEM typically involves the spinal cord and does not cause thickened enhancing roots. Sarcoidosis, GBS, and CIDP all should remain in the differential diagnosis.

2. **D.** Intrathecal nerve root enlargement and enhancement are more common in CIDP than GBS. Although enhancement of nerve roots may be seen in both CIDP and GBS, enlargement of the nerve roots is not a feature of GBS, and the combination of enhancing and enlarged nerve roots should favor CIDP over GBS. Illness in GBS is usually more acute. GBS tends not to relapse after resolution. CIDP may relapse not infrequently. Motor involvement is seen in both.

3. **B.** Radiculopathy secondary to focal disc herniation may be associated with nerve root enhancement. Nerve root enhancement secondary to disc herniation may affect a single compressed root over multiple levels. Patients with Charcot-Marie-Tooth disease show little or no nerve root enhancement. Intraforaminal enhancement is a normal finding, because there is no blood-nerve barrier in the dorsal root ganglia. Leptomeningeal or pial infiltration with tumor typically manifests as a coated enhancement pattern of the nerve, cord, or conus, which appears enlarged.

4. **D.** Diabetic amyotrophy. There is no nerve root enhancement in diabetic polyradiculoneuropathy (diabetic amyotrophy). Spinal nerve root enhancement can occur in the setting of radiation-induced polyradiculopathy. Lymphoma may cause nerve root infiltration and enhancement. Spinal nerve root enhancement can occur in the setting of infectious polyradiculopathy, such as that caused by CMV.

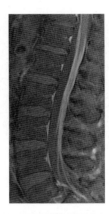

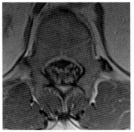

Comment

Background

CIDP is an immune-mediated, acquired demyelinating disorder of the peripheral nervous system characterized by either a relapsing and remitting course or a progressive course. It is characterized by progressive motor weakness or sensory dysfunction, or both, in more than one limb, with loss or reduction of reflexes. Diagnostic criteria have been based on clinical features, electrodiagnostic findings, cerebrospinal fluid results, and nerve biopsy findings. The criteria have been modified over the years and include imaging characteristics as supportive diagnostic criteria for CIDP.

Histopathology

The immunopathogenesis of CIDP is not fully understood. Breakdown of the blood-nerve barrier likely plays a cardinal role, allowing macrophages and T cells to enter the endoneurium and initiate an immune reaction involving antimyelin antibodies and other elements that cause demyelination and axonal loss. Biopsy of the sural nerve may demonstrate evidence of segmental demyelination and remyelination with occasional onion bulb formation, particularly in relapsing cases.

Imaging

Enlargement and enhancement of the spinal nerve roots (Figures 94-1 and 94-2), cauda equina (Figures 94-3 and 94-4), brachial and lumbosacral plexuses, cranial nerves, and sciatic nerve are well documented in CIDP. Central spinal canal stenosis, spinal cord compression, and spinal cord atrophy secondary to nerve root hypertrophy can also be seen. Nerve root enhancement, as shown in this case (see Figures 94-1 through 94-4), may be observed in GBS; sarcoidosis; postradiation injury; CMV infection; and, less commonly, hereditary motor and sensory neuropathy, infectious (pyogenic or granulomatous) disease, or neoplastic disease involving the leptomeninges (carcinomatosis, lymphoma, leukemia).

Management

Corticosteroids, intravenous immunoglobulin, and plasmapheresis provide clinical improvement in most patients with CIDP.

References

Midroni G, de Tilly LN, Gray B, et al. MRI of the cauda equina in CIDP: clinical correlations. *J Neurol Sci.* 1999;170(1):36-44.

Toyka KV, Gold R. The pathogenesis of CIDP: rationale for treatment with immunomodulatory agents. *Neurology.* 2003;60(8 suppl): S2-S7.

Cross-Reference

Neuroradiology: THE REQUISITES, 4th ed, p 578.

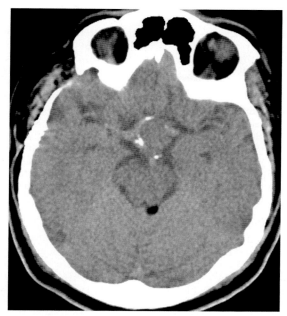

Figure 95-1

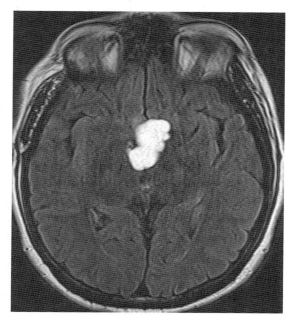

Figure 95-3

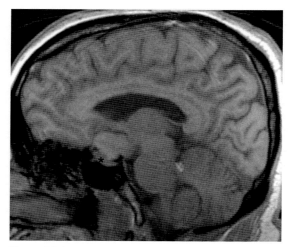

Figure 95-2

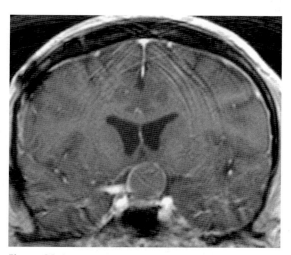

Figure 95-4

HISTORY: Child with endocrinopathy.

1. Which of the following is the single best diagnosis?
   A. Suprasellar craniopharyngioma
   B. Macroadenoma
   C. Hypothalamic astrocytoma
   D. Epidermoid

2. What is the typical age of presentation for this entity?
   A. Second and third decades of life
   B. Fourth decade of life
   C. Older than 80 years
   D. Bimodal, between 5 and 10 years and in the fifth and sixth decades

3. What other congenital midline lesion is present as shown on the axial computed tomography (CT) (Figure 95-1) and the sagittal T1-weighted image (Figure 95-2), located near the dorsal brainstem?
   A. Teratoma
   B. Lipoma
   C. Pontine cap dysplasia
   D. Pineal cyst

4. When transferring images from the scanner to the image archive, what technique can speed up transfer as well as decrease storage needs but not degrade image quality?
   A. Lossy compression
   B. Lossless compression
   C. Spectral waveform compression with redundancy
   D. Direct transfer without compression

CASE 95

Craniopharyngioma—Recurrent Adamantinomatous Type

1. **A.** Suprasellar craniopharyngioma. The cystic appearance of the lesion and peripheral calcifications are most consistent with a craniopharyngioma. A separate pituitary gland is noted, making macroadenoma unlikely. Cystic meningioma of the tuberculum sellae is cystic in appearance and can be associated with peripheral calcification and enhancement, which could have been a correct answer. Epidermoid and dermoid cysts can have peripheral calcification and enhancement, although epidermoid should be less intense on T2 and fluid-attenuated inversion recovery (FLAIR) imaging.

2. **D.** Bimodal, between 5 and 10 years and in the fifth and sixth decades. The age distribution is bimodal. Craniopharyngiomas in children 5 to 10 years old are of the adamantinomatous type. A second peak occurs in the fifth and sixth decades of life.

3. **B.** Lipoma. There is a hypodense, high T1 signal lesion adjacent to the pontine tegmentum compatible with a lipoma.

4. **B.** Lossless compression. There are two main categories of data compression. In lossless compression, there is reversible loss of image detail although the compression is not as great. In lossy compression, there is irreversible loss of image detail although the storage space necessary is far less.

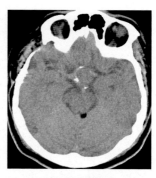

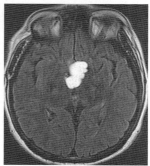

Comment

Craniopharyngiomas, seen in both children and adults, arise from metaplastic squamous epithelial rests (Rathke pouch) along the hypophysis or from ectopic embryonic cell rests. Histologically, they are characterized by palisading adamantinomatous epithelium, keratin, and calcification. They account for 1% to 3% of all intracranial neoplasms and 10% to 15% of all supratentorial tumors. They are more common in boys and men. Most craniopharyngiomas arise within the suprasellar cistern (80% to 90%), as in this case; however, they also may arise within the sella turcica and, occasionally, the third ventricle. Clinical presentation includes visual disturbances related to compression of the optic chiasm, pituitary hypofunction related to compression of the gland or hypothalamus, and symptoms of increased intracranial pressure.

Imaging

Imaging findings typically include a cystic or a solid and cystic mass lesion (Figures 95-1 through 95-4). Approximately 80% to 90% of all craniopharyngiomas have a cystic component. Smaller lesions may be purely solid. Most (90%) craniopharyngiomas have calcification (see Figure 95-1) or regions of avid homogeneous enhancement (in solid portions of tumor) or peripheral enhancement (around cystic portions). Because magnetic resonance imaging (MRI) may not be sensitive in detecting the presence of calcification, CT may be quite useful in establishing the diagnosis of craniopharyngioma (see Figure 95-1). On MRI, the signal characteristics can be variable, depending on the contents and viscosity within the cysts. The cystic portion is frequently hyperintense on T2-weighted and FLAIR imaging, whereas it may be hypointense, isointense, or hyperintense on T1-weighted imaging (see Figures 95-2 through 95-4). High signal intensity on T1-weighted images may reflect high concentrations of protein or methemoglobin (rather than cholesterol or lipid products).

Incidentally noted, there is a small lipoma in the perimesencephalic cistern on the left, adjacent to the tectum. It is hypodense on CT and hyperintense on the unenhanced sagittal T1-weighted images, typical of lipomas (see Figure 95-1).

References

Nagahata M, Hosoya T, Kayama T, et al. Edema along the optic tract: a useful MR finding for the diagnosis of craniopharyngiomas. *AJNR Am J Neuroradiol.* 1998;19:1753-1757.

Sartoretti-Schefer S, Wichmann W, Aguzzi A, et al. MR differentiation of adamantinous and squamous-papillary craniopharyngiomas. *AJNR Am J Neuroradiol.* 1997;18:77-87.

Cross-Reference

Neuroradiology: THE REQUISITES, 4th ed, pp 361-364.

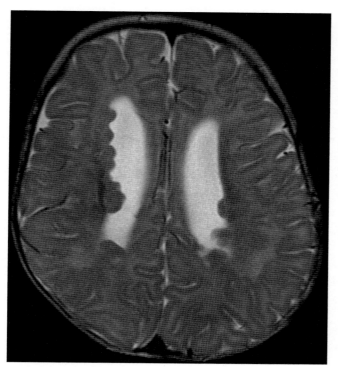

Figure 96-1

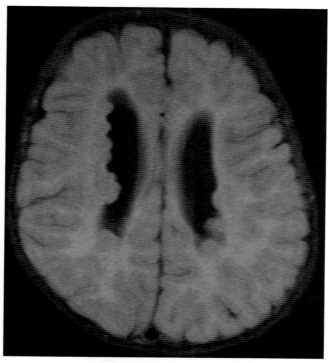

Figure 96-2

HISTORY: 5-month-old "doesn't seem right."

1. Which of the following is the single best diagnosis in this case?
   A. Subependymal heterotopia
   B. Subependymal giant cell tumor
   C. Neurocysticercosis
   D. Chronic cytomegalovirus infection

2. How did this 5-month-old infant present clinically?
   A. Seizure and developmental delay
   B. Developmental regression
   C. Obtundation
   D. Rash

3. What percentage of subependymal tubers in tuberous sclerosis is calcified?
   A. Greater than 90%
   B. 70% to 80%
   C. 50%
   D. 30%

4. What heritable pattern has been described in some cases of this entity?
   A. X-linked
   B. Y-linked
   C. Autosomal recessive
   D. Autosomal dominant

Subependymal Heterotopia

1. **A.** Subependymal heterotopia. There are multiple nodules protruding from the ventricular walls with imaging characteristics similar to cortical gray matter consistent with nodular heterotopias. Although they often calcify, the subependymal nodules of tuberous sclerosis may not calcify and can resemble heterotopias. There is no definite dominant lesion to suggest subependymal giant cell tumor. There is no evidence of cystic lesions to suggest neurocysticercosis. There is no evidence of periventricular calcifications to suggest prior cytomegalovirus exposure.

2. **A.** Seizure and developmental delay. Seizure and developmental delay are common presentations. Obtundation is not a clinical feature associated with nodular heterotopias. Although present in tuberous sclerosis (ash leaf spots), rash is not associated with nodular heterotopias.

3. **A.** Greater than 90%. Approximately 98% are calcified.

4. **A.** X-linked. Some cases have X-linked inheritance.

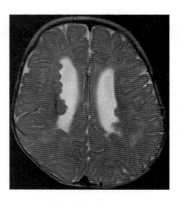

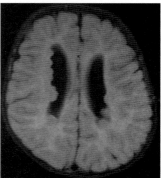

Comment

This case illustrates multiple subependymal heterotopias that consist of clusters of disorganized neurons and glial cells that are located in close proximity to the ventricular walls. In subependymal heterotopia, nodules are often bilaterally symmetric along the length of the lateral ventricles (Figures 96-1 and 96-2), or there may be just a few lesions. Heterotopias appear as masses that are isointense to gray matter on all pulse sequences and do not enhance. High signal intensity in the parenchyma surrounding the heterotopia should not occur.

Differential Diagnosis

The differential diagnosis for subependymal heterotopia is limited, and the diagnosis is usually easily established by the stereotypic imaging appearance. Subependymal nodules in tuberous sclerosis are readily differentiated because they do not follow the signal characteristics of gray matter and most are calcified (hypointense on T2-weighted and gradient echo susceptibility images and mildly hyperintense on unenhanced T1-weighted images). In addition, other sequelae of tuberous sclerosis are commonly present. Metastatic masses are uncommon and typically enhance after contrast agent administration. Other signs of metastatic disease are frequently present in the intracranial compartment.

Etiology

Periventricular heterotopia represents failed migration from the germinal region; however, some cases may result from abnormal proliferation of neuroblasts in the periventricular region, failure of regression, or apoptosis of neuroblasts within the germinal matrix.

Associations

Heterotopia may be associated with a spectrum of other congenital anomalies, including Chiari malformations, ventral induction defects (e.g., holoprosencephaly, dysgenesis of the corpus callosum), other migrational abnormalities, and encephaloceles. Some cases have X-linked inheritance, and early antenatal diagnosis is important for appropriate management. In this patient, there is ex vacuo enlargement of the occipital horns of the lateral ventricles (colpocephaly) as a result of underdevelopment of the surrounding deep white matter and dysgenesis of the splenium of the corpus callosum.

References

Barkovich AJ. Morphologic characteristics of subcortical heterotopia: MR imaging study. *AJNR Am J Neuroradiol.* 2000;21:290-295.

Mitchell LA, Simon EM, Filly RA, et al. Antenatal diagnosis of subependymal heterotopia. *AJNR Am J Neuroradiol.* 2000;21:296-300.

Cross-Reference

Neuroradiology: THE REQUISITES, 4th ed, p 275.

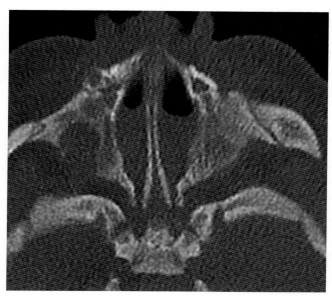

Figure 97-1

HISTORY: The patient is a 4-year-old child with nasal obstruction.

1. On the basis of the images, what should be included in the causes of this child's nasal obstruction?
   A. Membranous choanal atresia
   B. Fracture
   C. Nasal aperture stenosis
   D. Polyps

2. What percentage of choanal atresia is mixed bony-membranous?
   A. Less than 25%
   B. 26% to 50%
   C. 51% to 75%
   D. More than 75%

3. Which syndrome is associated with choanal atresia?
   A. CHARGE
   B. Gorlin syndrome
   C. Tuberous sclerosis
   D. VACTERL syndrome

4. What width of the vomer in a child suggests choanal stenosis or atresia?
   A. Greater than 3 mm
   B. 4 mm
   C. 5 mm
   D. 6 mm

CASE 97

Choanal Atresia

1. **A.** Membranous choanal atresia. Membranous choanal atresia and bony choanal atresia are the probable causes of the nasal obstruction. Soft tissue is obstructing the nasal cavity; this may represent secretions or membranous choanal atresia. Also, there is bony narrowing posteriorly. Probable causes do not include nasal aperture stenosis, inasmuch as the nasal aperture is normal in width, or polyps, inasmuch as there is nothing polypoid in the nose. There is no fracture.

2. **C.** 51% to 75%. Of all cases of choanal atresia, 70% are mixed bony-membranous.

3. **A.** CHARGE. CHARGE is associated with choanal atresia: *c*oloboma, *h*eart disease, choanal *a*tresia, *r*etardation, *g*enital abnormalities, and *e*ar anomalies. There are no associations between choanal atresia and Gorlin syndrome (nevoid basal cell carcinoma syndrome), tuberous sclerosis, or VACTERL syndrome (*v*ertebral anomalies, *a*nal atresia, *c*ardiac defects, *t*racheoesophageal fistula and/or *e*sophageal atresia, *r*enal anomalies, and *l*imb defects).

4. **D.** 6 mm. Vomer width of 6 mm in a child suggests choanal stenosis or atresia. The posteroinferior vomer normally measures less than 2.3 mm in width and should not exceed 5.5 mm in children younger than 8 years.

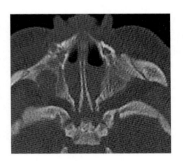

Comment

Incidence of Bilateral Choanal Atresia

Bilateral choanal atresia can lead to infantile respiratory distress because neonates are obligate nose breathers. The diagnosis is usually made clinically by the inability to pass a nasogastric tube in a newborn with a breathing disorder. Unilateral choanal atresia is twice as common as bilateral choanal atresia, but the diagnosis may, as a result, be delayed. Choanal atresia is twice as common in girls as in boys, but the overall incidence is 0.82 per 10,000 live births. The cause is failure of perforation of the buccopharyngeal membrane. Low levels of fetal thyroid hormones may be a factor in the development of this disorder.

Imaging Findings

In the past, 90% of cases of choanal atresias were said to be bony. Currently, most cases are thought to be combined membranous and bony (Figure 97-1). It is difficult to determine radiologically whether the soft tissue anterior to the bony narrowing is secondary to retained secretions in the nose or to membranous atresia. Suctioning should be performed immediately before scanning to reduce the likelihood that the soft tissue represents mucus as opposed to membranous choanal atresia. The posterior edge of the vomer is flared and widened in choanal atresia. It should not measure greater than 5.5 mm, but this depends in part on the overall stature of the child.

Reference

Cedin AC, Atallah AN, Andriolo RB, Cruz OL, Pignatari SN. Surgery for congenital choanal atresia. *Cochrane Database Syst Rev.* 2012;(2):CD008993.

Cross-Reference

Neuroradiology: THE REQUISITES, 4th ed, pp 415-416.

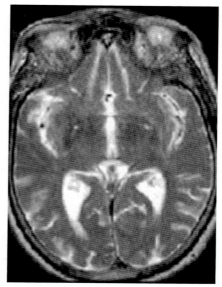

Figure 98-1

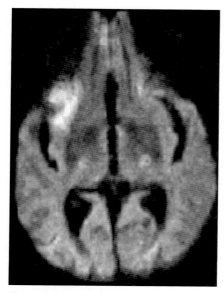

Figure 98-2

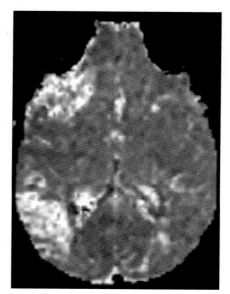

Figure 98-3

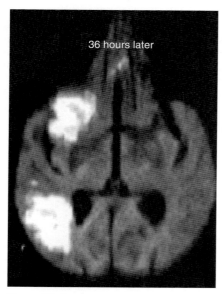

36 hours later

Figure 98-4

HISTORY: Altered mental status.

1. What specific symptom did this patient likely present with?
   A. Right-side neglect
   B. Right lower extremity paresis
   C. Expressive aphasia
   D. Receptive aphasia

2. Regarding the terms *infarct core, penumbra,* and *benign oligemia,* which of the following is the correct statement?
   A. Benign oligemia is brain tissue that will likely recover regardless of treatment.
   B. Penumbra is the region of brain tissue that shows cytotoxic edema without perfusion abnormality.
   C. The infarct core has decreased cerebral blood flow (CBF) but increased cerebral blood volume (CBV).
   D. Decreased mean transit time (MTT) is associated with the penumbra.

3. What technique in stroke imaging allows for the identification of increased deoxyhemoglobin in the vessel lumen?
   A. Arterial spin labeling
   B. Susceptibility-weighted imaging
   C. Dynamic susceptibility contrast perfusion
   D. Diffusion-weighted imaging

4. The concept of arterial spin labeling imaging is best reflected in which of the following statements?
   A. Contrast enhancement allows identification of poor perfusion.
   B. Changes in the volume of blood within a given volume of brain allow for identification of brain tissue at risk for injury.
   C. No contrast is administered, and the blood outside of a volume is labeled so that as it flows into the volume, changes in signal can be measured.
   D. No contrast is administered, and changes in free water motion are identified.

CASE 98

Acute Middle Cerebral Artery Stroke

1. **C.** Expressive aphasia. The infarct in the right middle cerebral artery territory involves the frontal operculum, which is where the Broca may be. Receptive aphasia would occur when the Wernicke area is affected, which is not clearly demonstrated here in the initial images. This right-side infarct would potentially result in left-side, not right-side, sensory or motor deficits.

2. **A.** Benign oligemia is brain tissue that will likely recover regardless of treatment. The infarct core is the dead brain tissue that will not recover. The penumbra is the area with abnormal perfusion characteristics but no restricted diffusion, at risk for infarct but not infarcted at the time of imaging. In the periphery of the perfusion abnormality is an area of oligemic tissue that will likely recover regardless of treatment. Core has decreased CBV and CBF. Increased MTT is seen in core and penumbra.

3. **B.** Susceptibility-weighted imaging. Changes in susceptibility as a result of changes in the concentrations of oxygenated and deoxygenated blood are detected with susceptibility-weighted imaging.

4. **C.** No contrast is administered, and the blood outside of a volume is labeled so that as it flows into the volume, changes in signal can be measured. The tissue to be evaluated is first imaged, then blood is labeled outside of the volume and it is imaged again; changes of signal are identified and the differences are detected, reflecting changes in CBF.

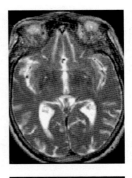

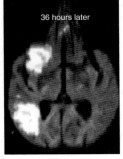

36 hours later

Comment

An unenhanced computed tomography (CT) scan of the head often remains the first imaging study for emergent evaluation of acute stroke because it is readily available, rapidly performed, and sensitive in identifying acute intracranial hemorrhage and mass effect that may require immediate and urgent surgical intervention. Magnetic resonance imaging (MRI) is more sensitive than CT in detecting acute infarcts and showing extension of infarctions on follow-up examinations, as in this case (Figures 98-1 and 98-4).

Perfusion Imaging

Tissue perfusion may be assessed with perfusion imaging. In one specific technique called dynamic susceptibility contrast (DSC) perfusion, rapid imaging is performed before and during the bolus intravenous injection of gadolinium. On first pass through the cerebral vasculature, there is a decrease in measured signal intensity because of the T2* effects of this agent. Mathematic models can be used to convert this decrease in signal intensity to concentration of contrast over time.

Diffusion Imaging

Diffusion-weighted imaging measures random Brownian movement of water molecules. Generally, densely cellular tissue or tissue with cellular edema results in lower diffusion coefficients. On the diffusion images, this correlates with high signal on the B1000 (diffusion-weighted imaging or diffusion trace) and lower signal on the apparent diffusion coefficient (ADC) map. Diffusion-weighted imaging is the most sensitive indicator of ischemia—the image becomes abnormal within minutes of onset.

Diffusion/Perfusion Mismatch

Mismatches between abnormal diffusion-weighted and perfusion imaging may indicate brain tissue at risk, as in this case (see Figures 98-1 through 98-4). Identification of this "penumbra" (brain tissue at risk for irreversible ischemia) is an area of further development of MRI techniques. It is important to protect this at-risk tissue from ischemia (see Figure 98-3) by applying appropriate interventions. To deliver protective agents, perfusion to this tissue is necessary.

References

Liu YJ, Chen CY, Chung HW, et al. Neuronal damage after ischemic injury in the middle cerebral arterial territory: deep watershed versus territorial infarction at MR perfusion and spectroscopic imaging. *Radiology*. 2003;229:366-374.

Neumann-Haefelin T, du Mesnil de Rochemont R, Fiebach JB, et al. Effect of incomplete (spontaneous and post-thrombolytic) recanalization after middle cerebral artery occlusion: a magnetic resonance imaging study. *Stroke*. 2004;35:109-114.

Cross-Reference

Neuroradiology: THE REQUISITES, 4th ed, pp 108-109.

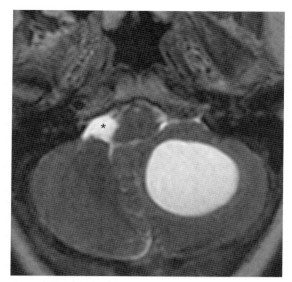

Figure 99-1 Patient A.

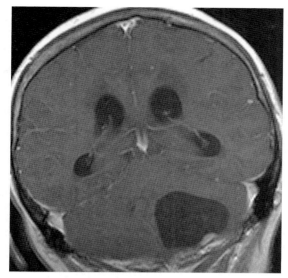

Figure 99-2 Patient A.

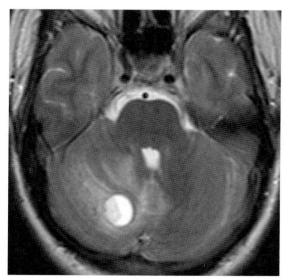

Figure 99-3 Patient B.

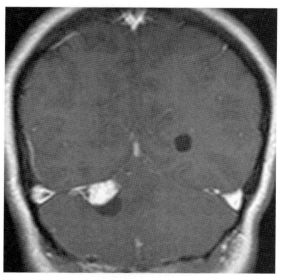

Figure 99-4 Patient B.

HISTORY: Patient A is a 45-year-old male and Patient B is a 59-year-old male. Both have the same diagnosis. They have no comorbid conditions.

1. Considering the history and imaging, what is the single best diagnosis for both of these patients?
   A. Hemangioblastoma
   B. Metastasis
   C. Astrocytoma
   D. Medulloblastoma

2. What neurocutaneous syndrome is associated with multiple hemangioblastomas?
   A. Tuberous sclerosis
   B. Neurofibromatosis type 1 (NF1)
   C. Neurofibromatosis type 2 (NF2)
   D. Von Hippel–Lindau disease

3. Which of the following clinical factors best helps to distinguish a hemangioblastoma from a pilocytic astrocytoma?
   A. Age
   B. Family history
   C. Headaches
   D. Symptoms of posterior fossa compression

4. Which of the following statements regarding gadolinium-based contrast in routine use is correct?
   A. Gadolinium can be used in chelated and nonchelated forms for imaging.
   B. Gadolinium is paramagnetic at body temperature.
   C. Gadolinium remains within the blood pool for 25 to 30 minutes, allowing for long acquisition time sequences.
   D. Gadolinium causes T1 prolongation.

CASE 99

Hemangioblastoma

1. **A.** Hemangioblastoma. In the adult population, metastatic disease is the most common cause of a posterior fossa mass. In patients with no comorbidities, hemangioblastoma is the most common primary cerebellar lesion in adults and often appears, as in these cases, as a small enhancing nodular mass with surrounding cystic component. Astrocytoma and medulloblastoma are more common in children than in adults.

2. **D.** Von Hippel–Lindau disease. Von Hippel–Lindau disease is associated with posterior fossa and spinal cord hemangioblastomas. Tuberous sclerosis is associated with subcortical tubers and subependymal nodules. NF1 is associated with neurofibromas and optic pathway gliomas. NF2 is associated with schwannomas, meningiomas, and ependymomas.

3. **A.** Age. Pilocytic astrocytomas tend to occur in children rather than adults. Family history is not associated with sporadic hemangioblastomas or astrocytoma. Symptoms cannot be used to discriminate between the two tumors.

4. **B.** Gadolinium is paramagnetic at body temperature. Free gadolinium is highly toxic and must be chelated. Most gadolinium for routine use is rapidly cleared from the intravascular space into the interstitial space, and most types are eliminated by renal excretion and some by both renal and hepatic pathways.

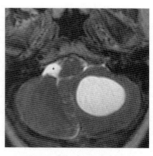

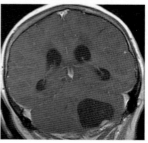

Comment

Cerebellar hemangioblastomas are benign neoplasms that represent the most common primary infratentorial neoplasm in adults. They are more common in men, and presentation is typically during adulthood (except when associated with von Hippel–Lindau disease, where symptoms can appear in late adolescence). Patients can present with headache, nausea, vomiting, ataxia, and vertigo. Although these neoplasms typically have a vascular nidus, subarachnoid hemorrhage is an uncommon presentation. More than 80% of posterior fossa hemangioblastomas occur in the cerebellum. They can also occur in the spinal cord or medulla (in the region of the area postrema). Cerebral hemangioblastomas are unusual, representing less than 2% of all hemangioblastomas, and they usually indicate von Hippel–Lindau disease (posterior fossa tumors are also usually present in this neurocutaneous syndrome).

Imaging

There are two characteristic imaging appearances of cerebellar hemangioblastomas. The first is that of a solid and cystic mass (more than 50% of cases). In most cases, there is no enhancement around the cyst wall. The solid vascular mural nodule associated with the cyst avidly enhances, and the nodule usually abuts the pial surface, as in these cases (Figures 99-1 through 99-4). Alternatively, hemangioblastomas appear as poorly demarcated, avidly enhancing masses typically associated with numerous vascular flow voids (up to 40% of cases). In Patient A, the *asterisk* marks an incidental arachnoid cyst in the right cerebellomedullary angle (see Figure 99-1).

Management

Management is typically surgical resection, which is considered curative. Recurrence can occur if the solid vascular nidus has been incompletely resected.

References

Quadery FA, Okamoto K. Diffusion-weighted MRI of hemangioblastomas and other cerebellar tumours. *Neuroradiology.* 2003;45: 212-219.

Slater A, Moore NR, Huson SM. The natural history of cerebellar hemangioblastomas in von Hippel–Lindau disease. *AJNR Am J Neuroradiol.* 2003;24:1570-1574.

Cross-Reference

Neuroradiology: THE REQUISITES, 4th ed, pp 70-72.

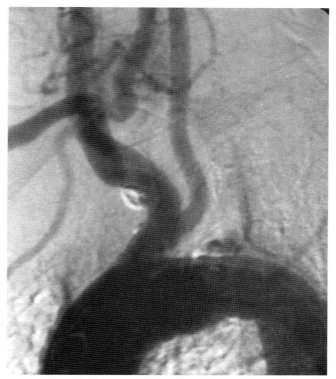

Figure 100-1

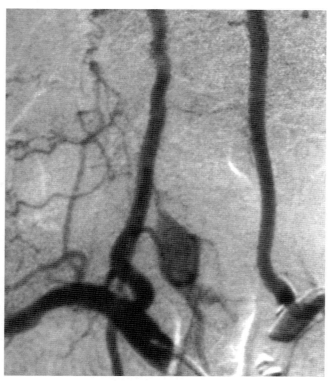

Figure 100-2

HISTORY: Dizziness and visual disturbances.

1. What is the single best diagnosis?
   A. Traumatic carotid dissection
   B. Subclavian steal
   C. Absence of the left subclavian artery
   D. Aberrant left subclavian artery

2. What vessel is selected by the angiographer on Figure 100-2?
   A. Brachiocephalic artery
   B. Subclavian artery
   C. Vertebral artery
   D. Right common carotid artery

3. To confirm the diagnosis of "subclavian steal" on two-dimensional time-of-flight magnetic resonance angiography (MRA), what is the best place to position the stationary saturation pulse?
   A. Superior to the sampling volume
   B. Inferior to the sampling volume
   C. At the level of the sampling volume
   D. "Subclavian steal" cannot be demonstrated on 2D time-of-flight.

4. What is an acceptable treatment for this patient?
   A. Ligation of the proximal left vertebral artery
   B. Subclavian endarterectomy
   C. Angioplasty and stenting of the left subclavian artery
   D. Blalock-Taussig shunt placement

CASE 100

Subclavian Steal

1. **B.** Subclavian steal. There is proximal occlusion of the left subclavian artery with retrograde filling just distal to the occluded segment via the left vertebral artery, consistent with subclavian steal.

2. **A.** Brachiocephalic artery. There is opacification of the right common carotid, subclavian, and vertebral arteries, consistent with injection of the right brachiocephalic artery.

3. **B.** Inferior to the sampling volume. This is opposite to the technique during the routine time-of-flight MRA of the neck, where a superior saturation band is used to suppress signal from the neck veins. The saturation pulse may be completely removed in these cases.

4. **C.** Angioplasty and stenting of the left subclavian artery. Ligation of the left vertebral artery would result in left upper extremity ischemia. Subclavian endarterectomy is not advocated, although there are multiple surgical options. Blalock-Taussig shunt placement is a systemic-to-pulmonary shunt procedure used to treat cyanotic congenital heart disease.

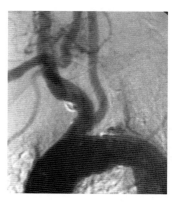

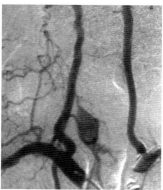

Comment

Subclavian steal results from occlusion or a hemodynamically significant stenosis of the subclavian artery proximal to the origin of the vertebral artery, or stenosis of the brachiocephalic artery. Subclavian steal occurs much more commonly on the left than on the right. There is retrograde flow of blood down the ipsilateral vertebral artery (stealing blood from the circle of Willis) to provide collateral blood supply to the arm, bypassing the occlusion or stenosis of the proximal subclavian artery (Figures 100-1 and 100-2).

Presentation

In patients with subclavian steal, symptoms and signs may be related to decreased blood flow to the arm (decreased pulse, reduced blood pressure, decreased temperature, or claudication) or to neurologic symptoms owing to periodic ischemia in the posterior circulation (as was the case in this patient) from decreased antegrade flow (not "stealing" of blood from the circle of Willis). Neurologic symptoms include transient attacks, dizziness, and visual symptoms. Similar neurologic symptoms can occur with high-grade stenoses or occlusions of the proximal vertebral artery; however, the arm is not symptomatic.

Diagnosis and Treatment

Subclavian stenosis can often be diagnosed on physical examination. Imaging studies that can help to confirm the diagnosis include Doppler ultrasound and MRA studies, which can correctly demonstrate retrograde flow down the involved vertebral artery. On arch aortography, early arterial films show occlusion or stenosis of the proximal left subclavian artery, whereas delayed films demonstrate retrograde flow. Neurointerventional techniques may be used to treat symptomatic patients and include percutaneous transluminal angioplasty with or without positioning of stents.

References

Al-Mubarak N, Liu MW, Dean LS, et al. Immediate and late outcomes of subclavian artery stenting. *Catheter Cardiovasc Interv.* 1999;46:169-172.

Malek AM, Higashida RT, Phatouros CC, et al. Treatment of posterior circulation ischemia with extracranial percutaneous balloon angioplasty and stent placement. *Stroke.* 1999;30:2073-2085.

Cross-Reference

Neuroradiology: THE REQUISITES, 4th ed, p 95.

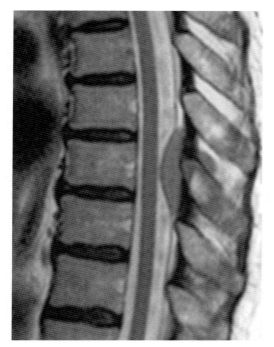

Figure 101-1

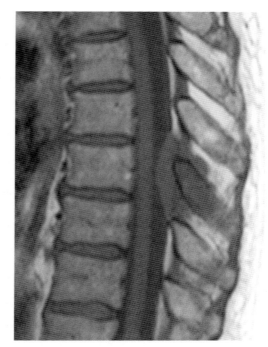

Figure 101-2

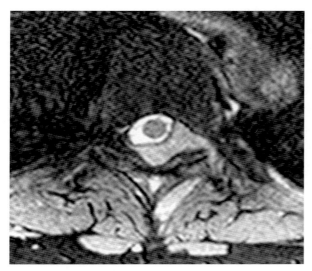

Figure 101-3

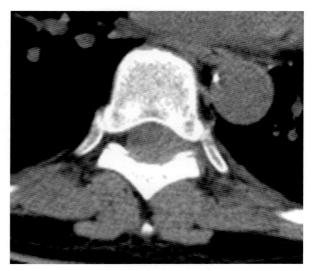

Figure 101-4

HISTORY: A 65-year-old woman presents with midback pain.

1. Aside from metastatic disease, what should be included in the differential diagnosis?
   A. Epidural hematoma
   B. Primary lymphoma
   C. Meningioma
   D. Astrocytoma

2. What is the predominate location of this lesion?
   A. Intramedullary
   B. Intradural extramedullary
   C. Epidural
   D. Paraspinal

3. What is the most common region of spinal involvement?
   A. Cervical spine
   B. Thoracic spine
   C. Lumbar spine
   D. Sacrum

4. Which of the following imaging features would correctly differentiate lymphoma from metastatic disease?
   A. Metastases are usually isointense relative to the spinal cord on T2-weighted images.
   B. Involvement of the posterior elements suggests metastatic disease rather than lymphoma.
   C. Lymphoma is usually more attenuating than metastasis on noncontrast computed tomography (CT).
   D. Lymphoma more commonly involves the thoracic spine, and metastasis more commonly involves the cervical spine.

CASE 101

Primary Epidural Lymphoma

1. **B.** Primary lymphoma. These findings are characteristic of primary epidural lymphoma. Identifying the soft tissue along the spinous process and decreased signal in the bone marrow on T1-weighted imaging makes hematoma less likely. Meningiomas are intradural, and astrocytomas are intramedullary.

2. **C.** Epidural. It replaces the epidural fat and, to a lesser extent, extends outside the spinal canal.

3. **B.** Thoracic spine. Order of frequency is thoracic, lumbar, cervical, sacrum.

4. **C.** Lymphoma is usually more attenuating than metastasis on noncontrast CT. Lymphoma is usually hyperdense on non–contrast-enhanced CT scan because of the hypercellularity and high nuclear-to-cytoplasmic ratio. Isointense T2-weighted signal would favor lymphoma. Metastases are typically hyperintense on T2-weighted images. Involvement of the posterior elements favors hematopoietic malignancy. Metastasis would typically involve the pedicles and vertebral body. Both primary epidural lymphoma and metastatic disease more frequently involve the thoracic spine.

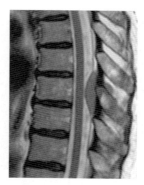

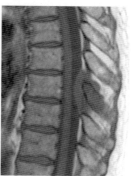

Comment

Background

Primary epidural lymphoma is a subset of lymphoma in which there are no other recognizable sites of lymphomas at the time of diagnosis. It occurs in 1% to 6% of patients with non-Hodgkin lymphoma. The most common region of involvement is the thoracic spine, followed by the lumbar and cervical spine. Patients usually present with backache followed by symptoms and signs of spinal cord and radicular compression.

Histopathology

Primary epidural lymphoma is often classified as a low-grade or intermediate-grade lesion histologically. In most cases of primary epidural lymphoma, the tumor is located posterior to the spinal cord and has a tendency to spread longitudinally, involving three to four vertebral levels.

Imaging

On magnetic resonance imaging, the lesion has homogeneous signal intensity on all pulse sequences (Figures 101-1 through 101-3) and homogeneous enhancement. Relative to cord signal intensity, the tumor is usually isointense on T1-weighted images (see Figure 101-2) and isointense to hyperintense on T2-weighted images (see Figure 101-1). Infiltrative growth through the foramen into the paravertebral space is frequent (Figure 101-4). Adjacent vertebral infiltration occurs in 50% of clinically diagnosed cases, appearing hypointense on T1-weighted images (see Figure 101-2).

Management

Patients have a potentially favorable outcome if diagnosed and treated early, because the lesions are very sensitive to radiation and chemotherapy.

References

Alameda F, Pedro C, Besses C, et al. Primary epidural lymphoma. Case report. *J Neurosurg*. 2003;98(2 suppl):215-217.

Boukobza M, Mazel C, Touboul E. Primary vertebral and spinal epidural non-Hodgkin's lymphoma with spinal cord compression. *Neuroradiology*. 1996;38(4):333-337.

Cross-Reference

Neuroradiology: THE REQUISITES, 4th ed, pp 74-76.

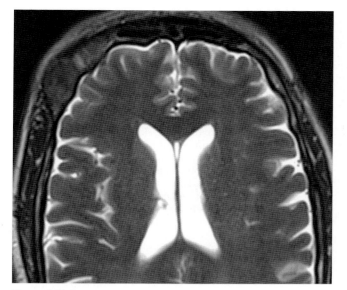

Figure 102-1

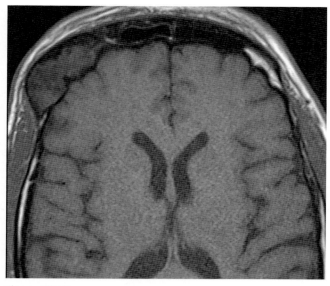

Figure 102-2

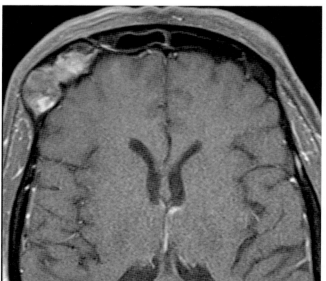

Figure 102-3

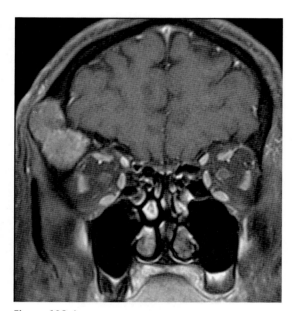

Figure 102-4

HISTORY: Painless swelling and deformity.

1. On computed tomography (CT), how would a lesion with hypointense T1 and T2 signal in the calvarium such as this one appear?
   A. Lytic
   B. Sclerotic
   C. Hemorrhagic
   D. Normal

2. What syndrome is associated with soft tissue myxoma and multiple bone lesions as seen here?
   A. McCune-Albright
   B. Mazabraud
   C. Carney complex
   D. Ollier

3. In what percentage of cases is this disease polyostotic?
   A. 0% to 10%
   B. 11% to 20%
   C. 21% to 30%
   D. 31% to 40%

4. Which bones are most commonly affected in polyostotic fibrous dysplasia?
   A. Femora and humeri
   B. Spine
   C. Calvarium and facial bones
   D. Scapulae, clavicles, and ribs

CASE 102

Fibrous Dysplasia of the Calvarium

1. **B.** Sclerotic. Generally, when bone appears hypointense on both T1 and T2, this correlates with a sclerotic or fibrous lesion. Lytic lesions tend to be hyperintense on T2. Hemorrhage may have variable signal intensity depending on the age of the blood product. Hemorrhagic lesions may also have fluid-fluid levels.

2. **B.** Mazabraud. Mazabraud syndrome is rare. It is an association of polyostotic fibrous dysplasia and intramuscular myxomas. McCune-Albright is a syndrome of polyostotic fibrous dysplasia, precocious puberty, and café-au-lait spots. Carney complex is a rare multiple endocrine neoplasia syndrome characterized by cardiac myxoma and blue nevi. Ollier disease is characterized by multiple enchondromas.

3. **C.** 21% to 30%. Fibrous dysplasia is polyostotic in approximately 25% of cases.

4. **C.** Calvarium and facial bones. The calvarium and facial bones are the most frequently involved skeletal structures in polyostotic fibrous dysplasia.

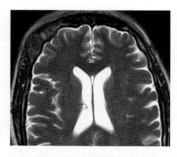

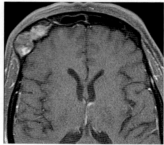

Comment

Background

Fibrous dysplasia is a developmental bone disorder in which osteoblasts do not undergo normal differentiation and maturation. The cause is unknown. Fibrous dysplasia may be monostotic (a solitary lesion) or polyostotic (multiple bones involved or multiple lesions in one bone). Approximately 75% of cases of fibrous dysplasia are monostotic (25% polyostotic). Polyostotic fibrous dysplasia involves the skull and facial bones more commonly than does monostotic disease. Common areas of calvarial involvement include the ethmoid, maxillary, frontal, and sphenoid bones. Involvement of these bones can result in orbital abnormalities such as exophthalmos, visual disturbances, and displacement of the globe. Involvement of the temporal bone can result in hearing loss or vestibular dysfunction.

Imaging

Fibrous dysplasia of the skull or facial bones on plain radiography can manifest as radiolucent or sclerotic lesions. Sclerotic lesions are more common in the calvaria, skull base, and sphenoid bones.

Differential Diagnosis

Although Paget disease can occur in these same locations of the calvaria, unlike fibrous dysplasia, concomitant involvement of the facial bones is less common. In this case, there is a mass in the right frontal bone, with associated focal expansion of the diploic space. There is preservation of the inner and outer cortical tables without destruction or significant thickening of the cortex (Figures 102-1 through 102-4). These features are typical of fibrous dysplasia. In contrast, although there may be expansion of the diploic space in patients with Paget disease, there is normally thickening of the cortex (which may be extensively involved).

Associations

Mazabraud syndrome is a rare disease presenting as fibrous dysplasia (which is usually polyostotic) and soft tissue myxomas. McCune-Albright presents as polyostotic fibrous dysplasia, café-au-lait spots, and precocious puberty.

References

Jee WH, Choi KH, Choe BY, et al. Fibrous dysplasia: MR imaging characteristics with radiopathologic correlation. *AJR Am J Roentgenol.* 1996;167:1523-1527.

Mazabraud A, Semat P, Roze R. Apropos of the association of fibromyxomas of the soft tissues with fibrous dysplasia of the bones. *Presse Med.* 1967;75:2223-2228.

Cross-Reference

Neuroradiology: THE REQUISITES, 4th ed, p 496.

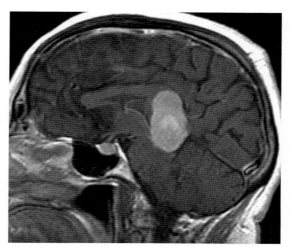

Figure 103-1

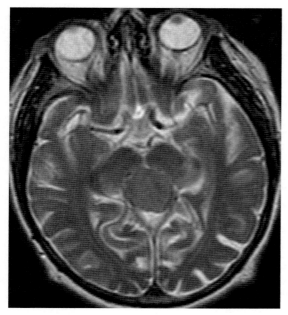

Figure 103-2

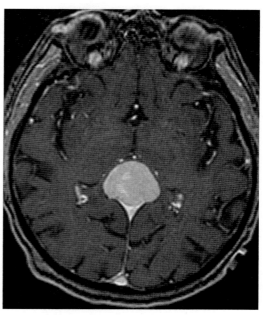

Figure 103-3

HISTORY: A 40-year-old woman presents with headache.

1. What is the single best diagnosis in this case?
   A. Intracranial lipoma
   B. Colloid cyst
   C. Meningioma
   D. Tectal astrocytoma

2. What vascular structure(s) course(s) above the pineal gland?
   A. Torcular Herophili
   B. Internal cerebral veins
   C. Straight sinus
   D. Basal vein of Rosenthal

3. What magnetic property does calcium have?
   A. Paramagnetic
   B. Diamagnetic
   C. Ferromagnetic
   D. Super paramagnetic

4. Which pineal neoplasm is *most frequently* associated with tumor seeding of the subarachnoid spaces?
   A. Pineocytoma
   B. Pineoblastoma
   C. Astrocytoma
   D. Germinoma

CASE 103

Peripineal Meningioma

1. **C.** Meningioma. This lesion is a well-defined dural-based mass isointense to cortex with homogeneous enhancement.

2. **B.** Internal cerebral veins. The internal cerebral veins and vein of Galen course above the pineal gland.

3. **B.** Diamagnetic. Calcium and water are diamagnetic. Gadolinium is paramagnetic. Iron is ferromagnetic. Super paramagnetic substances augment external fields but are not magnetic outside of a field.

4. **B.** Pineoblastoma. Pineoblastoma is the pineal neoplasm most frequently associated with subarachnoid seeding. When large enough, these neoplasms may directly invade the brain parenchyma.

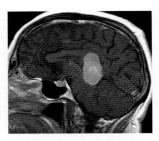

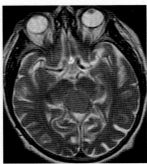

Comment

Case in Point

This case shows a well-demarcated, avidly enhancing cellular mass in the peripineal region (Figures 103-1 through 103-3). There is elevation of the internal cerebral veins and splenium of the corpus callosum (see Figure 103-1) and compression of the tectal plate. There is no acute hydrocephalus. On T2-weighted imaging, the mass is isointense to gray matter (see Figure 103-2) because of its dense cellularity.

Primary Pineal Tumors

Tumors of pineal cell origin (pineoblastoma and pineocytoma) account for only 15% of pineal region masses. In contrast to germ cell tumors, which show a marked predilection for boys and men, tumors of pineal cell origin occur equally among men and women. Tumors of pineal origin frequently calcify. Calcification of the pineal gland in a child younger than 7 years should raise suspicion of tumor until proven otherwise. After 7 years of age, the pineal gland begins to show calcification, which increases with age. By adolescence, 10% of people have calcification in the pineal gland, and 50% have pineal gland calcification by age 30. In cases in which the calcification is small and more central, it may be difficult to determine whether it is the natural calcification of the pineal gland or calcification within the tumor matrix. Pineal tumors of germ cell origin and pineoblastomas occur in children, whereas pineocytomas generally are seen in adults.

Imaging

Magnetic resonance imagining is most useful in characterizing masses in the pineal region. Tumors arising in the peripineal region in a child are usually gliomas arising from the tectal plate, whereas tumors arising in the peripineal region in adults may represent gliomas or meningiomas arising from the tentorium, as in this case. Imaging findings in the context of the age and sex of the patient may be useful in suggesting the correct histologic features of the tumor.

References

Nakamura M, Saeki N, Iwadate Y, et al. Neuroradiological characteristics of pineocytoma and pineoblastoma. *Neuroradiology*. 2000;42:509-514.

Smirniotopoulos JG, Rushing EJ, Mena H. Pineal region masses: differential diagnosis. *Radiographics*. 1992;12:577-596.

Cross-Reference

Neuroradiology: THE REQUISITES, 4th ed, pp 41-43.

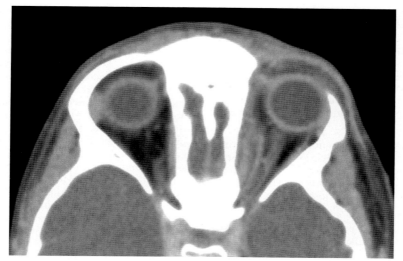

Figure 104-1

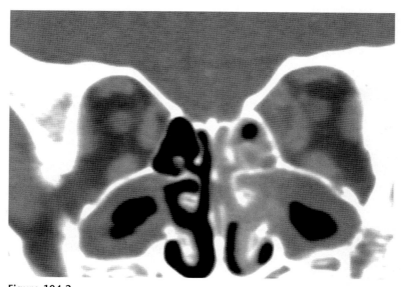

Figure 104-2

HISTORY: A teenager has had fever and left eye pain for 4 days.

1. What is *least* likely in the differential diagnosis in this case?
   A. Subperiosteal abscess
   B. Sinusitis
   C. Periorbital cellulitis
   D. Orbital trauma

2. What is *not* a risk factor for the development of subperiosteal abscesses?
   A. Sinusitis
   B. Pediatric age group
   C. Immunodeficiency
   D. Hypercalcemia

3. What percentage of patients with sinusitis has orbital manifestations?
   A. Less than 5%
   B. 6% to 10%
   C. 11% to 15%
   D. Greater than 15%

4. Why is ethmoid sinusitis most commonly associated with orbital complications?
   A. Thinness of the lamina papyracea and poor drainage
   B. Valveless veins and frequent obstruction of the posterior ethmoids
   C. Anterior and posterior ethmoid artery openings to the orbit and thinness of the lamina papyracea
   D. Proximity and poor drainage pathways

CASE 104

Orbital Subperiosteal Abscess

1. **D.** Orbital trauma. Sinusitis, visible on the images, may lead to a subperiosteal abscess and orbital cellulitis. Because of the edema in the retrobulbar fat and the swelling of the superficial soft tissues, periorbital and orbital cellulitis may be present.

2. **D.** Hypercalcemia. Sinusitis and immunodeficiency are risk factors for the development of subperiosteal abscesses. These abscesses are much more common in children than in adults because of the more dehiscent bone. There are no known associations between subperiosteal abscesses and hypercalcemia.

3. **A.** Less than 5%. Less than 5% of patients with sinusitis have orbital manifestations. The actual percentage is approximately 1% to 3%.

4. **C.** Anterior and posterior ethmoid artery openings to the orbit and thinness of the lamina papyracea. Ethmoid sinusitis is most commonly associated with orbital complications because of proximity, valveless veins, openings of the anterior and posterior ethmoid arteries to the orbit, thinness of the lamina papyracea, and propensity for dermal sinus tracts.

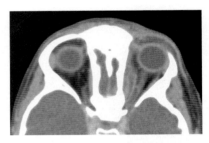

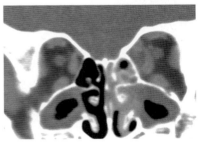

Comment

Imaging Findings

On imaging, the subperiosteal abscess of the orbit usually appears as a low-density, well-defined collection along the medial orbit adjacent to ethmoid sinusitis, which is the usual source of the infection (Figures 104-1 and 104-2). The walls of these collections often do *not* enhance and yet are mature abscess collections. Despite the excellent barrier function of the periorbita (i.e., the periosteum of the orbital walls), this disease may spread into the retroconal orbit. In about 20% of cases, sinusitis progresses to retrobulbar inflammatory optic neuritis, and its first indication may be stranding of the orbital fat or enlargement and low density of the extraocular muscles. Septic thromboses of veins or small arteries from the progressive infection have a well-known potential to cause necrosis of the nerve. Visual disturbance, culminating in diplopia, may be secondary to the effects on the medial rectus muscle. Visual blurring may also result from optic nerve injury by direct compression by the collection or by an ischemic vasculitic mechanism.

Treatment of Periorbital Subperiosteal Abscess

Loss of visual acuity, nonmedial abscess, intracranial spread, severe mass effect or pain, clinical deterioration, and failure to improve within 48 hours of antibiotic treatment are criteria for surgical treatment. Surgery may be performed via an endoscopic approach. The pathogens may be aerobic (more often streptococcal than staphylococcal) or anaerobic (*Bacteroides* organisms). After drainage, broad-spectrum antibiotic therapy is indicated. In decreasing order of frequency, the orbital complications of sinusitis include preseptal cellulitis, orbital cellulitis, subperiosteal abscess, and orbital abscess.

Reference

Liao JC, Harris GJ. Subperiosteal abscess of the orbit: evolving pathogens and the therapeutic protocol. *Ophthalmology*. 2015;122(3): 639-647.
Soon VT. Pediatric subperiosteal orbital abscess secondary to acute sinusitis: a 5-year review. *Am J Otolaryngol*. 2011;32(1):62-68.

Cross-Reference

Neuroradiology: THE REQUISITES, 4th ed, pp 338-339.

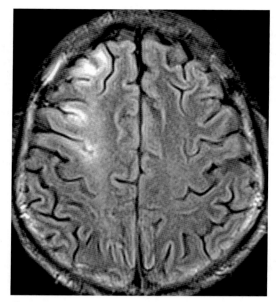

Figure 105-1

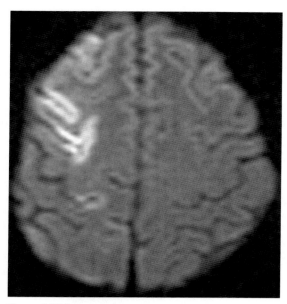

Figure 105-2

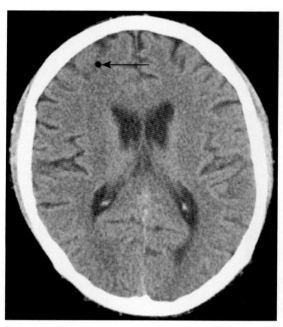

Figure 105-3

HISTORY: A 30-year-old man presents with a patent foramen ovale and confusion after central venous line manipulation.

1. What is the single best diagnosis?
   A. Lipoma
   B. Herpes encephalitis
   C. Acute right frontal infarct
   D. Cerebral contusion

2. What does the arrow point to on the computed tomography (CT) image?
   A. Blood
   B. Intracranial air
   C. Fat
   D. Cerebrospinal fluid

3. What does the term *pitch* in CT refer to?
   A. The rate of changes in dose in auto mA mode
   B. The angle of the gantry relative to the patient
   C. The speed at which the table moves through the bore
   D. Table feed per revolution divided by the collimated x-ray beam width

4. What type of technique is used in Figure 105-2?
   A. Fast or turbo spin echo
   B. Echo planar
   C. Gradient echo
   D. Magnetization transfer

CASE 105

Air Embolism with Acute Right Cerebral Infarct

1. **C.** Acute right frontal infarct. The correct diagnosis is acute right frontal infarction secondary to air embolism.

2. **B.** Intracranial air. This focus is extremely low attenuation, less than fat, compatible with air.

3. **D.** Table feed per revolution divided by the collimated x-ray beam width. Pitch is only a property of helical CT scanners.

4. **B.** Echo planar. Diffusion-weighted imaging (DWI) is performed utilizing echo planar technique, which is fairly resistant to motion artifacts but highly affected by magnetic field perturbations.

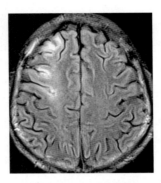

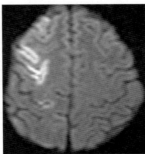

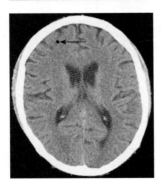

Comment

Causes

Cerebral air embolism is a known complication of trauma, surgical procedures, and central line catheterization. Cerebral and cardiac air emboli are also known complications of thoracic instrumentation, initially reported many years ago during pneumothorax therapy and pleurodesis for the treatment of tuberculosis. More recently, emboli have been associated with CT-guided percutaneous needle biopsy for pulmonary tumors. The mechanism by which air emboli occur in this scenario includes the presence of a fistula between a bronchus and a pulmonary vein and a transthoracic pressure gradient in which intrathoracic pressure is lower than atmospheric pressure, as when coughing or taking a deep breath, which allows air to flow into a pulmonary vein from the bronchus. From there, air may enter the systemic circulation.

Effects

Venous air embolism is an underrecognized, potentially fatal, but preventable complication of central lines. It can result in cardiovascular, pulmonary, and central nervous system infarcts (Figures 105-1 and 105-2) and dysfunction. Cerebral air embolism may result from a paradoxical intracardiac shunt (patent foramen ovale) or intrapulmonary right-to-left shunt. Insertion, accidental disconnection, or removal of a central venous catheter may result in cerebral air embolism, as it did in this patient.

Treatment

Cerebral air emboli (Figure 105-3) usually occur on the right side because air preferentially flows into the first branch of the aortic arch, the brachiocephalic artery. When a cerebral air embolism is suspected, the patient's head should be quickly lowered (to the Trendelenburg position), and the patient should be turned to the left lateral decubitus position. This keeps air within the left ventricle from being ejected into the coronary or systemic circulation and air within the right ventricle from entering the pulmonary artery or traversing through a potentially patent foramen ovale into the left ventricle. Oxygen should be administered. The best treatment is prevention. Central lines should be removed with the patient in the Trendelenburg position. An occlusive dressing should be applied.

References

Hiraki T, Fujiwara H, Sakurai J, et al. Nonfatal systemic air embolism complicating percutaneous CT-guided transthoracic needle biopsy. *Chest*. 2007;132:684-690.

Peter DA, Saxman C. Preventing air embolism when removing CVCs: an evidence-based approach to changing practice. *Medsurg Nurs*. 2003;12:223-228.

Cross-Reference

Neuroradiology: THE REQUISITES, 4th ed, p 190.

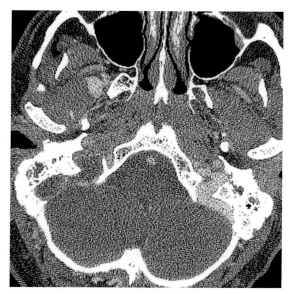

Figure 106-1 Patient A.

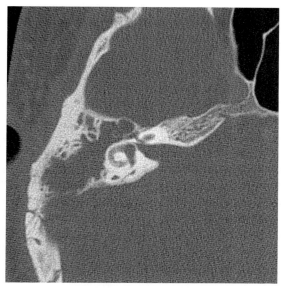

Figure 106-2 Patient A.

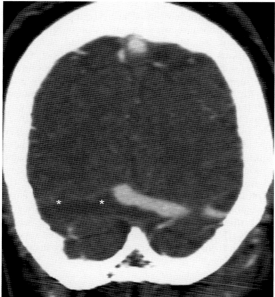

Figure 106-3 Patient B.

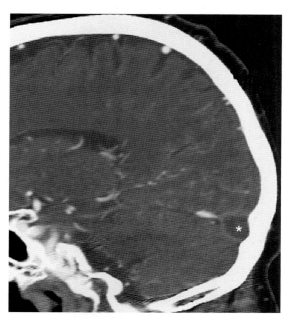

Figure 106-4 Patient B.

HISTORY:

Patient A: A 40-year-old man presents with ear infection and headache.

Patient B: A 45-year-old woman presents with seizures.

1. What is the single common diagnosis of these patients?
   A. Sinus thrombosis
   B. Congenital hypoplasia of the right transverse sinus
   C. Mastoiditis
   D. Intracranial hemorrhage

2. What is the cause of this condition in Patient A?
   A. Langerhans cell histiocytosis
   B. Otomastoiditis
   C. Metastasis
   D. Glomus jugulare

3. What is the most serious complication associated with venous thrombosis?
   A. Focal edema
   B. Hemorrhagic venous infarction
   C. Cerebritis
   D. Seizures

4. What structure transmits through the pars nervosa of the jugular foramen?
   A. Jugular bulb
   B. Cranial nerve (CN) X
   C. CN XI
   D. Inferior petrosal sinus

CASE 106

Venous Sinus Thrombosis Complicating Otomastoiditis

1. **A.** Sinus thrombosis. Sinus thrombosis of the right sigmoid and distal transverse sinuses is seen in Patient A. Thrombosis of the right transverse sinus is seen in Patient B. In Patient B, the filling defect in the sinus is shown *(asterisk)*. Otomastoiditis is the cause for thrombosis in Patient A but is not present in Patient B.

2. **B.** Otomastoiditis. The right mastoid air cells are opacified, and there is osseous destruction.

3. **B.** Hemorrhagic venous infarction. Hemorrhagic venous infarction is the most serious complication associated with venous thrombosis.

4. **D.** Inferior petrosal sinus. The pars nervosa of the jugular foramen transmits the inferior petrosal sinus and CN IX. The pars vascularis of the jugular foramen transmits the jugular bulb, CN X, and CN XI.

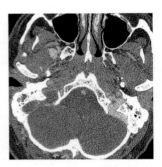

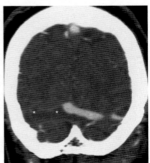

Comment

Dural sinus thrombosis and venous infarction are commonly underdiagnosed because physicians do not consider these entities.

Presentation

Sinus thrombosis has a spectrum of clinical presentations, including headache and papilledema related to increased intracranial pressure and focal neurologic deficits and seizures in cases complicated by intraparenchymal hemorrhage or venous infarction.

Associations

Venous thrombosis is associated with various underlying systemic disorders. There are many causes of hypercoagulable states. In the differential diagnosis of intracerebral hemorrhage in the absence of known risk factors (e.g., trauma, hypertension), the presence of bilateral or subcortical hemorrhages that are not in arterial vascular distributions should raise suspicion for sinus thrombosis complicated by venous infarction.

Diagnosis

Diagnosing venous thrombosis has become easier with noninvasive techniques (Figures 106-1 and 106-2, Patient A), especially with advanced magnetic resonance imaging (MRI) sequences and computed tomography venography (CTV) performed using multidetector computed tomography. On CTV, thromboses are readily identified as filling defects in the affected venous sinuses (Figures 106-3 and 106-4, Patient B). CTV is preferable to MRI, which is an excellent technique but requires more experience and an understanding of some physics. In the setting of acute thrombosis, deoxyhemoglobin is hypointense on T2-weighted imaging and may be mistaken for normal blood flow. In the acute setting, flow-sensitive gradient echo imaging may distinguish normal blood flow, which is of high signal intensity, from acute thrombosis, which is hypointense because of lack of flow. In subacute thrombosis, methemoglobin within the clot appears hyperintense on T1-weighted and T2-weighted images. Flow-sensitive time-of-flight gradient echo images often are not helpful because the methemoglobin in the thrombus and blood flow are hyperintense. In this situation, phase-contrast magnetic resonance angiography (MRA) is helpful because it provides suppression of high signal from the hemorrhage so that only flow is shown on these images.

References

Rodallec MH, Krainik A, Feydy A, et al. Cerebral venous thrombosis and multidetector CT angiography: tips and tricks. *Radiographics.* 2006;26(suppl 1):S5-S18.

Stolz E, Trittmacher S, Rahimi A, et al. Influence of recanalization on outcome in dural sinus thrombosis: a prospective study. *Stroke.* 2004;35:544-547.

Cross-Reference

Neuroradiology: THE REQUISITES, 4th ed, pp 134-137, 386.

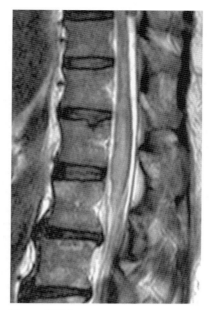

Figure 107-1

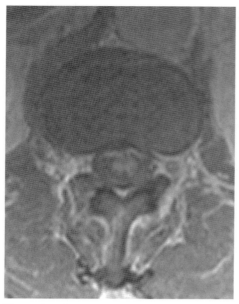

Figure 107-2

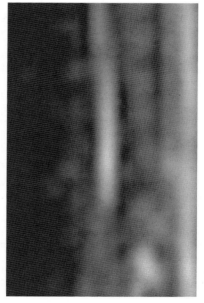

Figure 107-3

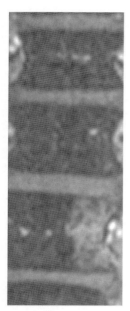

Figure 107-4

HISTORY: A 67-year-old man with vascular risk factors develops sudden onset of low back pain followed by immediate weakness and sensory disturbance in the bilateral lower extremities.

1. What is the single best diagnosis?
   A. Multiple sclerosis
   B. Guillain-Barré syndrome
   C. Conus infarction
   D. Meningitis

2. The findings are most likely due to involvement of which of the following arteries?
   A. Artery of Adamkiewicz
   B. Posterior spinal artery
   C. Radicular artery
   D. Posterior medullary artery

3. Which of the following imaging findings is the most reliable indicator of ischemia of the spinal cord in the acute phase?
   A. Spinal cord enlargement on T1-weighted images
   B. "Pencil-like" sign on sagittal T2-weighted images
   C. Hyperintense signal on diffusion-weighted imaging with corresponding low apparent diffusion coefficient
   D. "Snake eyes" configuration on axial T2-weighted images

4. Infarction of which of the following structures is most closely associated with cord infarction?
   A. Brain
   B. Vertebral body
   C. Bowel
   D. Lower extremity

CASE 107

Conus Infarction

1. **C.** Conus infarction. The involvement of the central gray matter and location in the conus are characteristic of conus medullaris spinal cord infarction. The abnormality involves the gray matter, whereas multiple sclerosis involves predominately the white matter. Guillain-Barré syndrome may manifest with enhancement of the ventral roots of the cauda equina, and meningitis may manifest with leptomeningeal enhancement; however, involvement of the spinal cord is unusual.

2. **A.** Artery of Adamkiewicz. The anterior spinal artery is the most common artery involved in cord infarctions. The findings in this case are most consistent with ischemia in the distribution of the artery of Adamkiewicz. Two posterior spinal arteries supply the posterior one third of the cord and are less commonly involved in cord infarction. The radicular artery supplies the nerve root at each spinal segment and does not supply the cord. The posterior medullary artery may communicate directly with the posterior spinal artery and is less commonly involved in cord infarction.

3. **C.** Hyperintense signal on diffusion-weighted imaging with corresponding low apparent diffusion coefficient. Restricted diffusion is the most reliable indicator of ischemia of the spinal cord. Spinal cord enlargement is frequently observed; however, it is nonspecific and may be observed in other conditions. Linear increased signal intensity on T2-weighted images is characteristic of cord infarction; however, it may be present in other conditions, such as transverse myelitis, demyelinating disease, and venous infarction. "Snake eyes" configuration corresponding to ischemic change in the region of the anterior horns is characteristic of cord ischemia; however, viral infections or neurodegenerative diseases affecting the central gray matter can mimic this pattern of signal abnormality.

4. **B.** Vertebral body. Vertebral body infarction is most associated with cord infarction and is seen at a level supplied by the same segmental artery as the affected region of the cord. The direct blood supply to the brain, bowel, and lower extremities is different from that to the spinal cord.

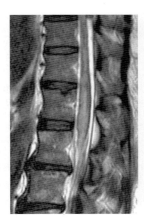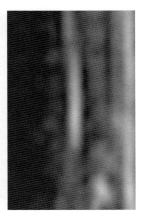

Comment

Background

Spinal cord infarction is uncommon and accounts for approximately 1% of all strokes.

Histopathology

Blood is supplied to the cord by the sulcal branches of the anterior spinal artery, which is primarily supplied by the artery of Adamkiewicz in the conus region and by radial perforating branches of the pial arterial plexus on the cord surface. The anterior spinal artery supplies approximately the anterior two thirds of the cord and most of the central gray matter. Hypoperfusion in this vascular distribution, as may occur from pathologic changes in the descending aorta (aneurysm, thrombosis, dissection) or from various causes (small vessel vasculitides, hypotension, pregnancy, sickle cell disease, caisson disease, diabetes, degenerative disease of the spine), can result in conus infarction.

Imaging

Spin echo magnetic resonance imaging findings include cord enlargement and hyperintense signal on T2-weighted images (Figure 107-1) in the first few days, with or without gadolinium enhancement (Figure 107-2). Diffusion-weighted imaging is particularly sensitive to the ischemic change (Figure 107-3). Abnormal signal and enhancement may demonstrate a double-dot ("owl's eyes" or "snake eyes") pattern in the region of the anterior horns, an H-shaped pattern involving the central gray matter, or a more diffuse pattern involving both gray matter and white matter. Amano and colleagues (1998) reported enhancement of the ventral part of the cauda equina, which is composed of motor fiber bundles, in association with conus enhancement (see Figure 107-2). When infarction results from compromise of a segmental artery, branches supplying the ipsilateral half of the vertebral body may also be affected (Figure 107-4). Cord atrophy and lack of contrast enhancement are found later (months) in the course of cord infarction.

Management

Treatment includes aspirin and management of the complications of acute paraplegia.

References

Amano Y, Machida T, Kumazaki T. Spinal cord infarcts with contrast enhancement of the cauda equina: two cases. *Neuroradiology*. 1998;40(10):669-672.

Masson C, Pruvo JP, Meder JF, et al.; Study Group on Spinal Cord Infarction of the French Neurovascular Society. Spinal cord infarction: clinical and magnetic resonance imaging findings and short term outcome. *J Neurol Neurosurg Psychiatry*. 2004;75(10): 1431-1435.

Shinoyama M, Takahashi T, Shimizu H, et al. Spinal cord infarction demonstrated by diffusion-weighted magnetic resonance imaging. *J Clin Neurosci*. 2005;12(4):466-468.

Cross-Reference

Neuroradiology: THE REQUISITES, 4th ed, p 588.

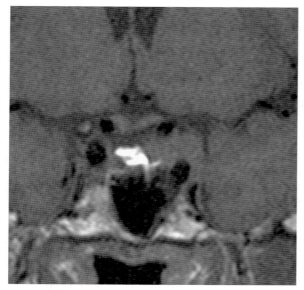

Figure 108-1

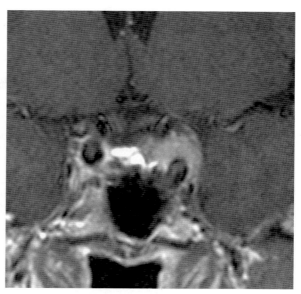

Figure 108-2

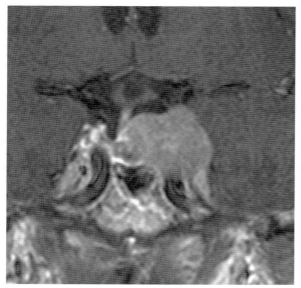

Figure 108-3

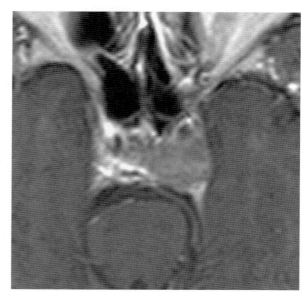

Figure 108-4

HISTORY: Withheld.

1. This mass primarily involves what anatomic area?
   A. Sphenoid sinus
   B. Cavernous sinus
   C. Planum sphenoidale
   D. Orbital apex

2. What was the clinical presentation of this patient? (Choose the single *best* answer.)
   A. Transient ischemic attack
   B. Third and sixth nerve palsy
   C. Fourth nerve palsy
   D. Right temporal visual field defect

3. What is the preferred first-line management for nonfunctional tumors with invasion of the cavernous sinus?
   A. Anticoagulation
   B. Bromocriptine
   C. Resection
   D. Radiation therapy

4. Which of the following is the most specific sign on magnetic resonance imaging (MRI) to identify cavernous sinus invasion by an adenoma?
   A. The mass encases the internal carotid artery
   B. The mass crosses the lateral intercarotid line
   C. Bulging of the lateral dural wall of the cavernous sinus
   D. Displacement of the internal carotid artery

CASE 108

Pituitary Macroadenoma Invading the Left Cavernous Sinus

1. **B.** Cavernous sinus. The mass primarily involves the left cavernous sinus arising from the pituitary gland in the sella turcica.

2. **B.** Third and sixth nerve palsy. This patient presented with third and sixth cranial neuropathies caused by invasion of the left cavernous sinus. The sixth nerve is usually the first affected as it traverses the venous compartment proper.

3. **C.** Resection. Although the approach may vary depending on patient and tumor characteristics, the mainstay of treatment and first line most often is surgical resection.

4. **A.** The mass encases the internal carotid artery. This MRI finding is 100% specific.

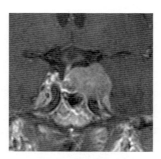

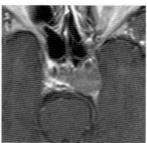

Comment

Pituitary adenomas arise from epithelial pituitary cells and account for 10% to 15% of all intracranial tumors. Tumors 10 mm and larger are defined as macroadenomas, and tumors smaller than 10 mm are microadenomas. Most pituitary adenomas are microadenomas. The exact pathophysiology leading to the development of pituitary adenomas is unknown.

Presentation

Approximately 75% of pituitary adenomas manifest because of endocrine dysfunction. Macroadenomas often manifest with compressive signs and symptoms related to mass effect, including headache, visual symptoms (characteristically bitemporal hemianopsia), increased intracranial pressure, and cranial nerve palsies, as in this case.

Case in Point

The challenging part of this case is determining where the mass arises, because this case illustrates predominantly lateral growth into the cavernous sinus of a macroadenoma (Figures 108-1 through 108-4), with a small portion in the left lateral sella (see Figures 108-1 and 108-2) and mild deviation of the pituitary stalk from left to right (see Figure 108-3).

Cavernous Sinus Invasion

Pituitary macroadenomas may encase the cavernous internal carotid artery, but in contrast to meningiomas, they usually do not result in significant narrowing. In a study examining cavernous sinus involvement by pituitary adenomas, Scotti and colleagues (1988) found that invasion was unilateral in all cases and most commonly occurred with prolactin-secreting or adrenocorticotropic hormone–secreting adenomas located laterally in the gland. The most specific sign of cavernous sinus invasion is encasement of the internal carotid artery.

Syndrome Associations

Some pituitary tumors may occur as part of a clinical syndrome. In multiple endocrine neoplasia type I, an autosomal dominant genetic disorder, pituitary adenomas (most often prolactinomas) occur in association with tumors of the parathyroid and pancreatic islet cells. In McCune-Albright syndrome, skin lesions and polyostotic fibrous dysplasia occur with hyperfunctioning endocrinopathies (most commonly somatotropinomas resulting in acromegaly).

Treatment

The goal of treatment is cure. When this is not attainable, reducing tumor size, restoring hormone function, and restoring normal vision are attempted using drug therapy, surgery, and radiation therapy. Macroadenomas often require surgical intervention; however, macroprolactinomas frequently have an excellent response to medical therapy.

References

Cottier JP, Destrieux C, Brunereau L, et al. Cavernous sinus invasion by pituitary adenoma: MR imaging. *Radiology*. 2000;215(2): 463-469.

Riedl M, Clodi M, Kotzmann H, et al. Apoplexy of a pituitary macroadenoma with reversible third, fourth, and sixth cranial nerve palsies following administration of hypothalamic releasing hormones: MR features. *Eur J Radiol*. 2000;36:1-4.

Scotti G, Yu CY, Dillon WP, et al. MR imaging of cavernous sinus involvement by pituitary adenomas. *AJR Am J Roentgenol*. 1988;151:799-806.

Cross-Reference

Neuroradiology: THE REQUISITES, 4th ed, p 353.

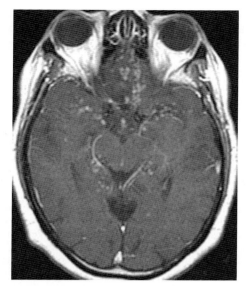

Figure 109-1 Patient A.

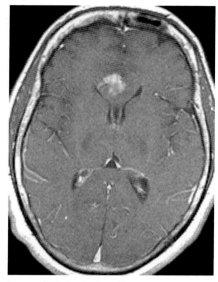

Figure 109-2 Patient B.

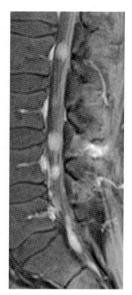

Figure 109-3 Patient C.

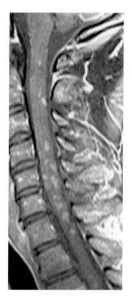

Figure 109-4 Patient D.

HISTORY:

Patient A (Figure 109-1): Left facial nerve palsy.

Patient B (Figure 109-2): Headache.

Patient C (Figure 109-3): Bilateral lower extremity pain, weakness, and sensory loss.

Patient D (Figure 109-4): Recurrent optic neuritis and mild spastic upper extremity paresis.

1. What is the most likely unifying diagnosis for these four patients?
   A. Meningiomatosis
   B. Melanoma
   C. Sarcoidosis
   D. Ruptured dermoid

2. Which of following cerebrospinal fluid (CSF) findings is likely to be common among the four patients?
   A. Low total protein
   B. Normal white blood cell count
   C. Presence of oligoclonal bands
   D. Elevated red blood cell count

3. What spinal region is most commonly involved in this disease?
   A. Cervical
   B. Thoracic
   C. Lumbar
   D. Sacral

4. Which of the following is the correct statement regarding this disease?
   A. Spinal cord involvement is usually the initial imaging manifestation of this disease.
   B. Dural-based granulomatous involvement is seen more than 50% of the time.
   C. Diagnosis and early treatment with steroids can minimize neurologic complications.
   D. Full response and cure are often achieved with steroids and immunotherapy.

CASE 109

Central Nervous System Sarcoidosis

1. **C.** Sarcoidosis. These are cases of sarcoidosis. The images provided are contrast-enhanced T1-weighted images with nodular enhancement in predominately leptomeningeal distributions with some parenchymal lesions, such as in Patient B and Patient D. Lymphoma may present in a magnitude of ways as well, but this is more fitting of sarcoidosis, especially considering the patients' histories.

2. **C.** Presence of oligoclonal bands. Oligoclonal bands are often identified in the CSF of patients with sarcoidosis. Protein and white blood cell counts are often elevated. Red blood cell elevation is not associated with sarcoidosis.

3. **A.** Cervical. The cervical spine is the most commonly affected spinal region.

4. **C.** Diagnosis and early treatment with steroids can minimize neurologic complications. Spinal cord involvement is usually late or absent in neurosarcoidosis. Dural-based involvement is rare. Full response and cure are not often achieved.

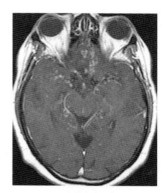

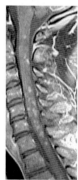

Comment

These cases are examples of central nervous system (CNS) sarcoidosis:

Patient A: Basilar leptomeningeal nodular enhancement with enhancement of the infundibulum and the optic nerves is demonstrated (Figure 109-1).

Patient B: There is solid, ill-defined enhancing tissue along the medial right frontal lobe (Figure 109-2). On initial inspection, the clinician might suspect a high-grade primary glial neoplasm or lymphoma as the cause of these findings.

Patient C: Nodular enhancement and linear enhancement along the nerve roots of the cauda equina are demonstrated (Figure 109-3).

Patient D: Nodular enhancement within and along the cervical and upper thoracic spinal cord is demonstrated (Figure 109-4).

Background

Sarcoidosis manifests histopathologically as noncaseating granulomas of unknown cause. Typical presentation is in the third and fourth decades of life. African Americans and whites of northern European descent have the highest disease incidence, and women are more frequently affected than men. CNS involvement has been reported in 5% to 15% of cases, but isolated CNS involvement occurs in less than 2% to 4% of cases.

Patterns of Involvement

Multiple patterns of CNS involvement in sarcoidosis have been described. The most common of these is chronic meningitis with a predilection for the leptomeninges of the basal cisterns. These patients may present with chronic meningeal symptoms, cranial neuropathies (especially involving the facial and optic nerves), or symptoms related to involvement of the hypothalamus and pituitary stalk. Imaging findings are best shown with magnetic resonance imaging (MRI) and include thick, nodular enhancement of the involved leptomeninges. There may be enhancing tissue around the hypothalamus and pituitary stalk. Parenchymal brain involvement with regions of abnormality may occur as a result of direct extension from leptomeningeal disease or disease along the Virchow-Robin spaces, or, less commonly, there may be granulomas in the brain. White matter lesions mimicking multiple sclerosis may be present because of disease extension along the perivascular spaces or related to sarcoid-induced small vessel vasculitis. Less commonly, dural-based disease may be the predominant imaging finding and may be mistaken for a meningioma.

The spinal manifestations of sarcoidosis are similar to intracranial findings and can have both intramedullary and extramedullary involvement. Involvement of the cord can be extensive and infiltrative, with cord enlargement and associated hyperintensity on T2-weighted images and hypointensity on T1-weighted images. The enhancement pattern may be patchy, circumscribed focal enhancement or broad-based and peripheral, extending from the spinal cord surface to the center of the cord, suggesting inflammation extending from the leptomeninges via perivascular spaces inward. In the chronic stages, cord atrophy without enhancement and gliosis may be present. In cases involving the cauda equina, enhancement is leptomeningeal with linear enhancement or small nodules, which are often dural-based and demonstrate intense enhancement. The lesions are hypointense or isointense in signal on T1-weighted images and isointense or hyperintense on T2-weighted images.

Treatment

Patients with CNS sarcoidosis are managed with steroid therapy. Response patterns over 1- to 2-year follow-up intervals show a spectrum of MRI findings ranging from regression to progression, including stable disease without significant imaging changes. Often, treatment recurrence after long-term therapy occurs. There is no cure.

References

Dumas JL, Valeyre D, Chapelon-Abric C, et al. Central nervous system sarcoidosis: follow-up at MR imaging during steroid therapy. *Radiology*. 2000;214:411-420.

Smith JK, Matheus MG, Castillo M. Imaging manifestations of neurosarcoidosis. *AJR Am J Roentgenol*. 2004;182:289-295.

Spencer TS, Campellone JV, Maldonado I, et al. Clinical and magnetic resonance imaging manifestations of neurosarcoidosis. *Semin Arthritis Rheum*. 2005;34(4):649-661.

Cross-Reference

Neuroradiology: THE REQUISITES, 4th ed, pp 202-204.

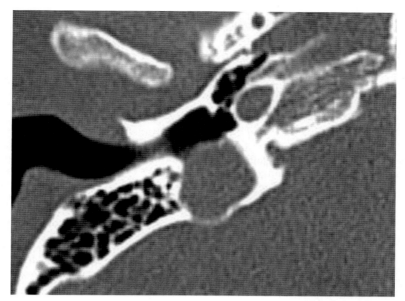

Figure 110-1

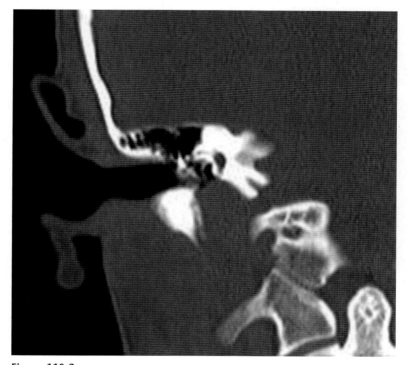

Figure 110-2

HISTORY: Abnormality on routine otoscopy.

1. Which of the following is the single best diagnosis?
   A. Glomus jugulare
   B. Aberrant internal carotid artery
   C. Cholesteatoma
   D. Dehiscent jugular bulb

2. How do these entities most often manifest?
   A. Pulsatile tinnitus
   B. Neck mass
   C. Hemotympanum
   D. Fistula

3. During surgery for middle ear disease, in what percentage of cases is this entity discovered?
   A. 0% to 10%
   B. 11% to 25%
   C. 26% to 50%
   D. More than 50%

4. In what percentage of cases is the right jugular bulb larger than the left?
   A. 0% to 20%
   B. 21% to 40%
   C. 41% to 60%
   D. More than 60%

CASE 110

Jugular Bulb Dehiscence

1. **D.** Dehiscent jugular bulb. Incompleteness of the wall of the jugular bulb is characteristic of dehiscent jugular bulb. There is no mass here, and so glomus jugulare and cholesteatoma would not be included. Also, the structure is not the carotid artery, and so aberrant internal carotid artery could not be a diagnosis.

2. **A.** Pulsatile tinnitus. Dehiscent jugular bulbs manifest as pulsatile tinnitus with transmitted vascular sounds.

3. **A.** 0% to 10%. A dehiscent jugular bulb is discovered only about 8% of the time as a normal variant.

4. **D.** More than 60%. The right jugular bulb is larger than the left in about 75% of individuals.

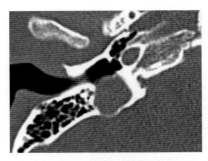

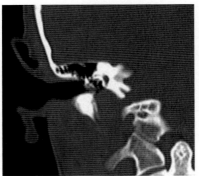

Comment

Types of Jugular Vein Anomalies

There are many different varieties of jugular vein anomalies in the temporal bone. The simplest is a high-riding jugular vein without dehiscence, which occurs when the jugular vein reaches the level of the internal auditory canal, above the inferior tympanic annulus, or above the basal turn of the cochlea (8.2%). These are more common on the right side than on the left. In the second simplest variety, the jugular bulb is dehiscent, and the sigmoid plate overlying the jugular vein's anterior wall is deficient (Figures 110-1 and 110-2). This anomaly may be observed at otoscopy as a retrotympanic, red, vascular mass. The more complex varieties include dehiscent jugular bulbs that communicate with structures other than the middle ear cavity, such as the endolymphatic sac, the facial nerve canal, or the semicircular canals. A diverticulum may protrude into the middle ear cavity and appear as a more focal mass, which is more common on the left side. On otoscopy, this lesion may be mistaken for a paraganglioma or another vascular tumor. The jugular venous pulsation wave may not be evident at otoscopy to suggest a normal variant diagnosis.

Reference

Friedmann DR, Eubig J, Winata LS, Pramanik BK, Merchant SN, Lalwani AK. Prevalence of jugular bulb abnormalities and resultant inner ear dehiscence: a histopathologic and radiologic study. *Otolaryngol Head Neck Surg.* 2012;147(4):750-756.

Cross-Reference

Neuroradiology: THE REQUISITES, 4th ed, pp 393-395.

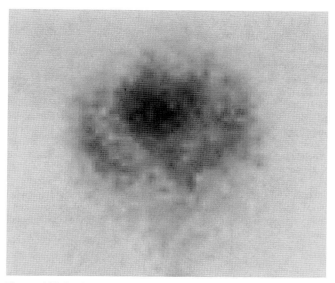

Figure 111-1   Anterior-posterior.

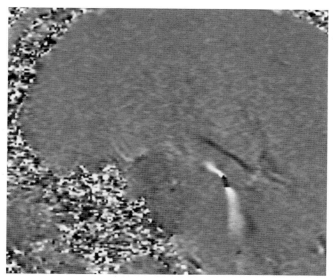

Figure 111-2

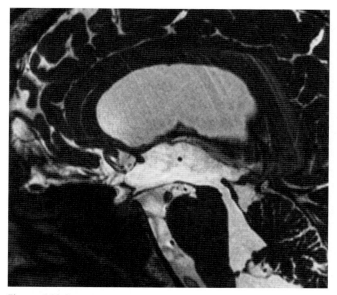

Figure 111-3

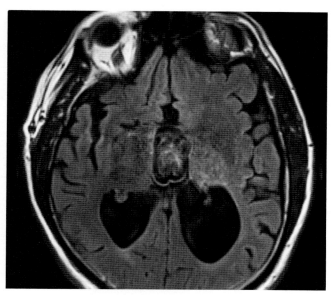

Figure 111-4

HISTORY: A 65-year-old man presents with ataxia and urinary incontinence.

1. What is the most likely diagnosis of this case?
   A. Noncommunicating obstructive hydrocephalus
   B. Normal-pressure hydrocephalus
   C. Alzheimer dementia
   D. Aqueductal stenosis

2. What is the preferred treatment for this entity?
   A. Acetazolamide
   B. Ventriculostomy shunt placement
   C. Memantine
   D. Endoscopic third ventriculostomy

3. In this entity, what statement best describes expected findings on indium-DTPA cisternography (Figure 111-1)?
   A. Radiotracer over the cerebral convexities without ventricular reflux within 2 to 24 hours
   B. Radiotracer over the cerebral convexities with ventricular reflux within 2 to 24 hours
   C. Reflux of radiotracer into the ventricular system that clears rapidly
   D. Reflux of radiotracer into the ventricular system and, to a lesser extent, the sylvian cisterns, without ascent of the radiotracer over the cerebral convexities at 24 hours

4. What is the most probable stochastic effect of radiation exposure?
   A. Genetic mutations
   B. Cancer incidence
   C. Temporary erythema of the skin
   D. Permanent hair loss

CASE 111

Normal-Pressure Hydrocephalus

1. **B.** Normal-pressure hydrocephalus (NPH). NPH is the most likely diagnosis. No point of obstruction is identified. There are no overwhelming signs of Alzheimer dementia. The cerebral aqueduct is patent.

2. **B.** Ventriculostomy shunt placement. Shunting is the preferred method of treatment, but response is variable.

3. **D.** Reflux of radiotracer into the ventricular system and, to a lesser extent, the sylvian cisterns, without ascent of the radiotracer over the cerebral convexities at 24 hours. In cases of communicating hydrocephalus and NPH, reflux of radiotracer into the ventricles is seen without radiotracer accumulation over the convexities 24 to 48 hours after administration. Normally, radiotracer is not present in the ventricles and is seen over the convexities.

4. **B.** Cancer incidence. The most probable stochastic effect (an effect of chronic, low-dose radiation) is cancer incidence (8% to 15% increased risk/Gy). Skin injury, including hair loss, is a deterministic effect. Genetic mutations occur at approximately 0.5%/Gy.

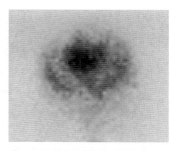

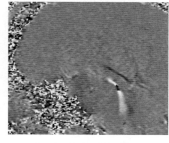

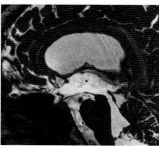

Comment

Definition and Imaging

NPH, a form of communicating hydrocephalus, is characterized by normal mean cerebrospinal fluid (CSF) pressure. The clinical triad is ataxia, urinary incontinence, and dementia. In NPH, the lateral and third ventricles are enlarged compared with the fourth ventricle. Distention of the lateral ventricles may result in thinning and elevation of the corpus callosum, whereas enlargement of the third ventricle may result in dilation of the infundibular and optic recesses, which may be displaced inferiorly (Figure 111-3). Patients typically have accentuation of flow-related artifacts in the aqueduct of Sylvius and possibly the third ventricle or near the foramina of Monro on spin echo images (Figure 111-4), and CSF flow in the aqueduct may be seen on flow-sensitive imaging (Figure 111-2), as in this case. Transependymal interstitial edema may be present, or on magnetic resonance imaging (MRI), NPH may show a more chronic, compensated communicating hydrocephalus.

Cause and Treatment

Although the cause of NPH is still debated, it is believed to result most often from remote intracranial hemorrhage or meningeal infection. Some investigators have suggested that ischemic injury or edema in the periventricular white matter reduces the tensile strength of the ventricles, resulting in their enlargement. Some patients with NPH have marked improvement of symptoms after shunting. Response to shunting is most favorable when ataxia is the predominant symptom, the patient has had symptoms for only a short time, findings on isotope cisternography (Figure 111-1) are positive, the patient has a known history of intracranial hemorrhage or infection, MRI shows a prominent CSF flow void in the aqueduct, and there is relative absence of deep periventricular white matter atrophy. Lumbar puncture with removal of 15 mL or more of CSF and subsequent improvement of clinical symptoms may also indicate a patient who may have a favorable response to shunting.

Outcome of Treatment

No MRI findings have been reliably shown to predict the outcome of shunt surgery in patients with NPH. It is unclear if the presence of foci of high signal intensity in the deep and subcortical white matter (small vessel ischemic disease) in patients with NPH can predict a lesser outcome from shunt surgery; however, when there is associated significant white matter volume loss, long-term outcomes may be diminished. Care must be used to separate foci of high signal intensity related to small vessel ischemic disease from irregular hyperintensity around the frontal and occipital horns that may be attributable to transependymal flow of CSF. The major diagnostic challenge is to differentiate NPH from cerebral atrophy and deep white matter ischemia, which are far more common causes of the clinical triad than NPH. The decision to perform shunt surgery should be based largely on clinical findings and MRI studies that indicate that brain atrophy is not responsible for the ventriculomegaly.

References

Fishman RA, Dillon WP. Normal pressure hydrocephalus: new findings and old questions. *AJNR Am J Neuroradiol.* 2001;22:1640-1641.

Sankey EW, Jusué-Torres I, Elder BD, et al. Functional gait outcomes for idiopathic normal pressure hydrocephalus after primary endoscopic third ventriculostomy. *J Clin Neurosci.* 2015;22(8): 1303-1308.

Tullerg M, Jensen C, Ekholm S, Wikkelso C. Normal pressure hydrocephalus: vascular white matter changes on MR images must not exclude patients from surgery. *AJNR Am J Neuroradiol.* 2001;22: 1665-1673.

Cross-Reference

Neuroradiology: THE REQUISITES, 4th ed, pp 234-236.

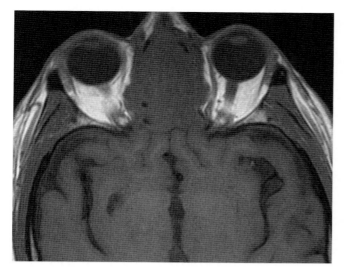

Figure 112-1

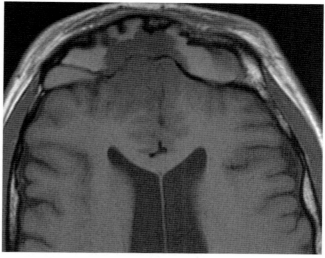

Figure 112-2

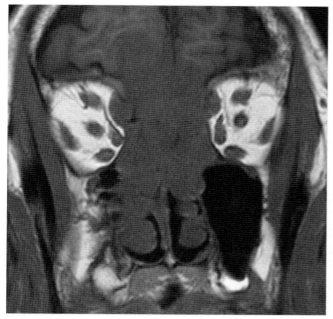

Figure 112-3

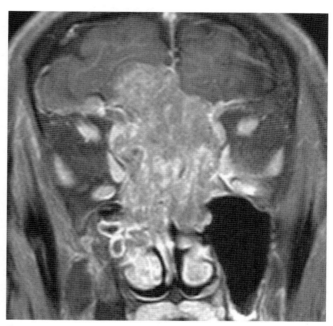

Figure 112-4

HISTORY: A 62-year-old with extensive smoking history and runny nose.

1. Regarding malignancy in the nasal cavity and paranasal sinuses, which statement is correct?
   A. The majority of malignancies arise in the sphenoid sinuses.
   B. Adenocarcinoma is the most common histologic type.
   C. Up to a fivefold increased risk of sinonasal carcinoma is observed with heavy smoking.
   D. Approximately 25% of all paranasal sinus tumors are T3 or T4 at the time of diagnosis.

2. What is the risk of malignant transformation of an inverting papilloma into squamous cell carcinoma?
   A. 0% to 10%
   B. 11% to 20%
   C. 21% to 30%
   D. 31% to 40%

3. What is the most common histology of maxillary sinus malignancies?
   A. Small cell adenocarcinoma
   B. Transitional cell carcinoma
   C. Squamous cell carcinoma
   D. Non–small cell adenocarcinoma

4. Which of the following is a possible effect of the static magnetic field in a patient lying still in a 1.5-tesla magnetic resonance imaging scanner?
   A. Dizziness
   B. Tingling and twitching of the hands
   C. Burns at skin-skin interfaces
   D. T-wave elevation of electrocardiogram (ECG) tracings

CASE 112

Sinonasal Undifferentiated Carcinoma with Intracranial Extension

1. **C.** Up to a fivefold increased risk of sinonasal carcinoma is observed with heavy smoking. The majority arise in the maxillary sinus, approximately 20% arise in the ethmoid sinuses, and the remainder (<1%) originate in the frontal and sphenoid sinuses. Squamous cell carcinoma is the most common histologic type. Up to 75% of all paranasal sinus tumors are stage T3 or T4 at the time of diagnosis.

2. **A.** 0% to 10%. The risk of malignant transformation of an inverting papilloma into squamous cell carcinoma is approximately 5% to 10%.

3. **C.** Squamous cell carcinoma. The most common histology of maxillary sinus malignancies is squamous cell carcinoma.

4. **D.** T-wave elevation of ECG tracings. Gradient switching has been implicated in tingling and twitching of the extremities and thermal injury at skin interfaces. Dizziness occurs in some patients as they enter or leave the magnetic field but is not reported when a patient is lying still.

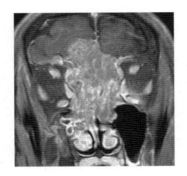

Comment

Case Description

This case shows a large, aggressive mass in the bilateral sinonasal cavity involving the nasal vault and ethmoid air cells (Figure 112-1), with extension into the frontal sinus (Figure 112-2). There is extension into the anterior cranial fossa through the cribriform plate, with elevation of the frontal lobes (Figures 112-3 and 112-4). T2-weighted images (not shown) showed no edema in the frontal lobes. There is lateral bowing of the bilateral lamina papyracea (see Figure 112-1), with findings highly suggestive of invasion of the periorbita. On the second unenhanced axial T1-weighted image (see Figure 112-2), the hyperintense material filling the frontal sinus is proteinaceous, inspissated secretions, whereas the central material isointense to muscle in the frontal sinus is neoplasm.

Sinonasal Malignancy

Malignant tumors of the sinonasal tract are rare, accounting for 3% of head and neck cancers. The majority arise in the maxillary sinus, approximately 20% arise in the ethmoid sinuses, and the remainder (<1%) originate in the frontal and sphenoid sinuses. Squamous cell carcinoma is the most common histologic type. Nickel and chrome refining processes have been implicated in the development of all types of malignancy of the paranasal sinuses, and exposure to wood dust has been associated specifically with adenocarcinoma of the ethmoid. Up to a fivefold increased risk of sinonasal carcinoma has been observed with heavy smoking. Clinical presentation of sinus malignancies is nonspecific and often mimics benign disease. Approximately 10% of patients are asymptomatic. Delay in diagnosis is common. Up to 75% of all paranasal sinus tumors are stage T3 or T4 at the time of diagnosis. Resectability and treatment are determined by the presence of orbital invasion, intracranial spread, dural invasion, and perineural spread.

Sinonasal Undifferentiated Carcinoma

Sinonasal undifferentiated carcinoma is a rare cancer of the sinonasal cavity. Initial symptoms may include bloody nose, rhinorrhea, diplopia, and proptosis. It has been associated with papillomas in the nasal cavity, which are benign, but can undergo malignant degeneration. A history of radiation therapy for other cancers has been associated with the development of sinonasal undifferentiated carcinoma, although most patients have not had previous radiation therapy.

References

Eisen MD, Yousem DM, Loevner LA, et al. Preoperative imaging to predict orbital invasion by tumor. *Head Neck*. 2000;22:456-462.

Loevner LA, Sonners A. Imaging of neoplasms of the paranasal sinuses. *Neuroimaging Clin N Am*. 2004;14:625-646.

Cross-Reference

Neuroradiology: THE REQUISITES, 4th ed, pp 435-436.

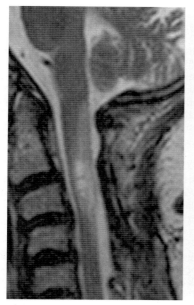

Figure 113-1

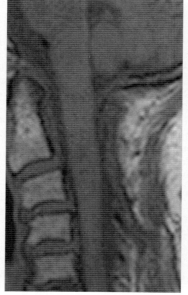

Figure 113-2

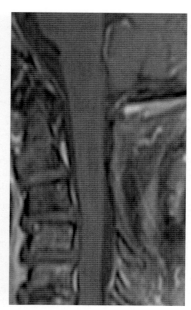

Figure 113-3

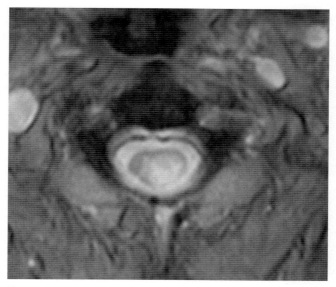

Figure 113-4

HISTORY: A 53-year-old woman presents with left-sided numbness, left arm and hand weakness, and imbalance.

1. What is the single best diagnosis?
   A. Ependymoma
   B. Sarcoid
   C. Lymphoma
   D. Astrocytoma

2. Which of the following is typically an imaging feature of this lesion?
   A. Avid contrast enhancement
   B. Lack of cord expansion
   C. Hyperintense T2 signal
   D. Hyperintense T1 signal

3. What is the most common primary intramedullary neoplasm in an adult?
   A. Ganglioglioma
   B. Lymphoma
   C. Astrocytoma
   D. Ependymoma

4. What is the most common location of spinal cord astrocytomas?
   A. Cervical
   B. Upper thoracic
   C. Lower thoracic
   D. Conus region

CASE 113

Astrocytoma of Cervical Cord

1. **D.** Astrocytoma. Ependymomas and intramedullary lymphomas typically enhance. There is asymmetric cord expansion supporting a tumor rather than inflammatory process.

2. **C.** Hyperintense T2 signal. Astrocytomas are typically hyperintense on T2-weighted images. No contrast enhancement is shown by 20% to 30% of astrocytomas in the cord, and when there is enhancement it is not frequently avid. Astrocytomas typically cause spinal cord expansion and are isointense to hypointense on T1-weighted imaging.

3. **D.** Ependymoma. In adults, ependymomas are the most common tumor type, accounting for 40% to 60% of all intramedullary spinal tumors, with the mean age of presentation being 35 to 40 years. Astrocytomas account for approximately 30% of spinal cord tumors. Gangliogliomas, lymphoma, and other tumors are rare.

4. **A.** Cervical. Order of frequency for location of astrocytoma in the spinal cord is top down—cervical, thoracic, conus.

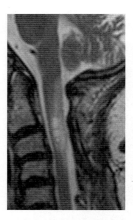

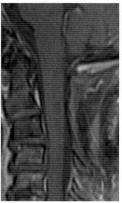

Comment

Background

Astrocytomas of the spinal cord are unusual and account for approximately 30% of spinal cord tumors. They are the most common childhood intramedullary neoplasms of the spinal cord and are second only to ependymomas in adults. Clinical presentation varies from nonspecific back pain to sensory and motor deficits, according to the size and location. The infiltrative nature of astrocytomas leads to a worse prognosis than is associated with ependymomas.

Histopathology

Astrocytomas arise from astrocytes in the spinal cord. Most astrocytomas (75%) are low-grade (World Health Organization grade II) fibrillary astrocytomas. They are most commonly found in the cervical spine.

Imaging

The classic magnetic resonance imaging appearance of intramedullary astrocytoma includes cord enlargement and poorly defined margins (Figures 113-1 through 113-4). Intramedullary astrocytoma is typically isointense to hypointense on T1-weighted images (see Figure 113-2) and hyperintense on T2-weighted images (see Figures 113-1 through 113-4). Peritumoral and tumoral cysts are frequently associated with astrocytomas (see Figure 113-1). Most intramedullary astrocytomas exhibit at least some enhancement, regardless of cell type or tumor grade. About 20% to 30% of intramedullary astrocytomas show no enhancement (see Figure 113-3).

Management

The optimal treatment of spinal astrocytomas is controversial. The goal of surgery is to remove the bulk of tumor where possible, especially for patients with low-grade astrocytomas. Radiation should be considered for high-grade tumors, inoperable tumors, tumors remaining after surgery, and recurring tumors.

Reference

Seo HS, Kim JH, Lee DH, et al. Nonenhancing intramedullary astrocytomas and other MR imaging features: a retrospective study and systematic review. *AJNR Am J Neuroradiol.* 2010;31(3):498-503.

Cross-Reference

Neuroradiology: THE REQUISITES, 4th ed, pp 571-572.

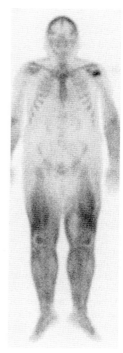

Figure 114-1

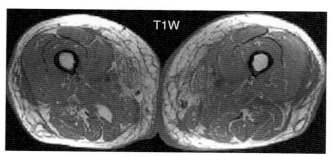

Figure 114-2

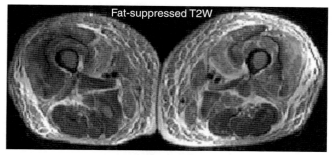

Figure 114-3

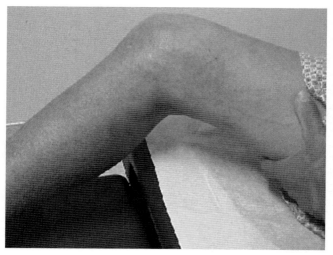

Figure 114-4

HISTORY: A 48-year-old woman with renal insufficiency and lower extremity weakness presents following a contrast-enhanced magnetic resonance imaging (MRI) scan.

1. What is the single best diagnosis?
   A. Sarcoidosis
   B. Nephrogenic systemic fibrosis (NSF)
   C. Osteomyelitis
   D. Abscess

2. What organ system does this disease primarily affect?
   A. Genitourinary
   B. Renal
   C. Skin
   D. Central nervous system

3. What systemic condition does this disease mimic?
   A. Scleroderma
   B. Systemic lupus erythematosus
   C. Dermatomyositis
   D. Chronic renal failure

4. What is the typical interval between gadolinium injection for MRI and the onset of symptoms in this disease?
   A. 1 to 2 days
   B. 3 to 4 days
   C. 1 to 2 weeks
   D. 2 to 8 weeks

CASE 114

Gadolinium-Associated Nephrogenic Systemic Fibrosis

1. **B.** Nephrogenic systemic fibrosis. This is a case of gadolinium-associated NSF.

2. **C.** Skin. Nephrogenic systemic sclerosis primarily affects the skin, but it can affect other organs.

3. **A.** Scleroderma. NSF mimics scleroderma.

4. **D.** 2 to 8 weeks. Symptoms develop within 2 to 8 weeks after gadolinium injection.

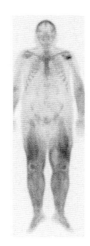

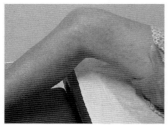

Comment

Background

NSF is a rare disorder that affects primarily the skin but can affect other organs in patients with renal insufficiency. More than 200 cases have been reported. Originally, this fibrosing skin condition was termed *nephrogenic fibrosing dermopathy* because it occurred exclusively in patients with renal failure. The skin changes can mimic progressive systemic sclerosis, or scleroderma, with a predilection for peripheral extremity involvement. Specific histologic findings include thickened collagen bundles with surrounding clefts, mucin deposition, and increased numbers of fibrocytes and elastic fibers. Systemic manifestations can include fibrosis of the skeletal muscle, bone, lungs, pleura, pericardium, myocardium, kidneys, and dura. Thus, the terminology has changed to *nephrogenic systemic fibrosis* to reflect this systemic involvement.

Cause

The exact cause of NSF is unclear. There is no convincing evidence that it is caused by specific drugs, infections, or dialysis itself. It has been specifically associated with intravenous gadodiamide injection in the setting of renal failure managed with dialysis and in patients with hepatorenal syndrome. The only gadolinium-based contrast agent to date reported to be associated with NSF is gadodiamide. It has been postulated that NSF might result from a toxic reaction to free gadolinium (Gd^{3+}) liberated from the chelate but not adequately excreted due to impaired renal function. Transmetallation, the release of free gadolinium from the chelate, with subsequent binding to endogenous ions, depends on the molecular conditional thermodynamic stability. Gadolinium agents with lower conditional stability constant values, such as gadodiamide, would be more likely to undergo transmetallation and result in NSF. It has been suggested that a combination of factors leads to the development of NSF, beginning with renal disease, followed by allergen deposition, leading to circulating fibrocyte deposition. The idea that endothelial damage and elevated levels of cytokines can lead to the development of NSF is supported by the fact that vascular surgery, deep venous thrombosis, and coagulopathies have been noted to occur in the interval between gadodiamide injection and the development of skin fibrosis.

Clinical Findings

In most reported cases, symptoms have developed within 2 to 8 weeks after gadolinium injection for MRI, although cases have been reported with longer time intervals. Lower extremity involvement is most common, followed by involvement of the upper extremities, as in this case. Less commonly, the torso may be affected. The face and neck appear to be spared. Early signs and symptoms seen within the first 2 weeks after gadolinium injection include extremity edema and swelling, arthralgias, myalgias, and extremity weakness. In this case, a bone scan (Figure 114-1) shows symmetric increased radionuclide skin and muscle uptake in the lower extremities and distal upper extremities. MRI of the thighs shows skin thickening and edema with soft tissue stranding in the subcutaneous fat and muscles (Figures 114-2 and 114-3). Late signs and symptoms (usually 2 to 8 weeks after gadolinium injection) include skin fibrosis, thickening, and tightening. Skin findings (Figure 114-4) include slightly raised and erythematous or brawny nodular plaques, linear striations, or confluent regions of fibrosis. Extremity contractures, myopathy, and weakness are common.

Mitigation of Risk

Most institutions now have policies regarding the use of these agents. Gadolinium is usually not given to patients with end-stage renal disease or to those receiving dialysis. To screen patients scheduled for contrast-enhanced MRI scans, glomerular filtration rate should be calculated in patients who have a history of kidney disease or diabetes and in those older than 60 years. Dialysis immediately after gadodiamide injection has not prevented NSF.

References

Broome DR, Girguis MS, Baron PW, et al. Gadodiamide-associated nephrogenic systemic fibrosis: why radiologists should be concerned. *AJR Am J Roentgenol.* 2007;188:586-592.

Kalb RE, Helm TN, Sperry H, et al. Gadolinium-induced nephrogenic systemic fibrosis in a patient with an acute and transient kidney injury. *Br J Dermatol.* 2008;158:607-610.

Cross-Reference

Neuroradiology: THE REQUISITES, 4th ed, p 427.

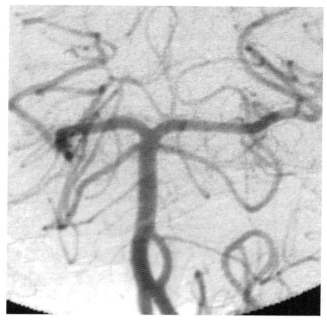

Figure 115-1 Patient A.

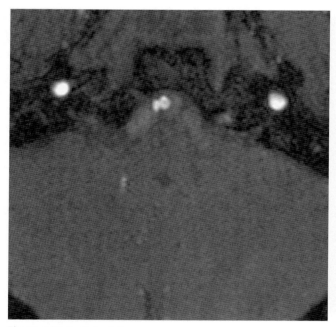

Figure 115-2 Patient B.

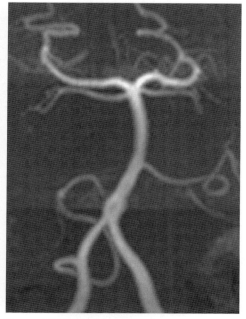

Figure 115-3 Patient B.

HISTORY:

Patient A (Figure 115-1): Incidental finding on magnetic resonance imaging for history of head trauma.

Patient B (Figures 115-2 and 115-3): Companion case, history withheld.

1. What is the single best diagnosis?
   A. Dissection
   B. Aneurysm
   C. Fenestration
   D. Traumatic injury

2. What posterior circulation vessel most often extends into the internal auditory canal?
   A. Superior cerebellar artery
   B. Anterior inferior cerebellar artery
   C. Posterior inferior cerebellar artery
   D. Posterior cerebral artery

3. What arteries of the posterior circulation give rise to midbrain perforating arteries?
   A. Posterior cerebral arteries
   B. Superior cerebellar arteries
   C. Anterior inferior cerebellar arteries
   D. Posterior inferior cerebellar arteries

4. What aneurysm can rupture directly into the fourth ventricle?
   A. Posterior communicating artery
   B. Posterior cerebral artery
   C. Posterior inferior cerebellar artery
   D. Posterior choroidal artery

CASE 115

Fenestration of the Basilar Artery

1. **C.** Fenestration. These are examples of a fenestration.

2. **B.** Anterior inferior cerebellar artery. This branch extends into the internal auditory canal.

3. **A.** Posterior cerebral arteries. The basilar artery and the proximal posterior cerebral arteries (P1 segments) give rise to midbrain perforating arteries.

4. **C.** Posterior inferior cerebellar artery. Aneurysms of the posterior inferior cerebellar artery can rupture into the fourth ventricle.

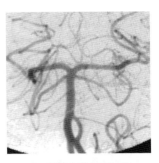

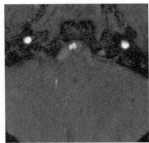

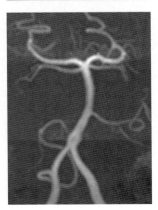

Comment

Fenestration of a cerebral artery is defined as a division of the vessel lumen that results in two separate vascular channels that are often not equal in size. Each of the channels is lined by endothelium. Pathologic evaluation of basilar artery fenestrations shows that the vascular channels might or might not share a common adventitial layer. Histologically, there are short segmental regions at both the proximal and distal ends of the fenestration in which there are defects in the media, similar to bifurcations of cerebral arteries.

Incidence

Fenestrations are more common in the posterior circulation (Figures 115-2 and 115-3, Patient B), reported in up to 0.6% of cerebral angiograms (Figure 115-1, Patient A). In comparison, the angiographic incidence of fenestrations in the anterior circulation has been reported in up to 0.2% of cases. On postmortem examination, fenestrations in the posterior and anterior circulation have been reported in 6% to 7% of cases. The discrepancy between pathologic and angiographic incidence is likely due to the increased sensitivity at pathology.

Embryology

The basilar artery is formed by early fusion of bilateral longitudinal neural arteries. Fenestrations occur along regions where there is failure of complete fusion of the medial aspects of these longitudinal arteries. The vertebral arteries are formed by fusion of primitive cervical segmental arteries and basivertebral anastomotic vessels. Extracranial duplications of a vertebral artery are most likely related to failure of regression of the cervical segmental arteries, whereas intracranial duplications likely arise as a result of persistence of basivertebral anastomoses.

Aneurysms

Aneurysms can arise from a fenestration; however, when considering all fenestrations (anterior and posterior circulation), the incidence is approximately 3%, not significantly different from the incidence of aneurysms arising at the circle of Willis. Aneurysms arising from fenestrations of the posterior circulation occur more often (in up to 7% of cases). Aneurysms arise most commonly at the proximal end of the fenestration.

Reference

Sanders WP, Sorek PA, Mehta BA. Fenestration of intracranial arteries with special attention to associated aneurysms and other anomalies. *AJNR Am J Neuroradiol.* 1993;14:675-680.

Cross-Reference

Neuroradiology: THE REQUISITES, 4th ed, pp 33-34.

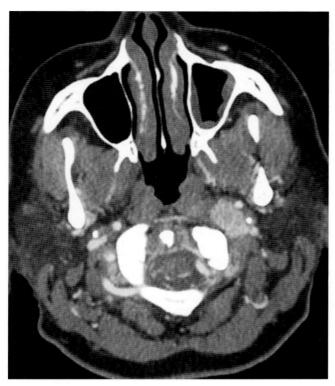

Figure 116-1

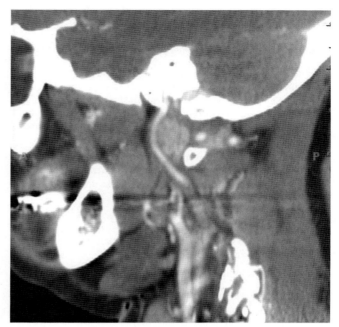

Figure 116-2

HISTORY: A 39-year-old man presents with hoarseness.

1. Which of the following is the single best diagnosis?
   A. Glomus jugulare
   B. Glomus vagale
   C. Carotid body tumor
   D. Meningioma

2. What percentage of head and neck paragangliomas are these tumors?
   A. 0% to 10%
   B. 11% to 25%
   C. 26% to 50%
   D. More than 50%

3. What percentage of these tumors secrete catecholemines?
   A. 0% to 10%
   B. 11% to 25%
   C. 26% to 50%
   D. More than 50%

4. Which of the following is *not* a component of the Carney triad?
   A. Gastric epithelioid leiomyosarcoma
   B. Pulmonary chondroma
   C. Pituitary adenoma
   D. Extra-adrenal paraganglioma

CASE 116

Glomus Vagale

1. **B.** Glomus vagale. This lesion does not enter the jugular foramen and therefore is unlikely to represent a glomus jugulare tumor; because of the lesion's location in the carotid space, it is more likely to be a glomus vagale tumor. Schwannomas and lymph nodes also populate the carotid space.

2. **A.** 0% to 10%. Glomus vagale tumors are the least common (only 2.5%) of the paragangliomas. Carotid body tumors outnumber glomus jugulare tumors; these are the two most common paragangliomas.

3. **B.** 11% to 25%. Of the paragangliomas, 12.5% of glomus vagale varieties secrete catecholamines, whereas 16.7% of glomus jugulare tumors secrete catecholamines (the highest rate among paragangliomas).

4. **C.** Pituitary adenoma. The Carney triad is gastric epithelioid leiomyosarcoma (which is now known to be malignant gastrointestinal stromal tumor), pulmonary chondroma, and extra-adrenal paraganglioma. Carney triad is a form of multiple endocrine neoplasia.

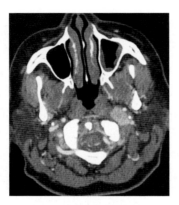

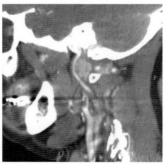

Comment

Characteristics of Glomus Vagale Tumors

Glomus vagale tumors are head and neck paragangliomas. They are the third most frequent such neoplasms, after carotid body tumors and glomus jugulare tumors, but they are more common than glomus tympanicum tumors. These tumors are found at the upper cervical regions below the jugular foramen but still in association with the carotid sheath (Figures 116-1 and 116-2). They may be distinguished from the other glomus tumors because they push carotid sheath and jugular vein structures anteriorly rather than splaying them (as do carotid body tumors) and they less commonly invade the jugular foramen or jugular vein (as do glomus jugulare tumors). Glomus vagale tumors can arise anywhere along the course of the vagus nerve, but the majority, including the one in this case, arise near the ganglion nodosum, located at C1. Typical manifestations may include pulsatile tinnitus, hoarseness (because they affect the vagus nerve in approximately 50% of cases), swallowing disorder, and, late in the disease process, a neck mass. More women than men are affected, and the incidence is highest among people aged 40 to 60 years. These tumors have a low rate of invasion into the jugular vein.

Secretion of Catecholamines

Glomus vagale tumors are hypervascular lesions, enhancing greatly on scans. In 12.5% of cases, they secrete catecholamine-like agents, and so hypertension may coexist. This characteristic may distinguish them from schwannomas of the vagus, which do not secrete any agents, enhance more variably, and have no flow voids within the tumor. Salt-and-pepper appearance on T2-weighted magnetic resonance imaging occurs when glomus vagale tumors are very large. The rate of surgical cure is 70% to 75%, but in the remainder of cases, the disease recurs or residual disease, distant disease, or metachronous new lesions occur.

Carney Triad

The Carney triad is gastric malignant gastrointestinal stromal tumor, pulmonary chondroma, and extra-adrenal paraganglioma. Carney triad is a form of multiple endocrine neoplasia.

Reference

Erickson D, Kudva YC, Ebersold MJ, et al. Benign paragangliomas: clinical presentation and treatment outcomes in 236 patients. *J Clin Endocrinol Metab.* 2001;86(11):5210-5216.

Cross-Reference

Neuroradiology: THE REQUISITES, 4th ed, pp 506-508.

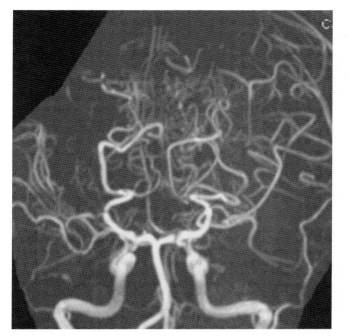

Figure 117-1

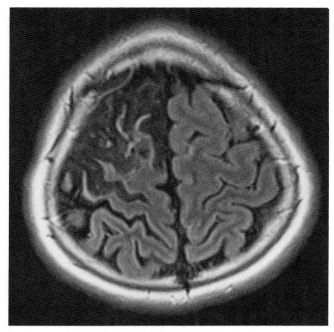

Figure 117-2

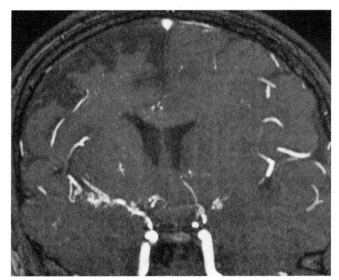

Figure 117-3

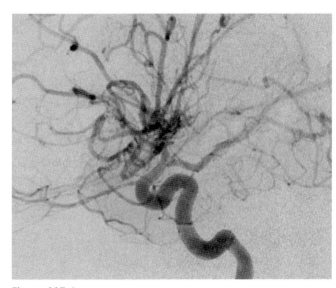

Figure 117-4

HISTORY: A 12-year-old with altered mental status.

1. What is the single best diagnosis if this child has sickle cell disease?
   A. Moyamoya disease
   B. Moyamoya syndrome
   C. Postoperative changes
   D. Effects of radiation therapy

2. What is the characteristic clinical presentation in children with this disorder?
   A. Transient ischemic attacks (TIAs)
   B. Intraparenchymal hemorrhage
   C. Intraventricular hemorrhage
   D. Subarachnoid hemorrhage

3. What is the most common clinical presentation in adults with this disorder?
   A. Seizure
   B. Intracranial hemorrhage
   C. Stroke
   D. Headache

4. What is the definitive treatment in the idiopathic form of this entity?
   A. Angioplasty and stenting
   B. Carotid endarterectomy
   C. Anticoagulation
   D. Revascularization with external carotid artery (ECA) grafting

CASE 117

Moyamoya Syndrome and Disease

1. **B.** Moyamoya syndrome. In a child with known sickle cell disease, the imaging findings of this case are most accurately called *moyamoya syndrome*. When the condition is idiopathic, the term *moyamoya disease* is most accurate.

2. **A.** Transient ischemic attacks (TIAs). Moyamoya has a progressive course in children, who present with symptoms of cerebral ischemia, including TIAs and stroke.

3. **B.** Intracranial hemorrhage. Adults with moyamoya most commonly present with intraparenchymal or subarachnoid hemorrhages. Over time, dementia develops as a result of progressive compromise of the vascular system and chronic hypoxia.

4. **D.** Revascularization with ECA grafting. This can either be direct or indirect by anastomosis of an ECA branch to a cortical branch of the middle cerebral artery or by placement of vascularized tissue in direct contact with the brain parenchyma to allow ingrowth.

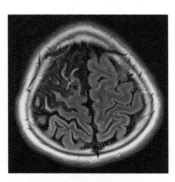
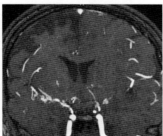

Comment

This case shows marked narrowing of the bilateral supraclinoid internal carotid arteries and occlusion of the proximal bilateral anterior and middle cerebral arteries (Figures 117-1, 117-3, and 117-4). There are collateral vessels from the external carotid circulation, leptomeningeal collaterals from the cerebral arteries, and collaterals from the perforators in the basal ganglia, best demonstrated in Figure 117-1.

Moyamoya refers to slow, progressive occlusive disease of the distal intracranial internal carotid arteries and their proximal branches, including the anterior and middle cerebral arteries. The posterior cerebral arteries also may be involved. Because of the slowly progressive development of high-grade stenoses or occlusions of the distal internal carotid arteries or their proximal branches, collateral circulation develops through a number of pathways, including leptomeningeal collaterals from the cerebral arteries; parenchymal collaterals through the perforating arteries (particularly the basal ganglia); and transdural collaterals, which most commonly arise from the ECA (ophthalmic and middle meningeal arteries).

Imaging

Findings include absent T2 flow voids in the distal internal carotid arteries and proximal middle and anterior cerebral arteries. Prominent collateral vascular flow voids around the circle of Willis and within the basal ganglia, thalamus, and hypothalamus are easily identified on magnetic resonance angiography. Leptomeningeal collateral vessels are often present, and this is associated with leptomeningeal enhancement and nonsuppression of signal on fluid-attenuated inversion recovery (FLAIR). Watershed infarcts are often present (Figure 117-2).

Disease

Moyamoya disease is predominantly an idiopathic arteriopathy. It is more prevalent in Japan with a bimodal presentation with median presentation at 5 years and 40 years of age. Moyamoya disease is more symptomatic when it occurs in childhood, typically with TIAs and stroke. In adults, the disease is less commonly symptomatic, but when it is, it more commonly presents with intracranial hemorrhage.

Syndrome

However, a moyamoya pattern has been associated with a variety of conditions, including neurofibromatosis type 1, sickle cell disease, radiation therapy, chronic infection, connective tissue disorders, and atherosclerosis. This is best termed *moyamoya syndrome*.

Treatment

In moyamoya syndrome, treatment of the underlying disease is critical in slowing the progression of the vasculopathy. Surgical treatment with either indirect or direct revascularization utilizing the external carotid circulation is performed in both moyamoya syndrome and moyamoya disease.

References

Bosemani T, Poretti A, Orman G, Tekes A, Pearl MS, Huisman TA. Moyamoya disease and syndrome in children: spectrum of neuroimaging findings including differential diagnosis. *J Pediatr Neuroradiol.* 2014;3:3-12.

Yamada I, Matsushima Y, Suzuki S. Moyamoya disease: diagnosis with three-dimensional time-of-flight MR angiography. *Radiology.* 1992;184:773-778.

Cross-Reference

Neuroradiology: THE REQUISITES, 4th ed, pp 118-121.

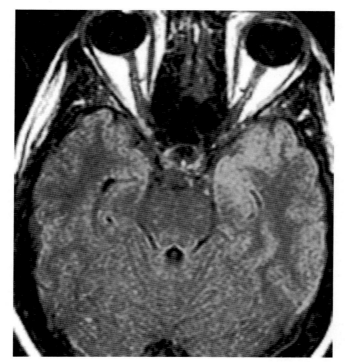

Figure 118-1

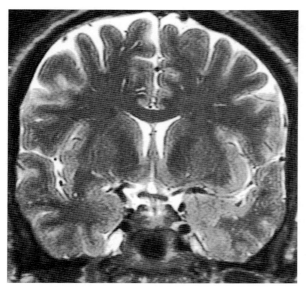

Figure 118-2

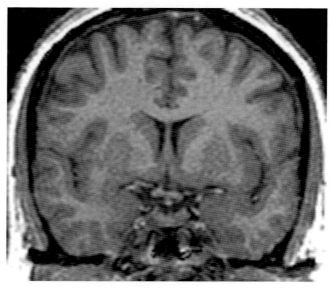

Figure 118-3

HISTORY: A 15-year-old with recurrent symptoms.

1. What is the single best diagnosis?
   A. Focal cortical dysplasia
   B. Ischemia
   C. High-grade neoplasm
   D. Infection

2. What was the patient's most likely clinical presentation?
   A. Headache
   B. Medically refractory epilepsy
   C. Subarachnoid hemorrhage
   D. Stroke

3. What embryologic term is accurate for both a primary and secondary brain vesicle?
   A. Telencephalon
   B. Diencephalon
   C. Mesencephalon
   D. Metencephalon

4. Along what path do neurons migrate from the germinal matrix along the lateral ventricles to the cerebral cortex?
   A. Cortical spinal tracts
   B. Radial glial fibers
   C. Longitudinal fasciculi
   D. Corona radiata

CASE 118

Focal Cortical Dysplasia

1. **A.** Focal cortical dysplasia. The differential diagnosis should include focal cortical dysplasia and low-grade infiltrating neoplasm in the medial left temporal lobe. Viral encephalitis may result in temporal lobe signal abnormalities, but the history of recurrent symptoms makes this less likely.

2. **B.** Medically refractory epilepsy. Many of these patients present with epilepsy.

3. **C.** Mesencephalon. The primary brain vesicles are the prosencephalon, mesencephalon, and rhombencephalon. The prosencephalon differentiates into the telencephalon and diencephalon. The rhombencephalon differentiates into the metencephalon and myelencephalon. The mesencephalon is a primary and secondary vesicle.

4. **B.** Radial glial fibers. Neurons migrate from the germinal matrix along the lateral ventricles to the cerebral cortex along radial glial fibers.

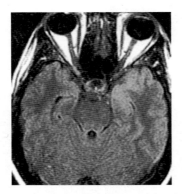

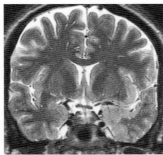

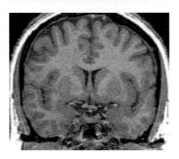

Comment

Focal cortical dysplasia (aberrant cortical lamination) is found in approximately 50% of patients with medically refractory epilepsy. These lesions have also been reported as an incidental finding in 1% to 2% of brain autopsies. These lesions might involve only mild disorganization of the cortex, but they can also contain abnormal neuronal elements. Advances in neuroimaging have allowed better identification of these lesions. Surgery often results in significant reduction or cessation of seizures, especially if the entire lesion is resected.

Classification

Focal cortical dysplasias are part of a spectrum of disorders that have been referred to as disorders of cortical development, cortical dysplasias, cortical dysgenesis, and neuronal migration abnormalities. Classification of these disorders has been based on their pathologic features or on the origin of their pathologic elements (i.e., neuronal migration). Histologic findings in cortical dysplasia include architectural abnormalities, such as cortical laminar disorganization. More severe forms are characterized by the presence of abnormal neuronal elements, such as immature neurons (round homogeneous cells with large nuclei), dysmorphic neurons (morphologically distorted cell bodies, axons, and dendrites), giant cells, and balloon cells. Balloon cells are considered a hallmark of focal cortical dysplasia, although they are not present in all cases. These cells have an eosinophilic cytoplasm and an eccentric nucleus.

Imaging

Magnetic resonance imaging findings associated with cortical dysplasia can include focal areas of increased cortical thickening (Figures 118-1 through 118-3), as in this case; reduced demarcation of the gray-white matter junction; T2-weighted hyperintensity of cortical gray matter and subcortical white matter (see Figure 118-2); T1-weighted hypointensity of subcortical white matter (see Figure 118-3); lobar underdevelopment; or extension of cortical tissue, with increased signal intensity from the brain surface to the ventricle.

References

Barkovich AJ. Morphologic characteristics of subcortical heterotopia: MR imaging study. *Am J Neuroradiol.* 2000;21:290-295.

Taylor DC, Falconer MA, Bruton CJ, et al. Focal dysplasia of the cerebral cortex in epilepsy. *J Neurol Neurosurg Psychiatry.* 1971;34:369-387.

Cross-Reference

Neuroradiology: THE REQUISITES, 4th ed, p 276.

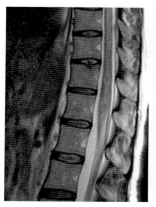
Figure 119-1

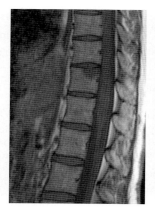
Figure 119-2

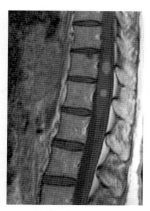
Figure 119-3

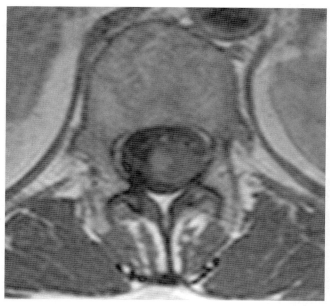
Figure 119-4

HISTORY: A 60-year-old woman presents with paraplegia and sphincter dysfunction.

1. What should be *excluded* from the differential diagnosis?
   A. Hemangioblastoma
   B. Schwannoma
   C. Sarcoidosis
   D. Metastases

2. Excluding primary central nervous system (CNS) neoplasms, which of the following is most commonly associated with intramedullary metastasis?
   A. Breast cancer
   B. Lung cancer
   C. Melanoma
   D. Lymphoma

3. What is the most likely route of spread for intramedullary metastasis?
   A. Cerebrospinal fluid (CSF) dissemination
   B. Lymphatic
   C. Hematogenous
   D. Direct

4. Which of the following statements regarding spinal cord metastasis is true?
   A. Based on autopsy results of patients with disseminated cancers, the number of patients with brain metastases is approximately 50 times more than the number of patients with spinal cord metastases.
   B. Because of its rich vascularization, the cervical cord is a more common site of intramedullary metastases than the thoracic spine.
   C. Intramedullary metastases with leptomeningeal disease most likely represent hematogenous spread of disease.
   D. Extra-CNS tumors can extend to the spinal cord by direct invasion from nerve roots or CSF.

CASE 119

Intramedullary Spinal Cord Metastases (Breast Cancer)

1. **B.** Schwannoma. These are typically extramedullary lesions. Hemangioblastomas may manifest as multiple, solid enhancing nodules. Sarcoidosis may manifest as enhancing cord lesions associated with edema. Intramedullary metastases may manifest as enhancing lesions associated with cord edema. This is a case of intramedullary metastases.

2. **B.** Lung cancer. Carcinoma of the lung is the most common tumor, accounting for approximately 50% of cases. Breast cancer is the second most common tumor, accounting for approximately 15% of cases. Melanoma accounts for approximately 7.5% of cases. Lymphoma is the third most common tumor, accounting for approximately 9% of cases.

3. **C.** Hematogenous. Given the intramedullary location and lack of leptomeningeal enhancement or nodularity, hematogenous spread is the most likely. CSF dissemination typically manifests as leptomeningeal enhancement. The lymphatics are not a common route of disease spread in the CNS. There is no evidence of tumor other than the intramedullary lesions to suggest direct spread.

4. **D.** Extra-CNS tumors can extend to the spinal cord by direct invasion from nerve roots or CSF. This explains some cases of coexistent intramedullary metastasis and leptomeningeal tumor. Brain metastases occur approximately 15 times more frequently than spinal cord metastases.

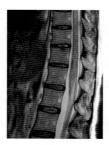

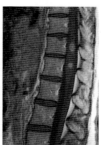

Comment

Background

Intramedullary metastases are rare; they are found in only 1% to 2% of cancer patients. Myelopathy is the first manifestation in most patients. Urinary and bowel dysfunction predominates in patients with conus medullaris metastasis.

Pathophysiology

Most studies suggest that intramedullary metastases from extra-CNS tumors reach the spinal cord mainly by two routes: (1) arterial circulation to the cord, and (2) vertebral venous plexus (Batson plexus). Extra-CNS tumors can also extend to the cord by direct invasion from nerve roots or CSF.

Imaging

On magnetic resonance imaging (MRI), intramedullary metastases are most frequently single, oval-shaped, and small, with little or no cord enlargement (Figures 119-1 through 119-4). They are typically isointense to cord on T1-weighted images before contrast agent administration and demonstrate homogeneous, nodular enhancement on images after contrast agent administration (see Figures 119-2 and 119-3). T2-weighted images show surrounding "pencil-shaped" hyperintensity, representing edema. Larger lesions are more likely to demonstrate central hypointensity on T1-weighted images, peripheral enhancement after contrast agent administration, extensive edema on T2-weighted images (see Figure 119-1), and cord enlargement. MRI of the brain should be recommended because of potential cerebral metastases and because mimickers of intramedullary metastasis, such as multiple sclerosis or sarcoid, may be favored based on the intracranial findings.

Management

Radiotherapy is the treatment of choice. Other treatment options include chemotherapy and surgery, especially in tumors that are highly radioresistant.

References

Crasto S, Duca S, Davini O, et al. MRI diagnosis of intramedullary metastases from extra-CNS tumors. *Eur Radiol*. 1997;7(5): 732-736.

Lee SS, Kim MK, Sym SJ, et al. Intramedullary spinal cord metastases: a single-institution experience. *J Neurooncol*. 2007;84(1):85-89.

Villegas AE, Guthrie TH. Intramedullary spinal cord metastasis in breast cancer: clinical features, diagnosis, and therapeutic consideration. *Breast J*. 2004;10(6):532-535.

Cross-Reference

Neuroradiology: THE REQUISITES, 4th ed, pp 527, 575.

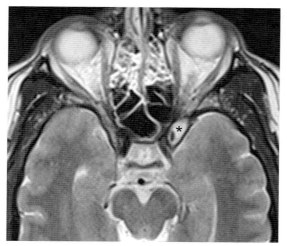

Figure 120-1

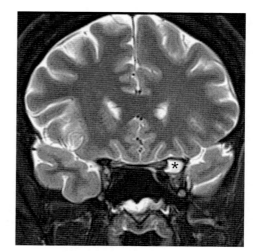

Figure 120-2

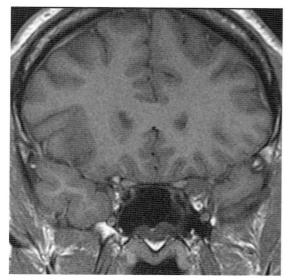

Figure 120-3

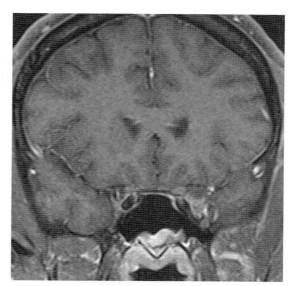

Figure 120-4

HISTORY: A 43-year-old with diplopia and chronic facial pain.

1. What is the single best diagnosis of this case?
   A. Mucus retention cyst
   B. Mucocele
   C. Paranasal sinus neoplasm
   D. Intracranial lipoma

2. What is most vulnerable to injury by processes involving the structure denoted by the asterisk?
   A. Trochlear nerve
   B. Internal carotid artery
   C. Optic nerve
   D. Trigeminal nerve

3. What is the most accurate definition of a commonly used eponym, "Onodi" cell?
   A. An infraorbital ethmoidal air cell
   B. A sphenoethmoidal air cell, superior to the sphenoid sinus proper
   C. Pneumatization of the anterior clinoid process
   D. A large lateral recess of the sphenoid sinus

4. Mucoceles occur *least* often in what paranasal sinus?
   A. Maxillary sinus
   B. Frontal sinus
   C. Ethmoid sinus
   D. Sphenoid sinus

CASE 120

Anterior Clinoiditis and Mucocele Formation Complicating Sinusitis

1. **B.** Mucocele. This is a case of an infected mucocele in the pneumatized anterior clinoid process, resulting in anterior clinoiditis.

2. **C.** Optic nerve. The optic nerve and the abducens nerves are most often affected by inflammation or tumor involving the anterior clinoid process.

3. **B.** A sphenoethmoidal air cell, superior to the sphenoid sinus proper. These are identified best on coronal and sagittal imaging planes as a horizontal septation within the sphenoid. The more superior air cells are ethmoid, and the inferior are sphenoid.

4. **A.** Maxillary sinus. Mucoceles are least common in the maxillary sinus. Mucoceles occur most commonly in the frontal or ethmoidal sinuses, followed by the sphenoid sinus.

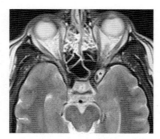

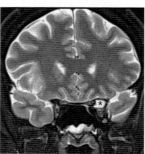

Comment

Imaging

These images show expansion of the left anterior clinoid process with material that is hyperintense on T2-weighted images (Figures 120-1 and 120-2) as well as T2-FLAIR (fluid-attenuated inversion recovery) images (not shown), consistent with proteinaceous or inspissated material. This demonstrates rim enhancement (Figure 120-4). The optic canal is mildly attenuated from the clinoid expansion. There is swelling in the orbital apex seen on the coronal images (Figures 120-2 through 120-4). The bony integrity along the medial margin of the left anterior clinoid or lateral margin of the optic canal cannot be assessed, and correlation with computed tomography (CT) is necessary.

The greater and lesser wings of the sphenoid bone form the floor and the roof of the orbital apex, respectively. When these structures become pneumatized in the course of normal development, like the paranasal sinuses, they may be affected by obstructive inflammatory disease and mucocele formation.

Mucocele versus Mucus Retention Cyst

A mucocele represents chronic expansion with mucoid secretions of a sinus or previously aerated bone lined by respiratory epithelium secondary to obstruction of the sinus ostium. Often the sinus is expanded, as in this case. Mucus retention cysts, commonly confused for mucoceles, are caused by obstruction of a seromucous gland, often not filling the sinus in which they are found. These are commonly found in the maxillary sinuses.

Mucoceles are uncommon in the posterior ethmoid and sphenoid sinuses but, when present, can manifest with signs and symptoms referable to cranial nerves II to VI. Vision loss, visual field defects, extraocular muscle palsies, and sensory deficits of the trigeminal nerve can occur. This patient presented with diplopia and chronic facial pain.

Onodi Cells

An Onodi cell is a posterior ethmoidal air cell, better termed a sphenoethmoidal air cell, that penetrates the sphenoid bone. The prevalence of sphenoethmoidal cells on CT studies varies from 8% to 13%. These are identified best on coronal and sagittal imaging planes as a horizontal septation within the sphenoid. The more superior air cells are ethmoid, and the inferior are sphenoid.

Pneumatization of the Anterior Clinoid Processes

The bones forming the orbital apex and anterior clinoid process may be aerated either by a sphenoethmoidal cell or by the sphenoid sinus proper.

In a patient with signs and symptoms referable to the orbital apex, a mucocele of a paranasal sinus should be considered in the differential diagnosis.

Reference

Lim CC, Dillon WP, McDermott MW. Mucocele involving the anterior clinoid process: MR and CT findings. *Am J Neuroradiol.* 1999;20: 287-290.

Cross-Reference

Neuroradiology: THE REQUISITES, 4th ed, p 427.

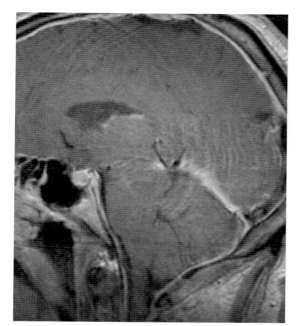

Figure 121-1

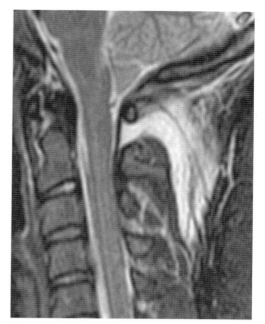

Figure 121-2

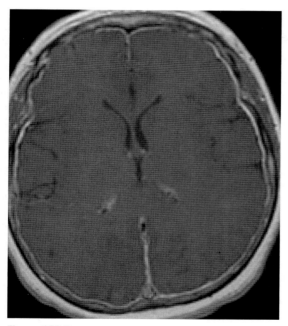

Figure 121-3

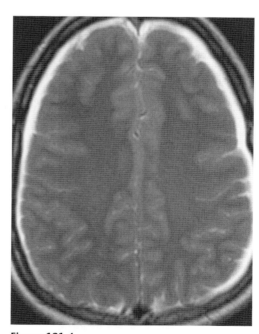

Figure 121-4

HISTORY: A 25-year-old woman with 4 months' duration of postural headaches.

1. What is the single best diagnosis in this case?
   A. Meningitis
   B. Intracranial hypotension
   C. Idiopathic intracranial hypertension
   D. Dandy-Walker variant

2. What is the mechanism of pachymeningeal enhancement in patients with this entity?
   A. Enlargement of the epidural space
   B. Dural thickening
   C. Dural inflammation
   D. Subdural hemorrhage

3. What is the next best step in imaging management for this patient?
   A. Contrast-enhanced computed tomography (CT) of the brain
   B. Myelogram and postmyelogram CT
   C. Magnetic resonance imaging (MRI) cine cerebrospinal fluid (CSF) flow study
   D. MRI of the lumbar spine

4. What is the best treatment option for this patient?
   A. Ventriculoperitoneal shunt placement
   B. Epidural blood patch
   C. Posterior fossa decompression
   D. Lumbar drain

CASE 121

Intracranial Hypotension

1. **B.** Intracranial hypotension. This constellation of findings—including subdural collections, downward sagging of the brain, and decreased CSF volume—is characteristic of intracranial hypotension. Although meningitis may be complicated by subdural collections, the constellation of findings is suggestive of a different diagnosis. There is no hypoplasia of the vermis. Idiopathic intracranial hypertension or pseudotumor cerebri manifests with increased fluid volume in the optic nerve sheaths and partially empty sella, which are not seen here.

2. **A.** Enlargement of the epidural space. The mechanism of pachymeningeal enhancement is low pressure resulting in enlargement of the epidural space. There is no thickening or inflammatory changes of the dura mater in intracranial hypotension. Subdural hemorrhage is not the underlying mechanism.

3. **B.** Myelogram and postmyelogram CT. In the absence of overshunting or skull base surgery or trauma, CSF hypotension is most commonly due to a spinal CSF leak. Myelography and postmyelography CT scan can be used to localize a leak. This study is commonly performed after, or in conjunction with, radionuclide cisternography to localize a leak.

4. **B.** Epidural blood patch. Epidural blood patch is commonly performed for treatment of spontaneous CSF leak refractory to conservative management (i.e., hydration, rest, and caffeine).

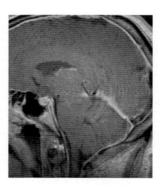

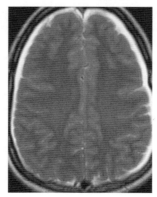

Comment

Presentation

The syndrome of intracranial hypotension is a single pathophysiologic entity of diverse origin. Usually, it is characterized by an orthostatic headache (a headache that occurs or worsens with upright posture), although patients with chronic headaches or even no headache have been described.

Pathophysiology

Most cases of intracranial hypotension result from a persistent CSF leak. This CSF leak most commonly occurs after dural puncture for a diagnostic lumbar puncture, myelography, or spinal anesthesia. In some cases, this syndrome may occur spontaneously. Evidence indicates that several of the abnormalities seen on imaging studies are the result of vascular dilation to compensate for reduced CSF volume.

Imaging

Imaging findings may be subtle and nonspecific such that, in the absence of providing a history of postural headaches, the diagnosis of intracranial hypotension is often overlooked. Imaging findings include sagging of the posterior fossa contents, with low-lying cerebellar tonsils, elongation of the fourth ventricle, engorgement of the dural venous sinuses, enlargement of the pituitary, bilateral subdural effusions, and diffuse dural enhancement (many of these findings are demonstrated in Figures 121-1 through 121-4). Intraspinal findings include collapse of the dural sac around the cord resulting in a paucity of CSF signal, a "festooned" appearance of the tethered dura mater, and dilation of the epidural venous plexus with marked enhancement on images after contrast agent administration. Another important finding is the C1-C2 sign, seen on MRI of the cervical spine as an area of fluid signal intensity between the spinous processes of C1 and C2 (see Figure 121-2). Visualization of this finding can lead to the diagnosis; however, this finding is not indicative of the leakage site.

Further Evaluation and Treatment

Symptoms of intracranial hypotension might resolve spontaneously; however, further work-up, including myelography and postmyelogram CT, may be necessary. MRI and nuclear scintigraphy may also play a role. If a source can be identified, an epidural blood patch can be performed and typically results in resolution of symptoms. Increasingly, prophylactic blood patches are being performed. Bed rest, intravenous caffeine, and theophylline are potential medical treatments.

References

Chiapparini L, Farina L, D'Incerti L, et al. Spinal radiological findings in nine patients with spontaneous intracranial hypotension. *Neuroradiology*. 2002;44(2):143-150, discussion 151-152.

Fishman RA, Dillon WP. Dural enhancement and cerebral displacement secondary to intracranial hypotension. *Neuroradiology*. 1993; 43:609-611.

Medina JH, Abrams K, Falcone S, et al. Spinal imaging findings in spontaneous intracranial hypotension. *AJR Am J Roentgenol*. 2010; 195(2):459-464.

Moayeri NN, Henson JW, Schaefer PW, Zervas NT. Spinal dural enhancement on magnetic resonance imaging associated with spontaneous intracranial hypotension. *J Neurosurg*. 1998;88: 912-918.

Cross-Reference

Neuroradiology: THE REQUISITES, 4th ed, pp 159-161.

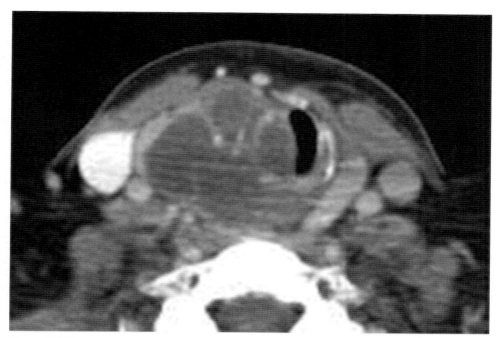

Figure 122-1

HISTORY: A 34-year-old patient presents with a 1-year history of voice changes.

1. Which of the following is the single best diagnosis?
   A. Chordoma
   B. Squamous cell carcinoma
   C. Chondrosarcoma
   D. Adenoid cystic carcinoma

2. What feature does *not* imply a higher grade of this lesion?
   A. Pain
   B. Size larger than 3 cm
   C. Rapid growth
   D. Enhancement

3. What part of the larynx is involved most commonly with chondroid tumors?
   A. Epiglottis
   B. Thyroid cartilage
   C. Arytenoid cartilage
   D. Cricoid cartilage

4. What cartilage is most commonly affected by squamous cell carcinoma?
   A. Epiglottis
   B. Thyroid cartilage
   C. Arytenoid cartilage
   D. Cricoid cartilage

CASE 122

Laryngeal Chondrosarcoma

1. **C.** Chondrosarcoma. This lesion is a submucosal mass, and therefore chondrosarcoma is the most likely diagnosis (although this lesion is without matrix). Lymphoma would also be on the differential (not an answer option). Because of the lack of mucosal mass, this is probably not squamous cell carcinoma or adenoid cystic carcinoma. Chordomas most commonly arise in the sacrococcygeal or spheno-occipital regions, less frequently in the vertebra, and almost never elsewhere.

2. **D.** Enhancement. Enhancement does *not* imply higher grade. Pain and rapid growth are signs of aggressiveness, hence higher grade. Larger size (>3 cm) is also a feature of higher grade.

3. **D.** Cricoid cartilage. The cricoid cartilage is involved in 70% of all laryngeal chondrosarcomas. The thyroid cartilage is second most commonly involved; the arytenoid cartilage is third most commonly involved; and the epiglottis is not usually involved.

4. **B.** Thyroid cartilage. The thyroid cartilage is most commonly affected by squamous cell carcinoma usually from a laryngeal or hypopharyngeal primary tumor. The epiglottis is second most commonly affected, by either oropharyngeal or laryngeal primary tumors. The arytenoid cartilage is third and the cricoid cartilage is fourth most commonly affected.

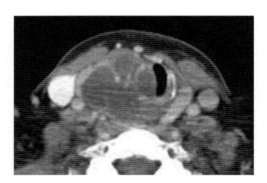

Comment

Implications of Chondrosarcomas

Squamous cell carcinoma is the dominant tumor of the larynx, but the most common sarcoma of the larynx is the chondrosarcoma. It may or may not have a chondroid matrix, and it is more a submucosal primary tumor (Figure 122-1). Although sarcomas usually have poor prognoses, chondrosarcomas of the cricoid cartilage are usually low-grade tumors that are not life-threatening. They metastasize infrequently and late in the course. The problem, of course, is that the voice cannot be preserved when these cricoid cartilage tumors are surgically removed. For this reason, these tumors are treated late in their course when all other treatment fails, including incomplete resection to preserve the airway, breathing, and voice.

Features of Aggressive Pathologic Processes

Features that suggest that such tumors are more aggressive and of higher grade are pain, rapid growth, and larger size. The grading system from I to III, first described by Evans, is based on mitotic rate, cellularity, and nuclear size. The most common symptom is dysphonia (hoarseness). Men are affected more than women by a 3:1 ratio.

Incidence

Chondrosarcomas are the second most common sarcoma overall after osteosarcoma. They may arise within benign chondromas and occur more commonly in syndromic conditions such as Ollier disease. The rate of 5-year survival is 70%.

Reference

Evans HL, Ayala AG, Romsdahl MM. Prognostic factors in chondrosarcoma of bone: a clinicopathologic analysis with emphasis on histologic grading. *Cancer.* 1977;40:818-831.

Policarpo M, Taranto F, Aina E, Aluffi PV, Pia F. Chondrosarcoma of the larynx: a case report. *Acta Otorhinolaryngol Ital.* 2008;28(1):38-41.

Cross-Reference

Neuroradiology: THE REQUISITES, 4th ed, pp 441, 474.

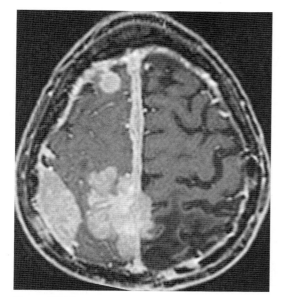

Figure 123-1

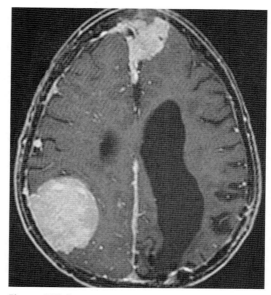

Figure 123-2

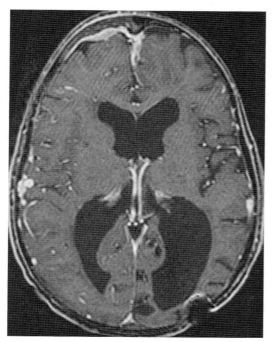

Figure 123-3

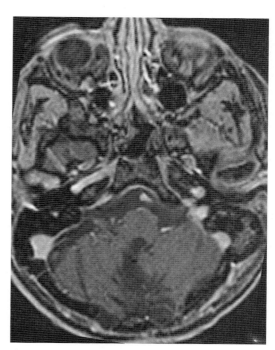

Figure 123-4

HISTORY: A 64-year-old woman with prior radiation therapy for childhood posterior fossa neoplasm.

1. What is the single best diagnosis in this case?
   A. Multiple meningiomas
   B. Metastases
   C. Neurosarcoidosis
   D. Leukemia

2. What percentage of these tumors are malignant?
   A. 0% to 10%
   B. 11% to 20%
   C. 21% to 30%
   D. 80% to 100%

3. Where are most intraventricular meningiomas located in adults?
   A. Third ventricle
   B. Fourth ventricle
   C. Frontal horn of lateral ventricle
   D. Atria of lateral ventricle

4. What non-neoplastic lesion is associated with whole-brain irradiation?
   A. Developmental venous anomaly
   B. Cavernous malformation
   C. Meningioma
   D. Cortical dysplasia

CASE 123

Multiple Meningiomas after Remote Whole-Brain Irradiation

1. **A.** Multiple meningiomas. These extra-axial enhancing lesions are found in this patient with the given history of whole-brain irradiation. Although dural metastases may look similar to meningiomas, they are an unlikely diagnosis given the appearance and the history. Sarcoid and lymphoma may have dural manifestations, but the extent and distribution as well as the given history make these less favored answers.

2. **A.** 0% to 10%. The percentage of meningiomas that are malignant is from 1% to 4%. Although meningiomas are more often found in women, malignant meningiomas are more often present in men.

3. **D.** Atria of the lateral ventricle. Intraventricular meningiomas in adults are most often found in the atria. In children, most intraventricular meningiomas are found in the fourth ventricle.

4. **B.** Cavernous malformation. Cavernous malformations are a slow-flow compact vascular malformation often induced in patients following whole-brain irradiation.

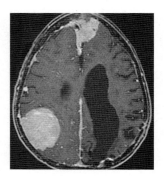

Comment

Balancing aggressive therapies that improve survival with efforts to decrease long-term side effects makes the treatment of brain tumors a major challenge in pediatric oncology. Pediatric brain tumors are a heterogeneous collection of lesions with 5-year survival rates ranging from 10% to 95%. Although standard care for most types of pediatric brain tumors continues to be surgery, often followed by radiation therapy with or without chemotherapy, there is increasing emphasis on trying to minimize the long-term effects of these treatments, such as cognitive deficits, as well as the risk of radiation-induced neoplasms.

Diagnostic Criteria

The criteria for diagnosis of radiation-induced meningiomas (tumors) are the following: a history of irradiation, tumors arising in a radiation field after a latency period of years, proof of histologic difference between the secondary tumor and the originally irradiated tumor, and no predisposition that could facilitate neoplastic growth. In the case of radiation-induced meningiomas, the patient cannot have other risk factors, such as neurofibromatosis type 2, that predispose to meningiomas. In this case, multiple extra-axial enhancing masses are demonstrated (Figures 123-1 through 123-3), and the patient had a fitting history with posttherapeutic findings of tumor resection (Figure 123-4).

Associations and Statistics

Meningiomas have been associated with low-dose irradiation treatment for tinea capitis and have a latency period of decades. Multiple meningiomas occur in up to 30% of patients with a remote history of radiation therapy and in 2% of nonirradiated patients with meningiomas. Recurrence rates are higher in radiation-induced tumors than in those occurring sporadically or in association with other entities, such as neurofibromatosis type 2. Radiation therapy induces up to five times as many meningiomas as it does sarcomas, schwannomas, or gliomas. The true risk of radiation-induced tumors is unknown.

Reference

Sadetzki S, Flint-Richter P, Ben-Thal T, Nass D. Radiation-induced meningiomas: a descriptive study of 253 cases. *J Neurosurg.* 2002;97:1078-1082.

Cross-Reference

Neuroradiology: THE REQUISITES, 4th ed, pp 42, 83-85.

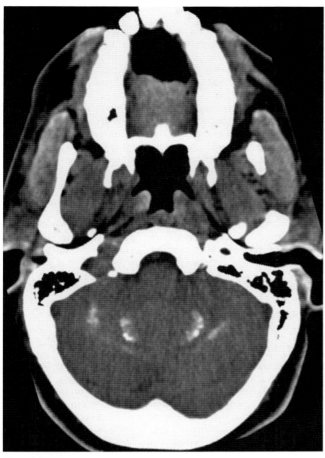

Figure 124-1

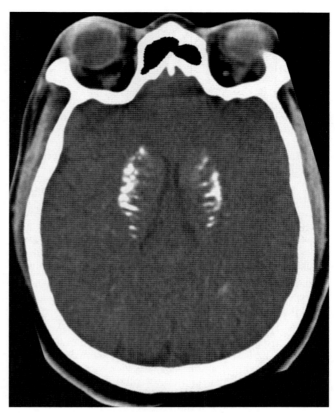

Figure 124-2

HISTORY: A 56-year-old man with progressive dementia and parkinsonism.

1. What is the single most likely diagnosis of this case?
   A. Physiologic basal ganglia calcifications
   B. Toxoplasmosis
   C. Fahr disease
   D. Down syndrome

2. What congenital infection is typically and most often associated with periventricular calcification?
   A. Toxoplasmosis
   B. Rubella
   C. Cytomegalovirus
   D. Herpes simplex virus

3. What location on imaging is most often affected by carbon monoxide poisoning?
   A. Putamen
   B. Globus pallidus
   C. Caudate
   D. Thalamus

4. What artery is implicated in infarcts involving the paramedian bilateral thalamus and/or bilateral paramedian midbrain?
   A. Adamkiewicz
   B. Percheron
   C. Heubner
   D. Wilkie

CASE 124

Fahr Disease (Familial Cerebrovascular Ferrocalcinosis)

1. **C.** Fahr disease. The clinical scenario of a patient with dementia and parkinsonism with extensive basal ganglia, thalamic, and dentate calcifications is most likely Fahr disease. Toxoplasmosis is often not limited to these locations and is often asymmetric. Calcifications may occur with normal aging and in Down syndrome, but this pattern is not likely.

2. **C.** Cytomegalovirus. This is the TORCH (*t*oxoplasmosis, *o*ther infections, *r*ubella, *c*ytomegalovirus, and *h*erpes simplex virus) infection typically associated with periventricular calcifications. Approximately 50% of patients have periventricular or parenchymal calcifications. Toxoplasmosis, rubella, and herpes simplex virus may also, although less characteristically, result in periventricular calcifications.

3. **B.** Globus pallidus. The globus pallidus is typically T2 hyperintense and demonstrates restricted diffusion acutely. Hemorrhage and necrosis are later findings.

4. **B.** Percheron. The artery of Percheron is the eponymous single trunk vessel arising from the P1 segment of a posterior cerebral artery which gives rise to paramedian thalamic and midbrain perforators. Adamkiewicz is an anterior spinal artery, and Heubner supplies the caudate head arising from the distal A1 or proximal A2 segments of the anterior cerebral artery. Wilkie is a supraduodenal artery.

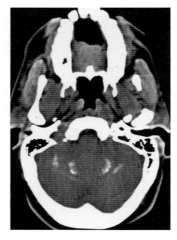

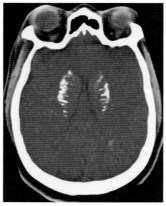

Comment

This case shows bilateral symmetric calcification within the dentate nuclei of the cerebellum (Figure 124-1) and in the basal ganglia (including the caudate and lentiform nuclei) (Figure 124-2) in a patient with progressive dementia. Mineral deposition is often noted to be hyperintense on unenhanced T1-weighted imaging.

Fahr disease represents a relatively uncommon spectrum of neurologic disorders characterized by extensive abnormal calcium deposition in characteristic locations, such as the bilateral basal ganglia, with associated cell loss. Calcification may also be seen in the dentate nuclei (as in this case), as well as within the white matter, including the centrum semiovale, corona radiata, and subcortical white matter.

Presentation

This condition has been referred to as idiopathic basal ganglia calcification. Variable neurologic manifestations, including movement disorders such as athetosis (slow, involuntary movements), and chorea, dementia, and psychological impairment, occur.

Familial patterns of Fahr disease have been commonly noted in the literature. Transmission may be as an autosomal recessive trait, or it can occur in large affected families as an autosomal dominant inheritance pattern.

Differential Diagnosis

The differential diagnosis of calcification within the deep gray matter of the cerebral hemispheres, particularly the basal ganglia, is extensive. Probably the most common cause is idiopathic. Calcification in the globus pallidus bilaterally may be noted as a normal finding, representing senescent calcification that occurs with advancing age. Hypoparathyroidism and a variety of endocrine disorders, including abnormalities in phosphate and calcium metabolism, can result in calcification in these locations. Symptomatic patients might respond to correction of serum calcium phosphate abnormalities. Another common cause of calcium deposition is in the postinflammatory setting. Specifically, calcification may be seen in infections, such as in utero cytomegalovirus exposure, tuberculosis, and cysticercosis, although in these instances, the pattern of calcification is not similar to that seen in Fahr disease. In recent years, calcification within the basal ganglia has been described in patients with in utero human immunodeficiency virus infection. Some experts believe that, in general, Fahr disease may be the result of in utero infections.

References

Holland BA, Kucharcyzk W, Brant-Zawadzki M, et al. MR imaging of calcified intracranial lesions. *Radiology*. 1985;157:353-356.
Scotti G, Scialfa G, Tampieri D, Landoni L. MR imaging in Fahr disease. *J Comput Assist Tomogr*. 1985;9:790-792.

Cross-Reference

Neuroradiology: THE REQUISITES, 4th ed, p 251.

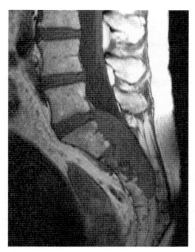

Figure 125-1

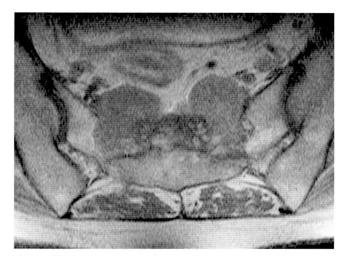

Figure 125-2

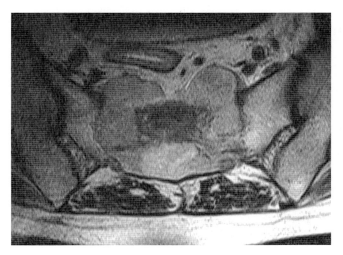

Figure 125-3

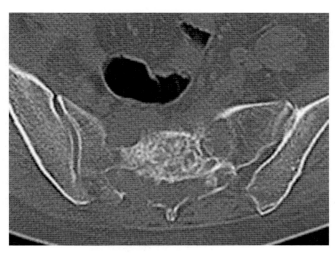

Figure 125-4

HISTORY: A 51-year-old woman with low back pain for the past 2 years presents with cauda equina syndrome.

1. Which is the *least* likely in the following differential diagnosis?
   A. Langerhans cell histiocytosis
   B. Chondrosarcoma
   C. Lymphoma
   D. Chordoma

2. What percentage of these tumors originate in the sacrococcygeal region?
   A. 65% to 75%
   B. 45% to 55%
   C. 25% to 35%
   D. 5% to 15%

3. Which of the following statements regarding sacral chordomas is true?
   A. Sacral chordomas are typically midline in location.
   B. Sacral chordomas usually extend posteriorly.
   C. Most sacral chordomas invade the rectum.
   D. Sacral chordomas are more common in women than in men.

4. Which joint is most commonly invaded by sacral chordoma?
   A. Facet joint
   B. Femoral joint
   C. Sacroiliac joint
   D. Discovertebral joint

CASE 125

Sacral Chordoma

1. **A.** Langerhans cell histiocytosis. Sarcoma, lymphoma, and chordoma can all involve the sacrum, all have paraspinal masses, and all have soft tissue components. The findings in this case are typical of a destructive neoplasm but are nonspecific. Sacral chordoma is typically midline in location and can involve the bone and have paraspinal and epidural extension.

2. **B.** 45% to 55%. Sacrococcygeal region involvement is seen in 50% of all chordomas. The clivus is involved in 35% and the spine in 15%.

3. **A.** Sacral chordomas are typically midline in location. Sacral chordomas usually extend anteriorly rather than posteriorly and may compress or invade the lower sacral nerves. Most sacral chordomas displace rather than invade the rectum. Sacral chordomas occur almost twice as frequently in men compared with women.

4. **C.** Sacroiliac joint. The sacroiliac joint is the most frequently involved, followed by the disc spaces.

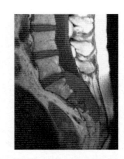

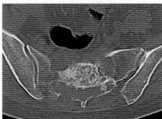

Comment

Background

Chordomas can occur at any age, but they are uncommon in patients younger than 40 years of age. Chordomas are typically slow growing but are locally aggressive. Metastasis is usually a late event and occurs in about one fourth of patients. The presenting symptom in most patients is local pain. Approximately one third of patients also have radiculopathy as a result of irritation of the sciatic nerve. Gluteal muscle infiltration secondary to lateral extension of tumor is common in sacral chordomas.

Histopathology

Because they originate from notochord remnants, chordomas may involve any segment of the craniospinal axis from the sphenoid to the coccyx. Two types are distinguished histopathologically: typical chordomas, which have a watery, gelatinous matrix, and chondroid chordomas, in which this matrix is replaced by cartilaginous foci.

Imaging

Magnetic resonance imaging (MRI) and computed tomography (CT) have complementary roles in evaluating chordomas. On MRI, chordomas are lobulated masses (Figures 125-1 through 125-3) and are typically low to intermediate in signal on T1-weighted images (see Figure 125-1) and heterogeneous in signal on T2-weighted images (see Figure 125-3). Enhancement is heterogeneous (see Figure 125-2). CT is helpful in assessing the degree of bone involvement and destruction (Figure 125-4) and in detecting a pattern of calcification within the lesion.

Management

Sacral chordomas are relatively resistant to radiation and chemotherapy. Radical resection is associated with a significantly longer disease-free interval compared with subtotal removal of the tumor. Radiation therapy after subtotal resection improves the disease-free interval.

References

Sung MS, Lee GK, Kang HS, et al. Sacrococcygeal chordoma: MR imaging in 30 patients. *Skeletal Radiol.* 2005;34(2):87-94.

York JE, Kaczaraj A, Abi-Said D, et al. Sacral chordoma: 40-year experience at a major cancer center. *Neurosurgery.* 1999;44(1):74-79, discussion 79-80.

Cross-Reference

Neuroradiology: THE REQUISITES, 4th ed, p 586.

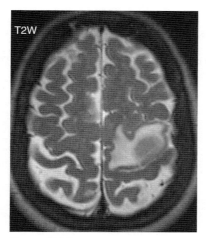

Figure 126-1

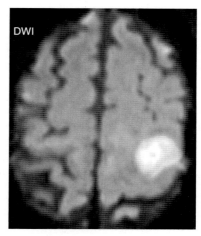

Figure 126-2

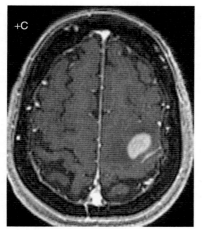

Figure 126-3

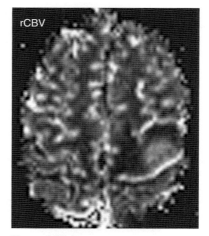

Figure 126-4

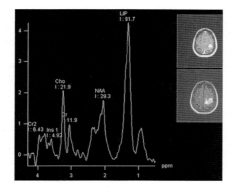

Figure 126-5

HISTORY: A 62-year-old man with right-sided weakness.

1. What is the single best diagnosis in this case?
   A. Metastatic disease
   B. Glioblastoma
   C. Central nervous system (CNS) lymphoma
   D. Abscess

2. What conditions predispose a patient to the development of primary CNS lymphoma?
   A. Prior radiation
   B. Immunocompetence
   C. Immunosuppression
   D. Diabetes

3. Why does this mass have restricted diffusion?
   A. Free water movement
   B. Low cellularity
   C. Dense cellularity
   D. High vascularity

4. What is the approximate resonance peak of glutamate/glutamine?
   A. 1.2 to 1.4 ppm
   B. 2.2 to 2.4 ppm
   C. 3.0 ppm
   D. 3.2 ppm

CASE 126

Central Nervous System Lymphoma in an Immunocompetent Patient

1. **C.** CNS lymphoma. CNS lymphoma is the best diagnosis in this case. This is a solid enhancing mass with restricted diffusion and elevated perfusion. The spectrum supports neoplasm.

2. **C.** Immunosuppression. Immunosuppression (particularly in patients with HIV infection) and immunosuppressive therapy for the treatment of cancer or after organ transplantation predispose a patient to the development of primary CNS lymphoma.

3. **C.** Dense cellularity. Lymphoma is a highly cellular mass with decreased extracellular spaces. There is restricted free water diffusion in these lesions.

4. **B.** 2.2 to 2.4 ppm. The glutamate/glutamine peak is at this level on 3.0-T magnetic resonance (MR) spectroscopy, myoinositol is at 3.3, choline is at 3.2, creatine is at 3.0, *N*-acetyl-aspartate is at 2.0, and lactate/lipid is at 1.3.

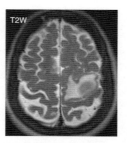

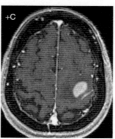

Comment

Primary CNS lymphoma is uncommon, but its incidence has increased significantly over the past decade as a result of its relatively common occurrence in patients with AIDS (affecting approximately 6%).

Histology

The origin of lymphoma is unknown because the CNS does not have lymphoid tissue. It has been postulated that CNS lymphoma arises from microglial cells. Histologic evaluation of primary CNS lymphoma almost always shows intermediate- to high-grade extranodal non-Hodgkin lymphoma of B-cell origin.

It is most commonly seen in immunocompromised patients, but it has been increasingly recognized in immunocompetent patients. It usually occurs in the sixth and seventh decades of life.

Common Locations of Involvement

The supratentorial compartment is most commonly involved, although involvement of the brainstem and cerebellum is not rare. The most common imaging presentation of primary CNS lymphoma is multiple masses. Focal masses in the basal ganglia, thalami, and periventricular white matter are common. Alternatively, patients present with a single mass with vasogenic edema, as in this case, in which a mass in the left precentral gyrus is seen (Figure 126-1).

Imaging

Conventional MR imaging, on a 3.0-T unit in this case, shows features that favor lymphoma, including restricted diffusion (Figure 126-2) and solid homogeneous enhancement (Figure 126-3). Advanced MR imaging shows moderate elevation in relative cerebral blood volume on the perfusion study (Figure 126-4). Spectroscopy (Figure 126-5) shows an elevated choline-to-creatine ratio, consistent with neoplasm, and decreased *N*-acetylaspartate. There is also marked elevation in the lipid and lactate peaks that have been described with lymphoma.

Although CNS lymphoma typically enhances solidly and avidly, in the setting of AIDS and other forms of immunosuppression, there is a spectrum of patterns of pathologic enhancement, ranging from solid to ringlike. The patient in this case is not immunocompromised. The T2-weighted signal intensity characteristics may be quite variable, ranging from hyperintensity to marked hypointensity (isointense to brain) in cases of very cellular neoplasms. Hemorrhage is uncommon in lymphomatous masses.

References

Erdag N, Bhorade RM, Alberico RA, et al. Primary lymphoma of the central nervous system: typical and atypical CT and MR imaging appearances. *AJR Am J Roentgenol.* 2001;176:1319-1326.

Lai R, Rosenblum MK, DeAngelis LM. Primary CNS lymphoma: a whole-brain disease? *Neurology.* 2002;59:1557-1562.

Vazquez E, Lucaya J, Castellote A, et al. Neuroimaging in pediatric leukemia and lymphoma: differential diagnosis. *Radiographics.* 2002;22:1411-1428.

Cross-Reference

Neuroradiology: THE REQUISITES, 4th ed, pp 74-76, 189-190.

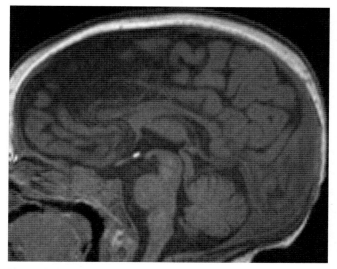

Figure 127-1

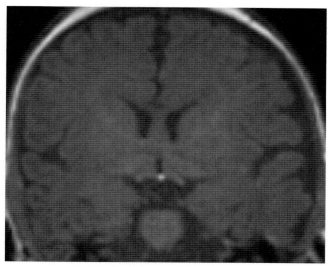

Figure 127-2

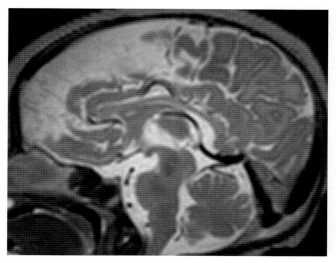

Figure 127-3

HISTORY: A 12-year-old with short stature.

1. What is the single best diagnosis of this case?
   A. Ectopic posterior pituitary
   B. Intracranial lipoma
   C. Pituitary hemorrhage
   D. Hamartoma

2. What is responsible for intrinsic T1 hyperintensity in the neurohypophysis?
   A. Blood
   B. Melanin
   C. Neuropeptides and lipids
   D. Dietary iodine

3. What structure is not visualized?
   A. Optic nerve
   B. Anterior pituitary
   C. Mammillary body
   D. Infundibulum

4. What structure regulates pituitary endocrine function?
   A. Thalamus
   B. Hypothalamus
   C. Globus pallidus
   D. Putamen

CASE 127

Ectopic Posterior Pituitary and Nonvisualization of the Infundibulum: Hypopituitarism

1. **A.** Ectopic posterior pituitary. The normal T1 hyperintense neurohypophysis is not within the sella turcica and there is absence of the infundibulum.

2. **C.** Neuropeptides and lipids. This hyperintensity has been attributed to lipids within pituicytes, the arginine vasopressin neurophysin complex, or phospholipids within the walls of the secretory vesicles containing the arginine vasopressin neurophysin complex.

3. **D.** Infundibulum. This is most evident on the coronal T1 sequence (Figure 127-2). The structures mentioned in the other answer options are present.

4. **B.** Hypothalamus. The hypothalamus regulates pituitary endocrine function.

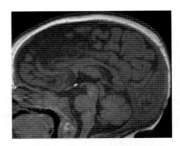

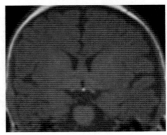

Comment

Structural Considerations

The posterior pituitary develops from the neuroectoderm of the diencephalon. Pituitary gland function is controlled by the hypothalamus via the infundibular stalk. Nerve fibers from nuclei in the hypothalamus course into the infundibulum to reach the posterior pituitary gland. Normally, the anterior pituitary gland and the pituitary stalk are well defined. The posterior pituitary is usually identified as a hyperintense focus on T1-weighted magnetic resonance (MR) images (Figures 127-1 and 127-2). This hyperintensity has been attributed to lipids within pituicytes, the arginine vasopressin neurophysin complex, or phospholipids within the walls of the secretory vesicles containing the arginine vasopressin neurophysin complex.

Cause

An ectopic posterior pituitary gland can result from aberrant neuronal migration during embryogenesis, transection of the pituitary, or an insult to the pituitary stalk resulting from ischemia, anoxia, or compression leading to reorganization of the proximal neurons of the neurohypophysis. Breech delivery and perinatal anoxia have been associated with transection of the pituitary stalk and hypopituitarism. However, many patients with hypopituitarism and ectopic posterior pituitary have uncomplicated perinatal courses.

Hormone Deficiencies

Growth hormone deficiency is a common cause of short stature. It may be idiopathic or acquired (tumors, instrumentation of the sellar region). Idiopathic growth hormone deficiency can occur in isolation or in association with other anterior pituitary hormone deficiencies. An ectopic posterior pituitary and nonvisualization of the stalk on MR imaging is associated with decreased function of the anterior pituitary (hypopituitarism). Posterior pituitary hormone deficiency in the presence of an ectopic posterior pituitary is uncommon, suggesting that this ectopic tissue functions normally to produce antidiuretic hormone. Nonvisualization of the pituitary stalk alone on MR imaging (Figure 127-3) is associated with anterior pituitary hormone deficiencies limited to growth hormone and thyrotropin.

References

Hamilton J, Blaser S, Daneman D. MR imaging in idiopathic growth hormone deficiency. *Am J Neuroradiol.* 1998;19:1609-1615.
Takahashi T, Miki Y, Takahashi JA, et al. Ectopic posterior pituitary high signal in preoperative and postoperative macroadenomas: dynamic MR imaging. *Eur J Radiol.* 2005;55:84-91.

Cross-Reference

Neuroradiology: THE REQUISITES, 4th ed, pp 350-353.

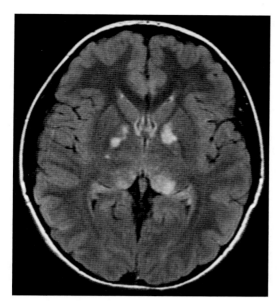

Figure 128-1

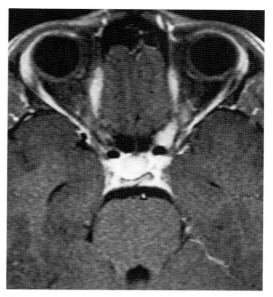

Figure 128-2

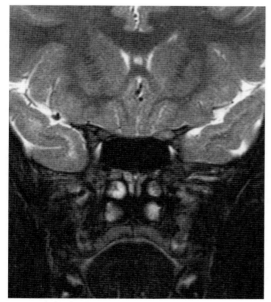

Figure 128-3

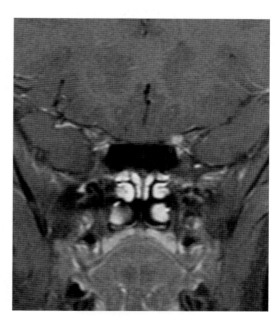

Figure 128-4

HISTORY: An 11-year-old with a pelvic mass.

1. What is the single best diagnosis of this case?
   A. Neurofibromatosis type 2
   B. Neurofibromatosis type 1
   C. Hypothalamic hamartomas
   D. Pituitary adenoma

2. Which of the following is a diagnostic criterion for this disease?
   A. More than two café-au-lait spots by age 10
   B. More than two plexiform neurofibromas
   C. One iris hamartoma
   D. Axillary or inguinal freckling

3. Regarding focal areas of signal abnormality in the brain parenchyma, which of the following is the most correct statement?
   A. These lesions are premalignant.
   B. These lesions are areas of ischemia.
   C. These lesions may regress spontaneously.
   D. These lesions enhance with contrast.

4. What chromosome has a mutation in this disease?
   A. Chromosome 22
   B. Chromosome 13
   C. Chromosome 17
   D. Chromosome 5

CASE 128

Neurofibromatosis Type 1: Pilocytic Astrocytoma of the Optic Pathway

1. **B.** Neurofibromatosis type 1. There are nonspecific foci of signal abnormality in the basal ganglia and thalami, and there is an enhancing left optic nerve glioma.

2. **D.** Axillary or inguinal freckling. Neurofibromatosis type 1 can be diagnosed when two or more of the following criteria are present: a first-degree relative with neurofibromatosis type 1, one plexiform neurofibroma or two or more neurofibromas of any type, six or more café-au-lait spots in 1 year, two or more Lisch nodules (iris hamartomas), axillary or inguinal freckling, optic pathway glioma, and a characteristic bone abnormality.

3. **C.** These lesions may regress spontaneously. Limited tissue specimens have confirmed many of these to represent spongiotic change or vacuolization. Serial T2-weighted imaging shows regression in both the number and size of lesions over a 2- to 3-year period.

4. **C.** Chromosome 17. Neurofibromatosis type 1 is caused by a mutation of chromosome 17 with locus at 17q11.2, which affects the protein neurofibromin, a tumor suppressor gene.

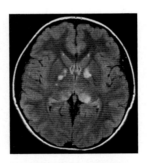

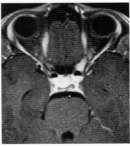

Comment

Diagnosis

Neurofibromatosis type 1 (von Recklinghausen disease) is a neurocutaneous disorder. It is the most common phakomatosis and is caused by a mutation of chromosome 17 with locus at 17q11.2, which affects the protein neurofibromin, a tumor suppressor gene. In one half of cases, this mutation is transmitted in an autosomal dominant pattern; in the other half, it is sporadic. Neurofibromatosis type 1 can be diagnosed when two or more of the following criteria are present: a first-degree relative with neurofibromatosis type 1, one plexiform neurofibroma or two or more neurofibromas of any type, six or more café-au-lait spots in 1 year, two or more Lisch nodules (iris hamartomas), axillary or inguinal freckling, optic pathway glioma, and a characteristic bone abnormality (dysplasia of the greater wing of the sphenoid, overgrowth of a digit or limb, pseudarthrosis, lateral thoracic meningocele, or dural ectasia with vertebral dysplasia).

The most common central nervous system tumor in neurofibromatosis type 1 is a low-grade optic nerve pilocytic glioma, reported in 15% to 28% of patients and demonstrated on the left in this case. Growth along the optic tract, the lateral geniculate, and the optic radiations can occur. Magnetic resonance imaging is the best choice for assessing the extent of these tumors.

Imaging

In this case, there are non-enhancing T2 hyperintense lesions in the basal ganglia and thalami (Figure 128-1). Neurofibromatosis type 1 may be associated with non-neoplastic hyperintense lesions on T2-weighted sequences within the basal ganglia, cerebellar peduncles, dentate nuclei, brainstem, and white matter and may be present in up to 60% of patients, especially in the pediatric age group. Mass effect is predominantly associated with lesions in the brainstem, thalamus, and cerebellar peduncles. Limited tissue specimens have confirmed many of these to represent spongiotic change or vacuolization. Serial T2-weighted imaging shows regression in both the number and size of lesions over a 2- to 3-year period. In this case, there is also enlargement and enhancement of the canalicular segment of the left optic nerve consistent with an optic pathway glioma (Figures 128-2 through 128-4). The clinical history of a pelvis mass is suggestive of a plexiform neurofibroma.

Associated Neoplasms

Neoplasms seen with increased incidence in neurofibromatosis type 1 include neurofibrosarcoma (malignant degeneration of a neurofibroma), seen in up to 5% of patients; leukemia; lymphoma; medullary thyroid carcinoma; pheochromocytoma; melanoma; and Wilms tumor.

References

DiMario FJ, Ramsby G. Magnetic resonance imaging lesion analysis in neurofibromatosis type 1. *Arch Neurol*. 1998;55:500-505.

Thiagalingam S, Flaherty M, Billson F, North K. Neurofibromatosis type 1 and optic pathway gliomas: follow-up of 54 patients. *Ophthalmology*. 2004;111:568-577.

Cross-Reference

Neuroradiology: THE REQUISITES, 4th ed, pp 291-293, 327.

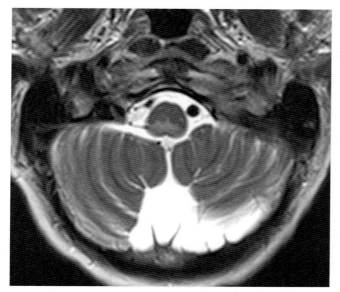

Figure 129-1

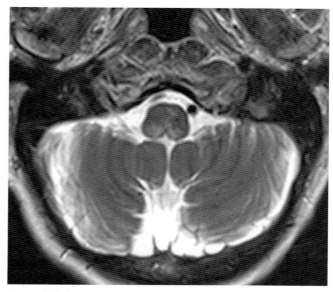

Figure 129-2

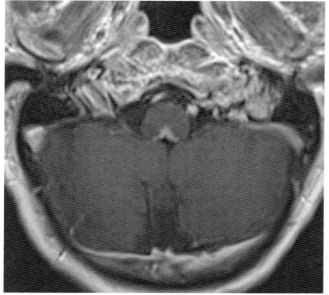

Figure 129-3

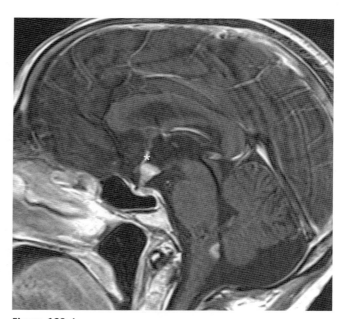

Figure 129-4

HISTORY: A 52-year-old male with emesis.

1. What area of the brainstem is involved with this entity?
   A. Pons
   B. Midbrain tectum
   C. Area postrema
   D. Medullary olives

2. What structure does the asterisk in Figure 129-4 indicate?
   A. Optic chiasm
   B. Infundibulum
   C. Lamina terminalis
   D. Hypothalamus

3. Considering the imaging findings, what is likely part of the patient's clinical presentation?
   A. Diabetes insipidus
   B. Ataxia
   C. Urinary incontinence
   D. Impaired speech

4. What non-primary central nervous system (CNS) malignancy most commonly seeds the cerebrospinal fluid (CSF) spaces in adults and happens to be the diagnosis in this case?
   A. Invasive ductal carcinoma of the breast
   B. Melanoma
   C. Prostate carcinoma
   D. Lymphoma/leukemia

CASE 129

Lymphoma Involving the Circumventricular Organs

1. **C.** Area postrema. The dorsal medulla at the level of the fourth ventricle outflow pathways is the location of the area postrema. It is located in the lateral reticular formation of the medulla oblongata.

2. **C.** Lamina terminalis. The asterisk in Figure 129-4 is overlying the lamina terminalis or the ventral margin of the third ventricle.

3. **A.** Diabetes insipidus. There is nodular enhancement and thickening of the infundibulum and infundibular recess of the third ventricle, which may result in disruption of the hypothalamic-hypophyseal communication.

4. **D.** Lymphoma/leukemia. This patient has lymphoma affecting the circumventricular organs. Lymphoma and leukemia are the most common non-primary CNS malignancies to result in subarachnoid seeding.

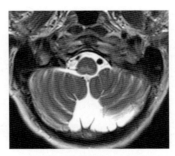

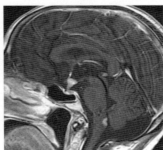

Comment

Imaging

This case shows abnormal T2-weighted signal intensity involving the posterior medulla in the region of the area postrema (Figures 129-1 and 129-2), with avid enhancement along the surface of the medulla (Figure 129-3). There is also an avidly enhancing mass along the hypothalamus and infundibulum (Figure 129-4). The imaging findings are not specific for a particular disease entity. Correlation with the patient's clinical history is essential.

Differential Diagnosis

Differential considerations include inflammatory disorders, such as sarcoidosis, and infectious causes, such as tuberculosis. Neoplastic conditions, such as lymphoma, and carcinomatosis from a systemic cancer, such as breast or lung carcinoma, must also be strongly considered.

Circumventricular Organs

Circumventricular organs, such as the area postrema and the lamina terminalis, play critical roles as transducers of information among the blood, the neurons, and the CSF. They permit both release and sensing of hormones without disrupting the blood-brain barrier and hence participate in the regulatory control of multiple physiologic functions. They have a documented role in the control of cardiovascular function, the regulation of body fluids, the mediation of the central immune response, and in aspects of reproductive function. The area postrema is the part of the brainstem that controls vomiting. It is located in the lateral reticular formation of the medulla oblongata. It is a circumventricular organ that detects toxins in the blood and, when necessary, induces vomiting. It connects to the nucleus of the solitary tract as well as other autonomic control centers in the brainstem. It is stimulated by visceral afferent sympathetic and vagal impulses arising from peripheral trigger areas, such as the gastrointestinal tract.

References

Danchaivijitr N, Hesselink JR, Aryan HE, Herndier B. Cerebello-pontine angle (CPA) lymphoma with perineural extension into the middle fossa: case report. *Surg Neurol.* 2004;62:80-85.

Nozaki M, Tada M, Mizugaki Y, et al. Expression of oncogenic molecules in primary central nervous system lymphomas in immunocompetent patients. *Acta Neuropathol.* 1998;95:505-510.

Cross-Reference

Neuroradiology: THE REQUISITES, 4th ed, pp 74-76.

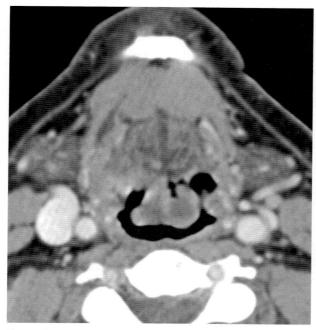

Figure 130-1

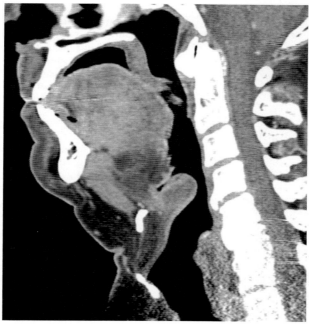

Figure 130-2

HISTORY: A young adult has fever, difficulty swallowing, and drooling.

1. Which of the following is the single best diagnosis?
   A. Croup
   B. Supraglottitis
   C. Tonsillitis
   D. Peritonsillar abscess

2. What is the stereotypical organism associated with epiglottitis in children?
   A. Adenovirus
   B. *Staphylococcus*
   C. *Streptococcus*
   D. *Haemophilus influenza*

3. What is one clinical or imaging sign of this disease suggesting the need for immediate airway support?
   A. Severe pain
   B. Lymphadenopathy
   C. Torticollis
   D. Diabetes mellitus

4. Why is computed tomography (CT) not used to diagnose acute epiglottitis in children?
   A. Airway compromise is possible during CT.
   B. Plain radiographs with the patient supine are just as efficacious as CT and deliver less radiation.
   C. The radiation dosage is too high with CT.
   D. Reactions to contrast are more severe in atopic patients.

CASE 130

Supraglottitis

1. **B.** Supraglottis. The epiglottis, which is part of the supraglottis, is swollen. The tonsil is not affected, and no abscess is present. Pain and dysphagia are uncommon in croup.

2. **D.** *Haemophilus influenzae*. *H. influenzae* is the organism stereotypically associated with this diagnosis in children, although infection with this organism has become less frequent because of immunizations. Streptococci are the most common pathogens in adults.

3. **D.** Diabetes mellitus. Signs that suggest a need for immediate airway support include drooling, diabetes mellitus, shorter onset of symptoms, epiglottic abscess, severe swelling of the epiglottis, and arytenoid swelling.

4. **A.** Airway compromise is possible during CT. CT should not be used to diagnose supraglottitis in children because of the risk of airway compromise. In pediatric patients, the inflamed airway can close when they are supine. In adults, the airway is wider with less lymphoid tissue therefore; airway compromise is less of a concern in adults.

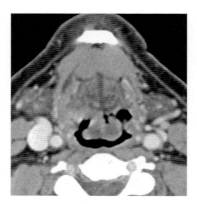

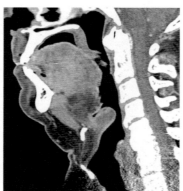

Comment

Background

Supraglottitis is reemerging in adults, possibly because of the acquired immunodeficiency syndrome (AIDS) epidemic. It is a more indolent infection in adults than pediatric epiglottitis because adults can tolerate more supraglottic and prevertebral swelling than children can. Epiglottitis occurs most commonly in the winter and has a bimodal age distribution of ages 0 to 8 years and 20 to 40 years. Vaccinations for *H. influenzae* type B have reduced the number of cases with that as a pathogen. Adults have more strep infections.

Signs and Symptoms

Fever, drooling, sore throat, dysphagia, stridor, and tachypnea are common in children. Most adult patients with epiglottitis have sore throat, odynophagia, and malaise. The diagnosis may be made by plain radiography (81.4% accurate) or flexible laryngoscopy (100%).

Imaging

The width of the epiglottis in an adult is normally less than one third the anteroposterior width of the C4 vertebral body (Figures 130-1 and 130-2). Likewise, the width of the prevertebral tissue in an adult is normally less than half the anteroposterior width of the C4 vertebral body. Two classical findings on lateral plain films are (1) the thumbprint appearance of the epiglottis, because of its thickness, and (2) hypopharyngeal distention, caused by airway obstruction. Anteroposterior plain radiographs are obtained only if croup is part of the differential diagnosis. Croup occurs in young children (younger than 2 years) and is usually caused by a viral illness. Pain is not a typical finding, and dysphagia is unusual with croup. The "steeple" sign of laryngeal narrowing can be seen on anteroposterior plain radiographic views of the airway of a patient with croup.

Management

Signs that suggest a need for immediate airway support include (1) drooling, (2) diabetes mellitus, (3) shorter onset of symptoms, (4) epiglottic abscess, (5) severe swelling of the epiglottis, and (6) arytenoid swelling.

Reference

Verbruggen K, Halewyck S, Deron P, Foulon I, Gordts F. Epiglottitis and related complications in adults. Case reports and review of the literature. *B-ENT*. 2012;8(2):143-148.

Cross-Reference

Neuroradiology: THE REQUISITES, 4th ed, pp 449-452.

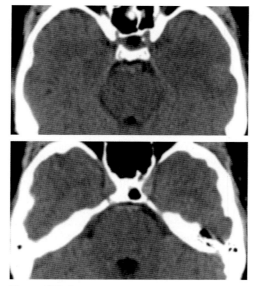

Figure 131-1

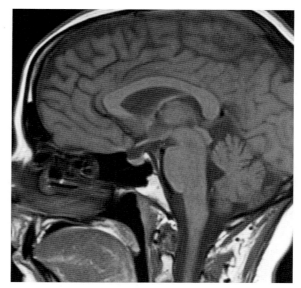

Figure 131-2

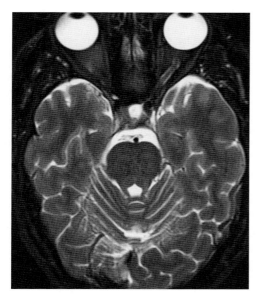

Figure 131-3

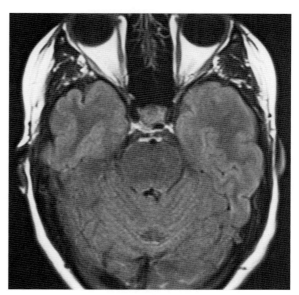

Figure 131-4

HISTORY: A 53-year-old with sudden onset of severe headache.

1. What is the single best diagnosis of this case?
   A. Subarachnoid hemorrhage
   B. Epidermoid
   C. Hypertensive hemorrhage
   D. Venous infarction

2. What is the next step in imaging management?
   A. Magnetic resonance imaging (MRI) with contrast
   B. Fluoroscopy-guided lumbar puncture
   C. Total spine MRI
   D. Cerebral angiogram

3. What is believed to be the cause of this entity when occurring at this location?
   A. Aneurysm rupture
   B. Rupture of small perforating arteries
   C. Increased intracranial pressure
   D. Rupture of small veins or capillaries

4. What is the correct statement regarding pulsation artifacts?
   A. Pulsation artifact and prepontine blood are easily distinguishable on T2-weighted fluid-attenuated inversion recovery (FLAIR).
   B. Pulsation artifact occurs in the phase encoding direction.
   C. Pulsation artifact occurs in the frequency encoding direction.
   D. Pulsation artifact occurs on computed tomography (CT) with contrast.

265

CASE 131

Nonaneurysmal Perimesencephalic Subarachnoid Hemorrhage

1. **A.** Subarachnoid hemorrhage. There is hyperdensity in the prepontine cistern on CT correlating with hyperintense T1, and T2-FLAIR signal and hypointense T2 signal on MRI.

2. **D.** Cerebral angiogram. Although this is likely benign, aneurysm must still be excluded.

3. **D.** Rupture of small veins or capillaries. Perimesencephalic hemorrhage is thought to be due to rupture of small veins.

4. **B.** Pulsation artifact occurs in the phase encoding direction. Nearly all artifacts occur in the phase encoding direction with the exception of chemical shift artifact occurring in the frequency encoding direction. Cerebrospinal fluid (CSF) pulsation artifact may mimic prepontine hemorrhage.

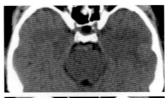

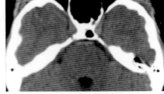

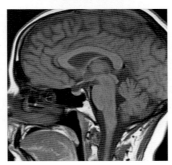

Comment

Benign, nonaneurysmal subarachnoid hemorrhage with a distinct radiographic appearance was identified by van Gijn and associates in 1985. Nonaneurysmal perimesencephalic subarachnoid hemorrhage is an increasingly recognized cause of nontraumatic subarachnoid hemorrhage. These patients typically present in adulthood with an acute headache.

Imaging

On CT, acute subarachnoid hemorrhage is present and has a somewhat characteristic location. Specifically, hemorrhage is noted predominantly in the cisterns around the brainstem, including the prepontine (as in this case), interpeduncular, and ambient cisterns. Note the small hyperdensity in the prepontine cistern on CT (Figure 131-1) and the T1 iso-hyperintense region on the MRI performed on the same day (Figure 131-2). This is again seen on T2 as hypointense signal and again on T2-FLAIR as hyperintense signal (Figures 131-3 and 131-4). A small amount of hemorrhage may be present in the dependent portion of the sylvian cisterns. Significant intraventricular hemorrhage should not be present, and blood is not usually localized in the anterior interhemispheric fissure. Flow artifacts of the CSF may sometimes be present in these CSF spaces and must not be confused for blood on MRI.

Management

Catheter angiography (which currently should still be performed, even in the presence of a characteristic localization of subarachnoid hemorrhage) shows no aneurysm. Subarachnoid hemorrhage in nonaneurysmal hemorrhage is believed to be related to venous or capillary rupture. In the presence of a characteristic pattern of subarachnoid hemorrhage and negative findings on high-quality conventional angiogram, follow-up angiography might not be necessary. Patients with this type of subarachnoid hemorrhage generally have an excellent prognosis.

Reference

Flaherty ML, Haverbusch M, Kissela B, et al. Perimesencephalic subarachnoid hemorrhage: incidence, risk factors and outcome. *J Stroke Cerebrovasc Dis.* 2005;14:267-271.

van Gijn J, van Dongen KJ, Vermeulen M, Hijdra A. Perimesencephalic hemorrhage: a nonaneurysmal and benign form of subarachnoid hemorrhage. *Neurology.* 1985;35(4):493-497.

Cross-Reference

Neuroradiology: THE REQUISITES, 4th ed, pp 140-141, 145.

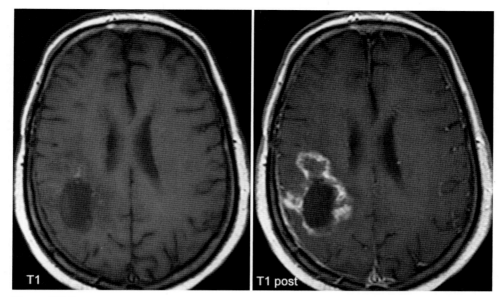

Figure 132-1

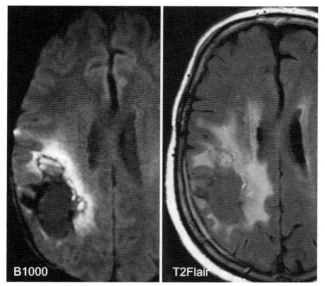

Figure 132-2

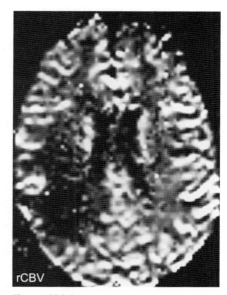

Figure 132-3

HISTORY: A 44-year-old with glioblastoma. Follow-up after treatment.

1. What is the most likely diagnosis?
   A. Residual neoplasm
   B. Radiation necrosis
   C. Abscess
   D. Acute infarct

2. When is the best time to image a patient after resection of a brain tumor to assess for residual neoplasm?
   A. Before postoperative day 2
   B. Between postoperative day 3 and day 5
   C. Between postoperative day 6 and 2 weeks
   D. 6 weeks after surgery or later

3. Regarding perfusion imaging, what is the most correct statement?
   A. Perfusion imaging using contrast can be performed using either gradient echo or spin echo pulse sequences.
   B. In dynamic susceptibility contrast perfusion, the signal intensity increases in areas of higher contrast concentration.
   C. In dynamic contrast-enhanced perfusion, T2-weighted sequences are used.
   D. Computed tomography (CT) perfusion techniques do not result in higher radiation doses to the patient compared to routine contrast-enhanced CT.

4. What finding on magnetic resonance (MR) spectroscopy would be associated with this finding and be supportive of the correct diagnosis?
   A. Increased Cho/NAA ratio
   B. Increased Cho/Cr ratio
   C. Decreased Cho/Cr ratio
   D. Elevated lipid/lactate peak

CASE 132

Radiation Necrosis after Treatment of High-Grade Glioma

1. **B.** Radiation necrosis. Although there is mass effect, enhancement, and edema, these findings are not specific for either tumor progression or treatment effects. The low relative cerebral blood volume (rCBV) is most consistent with radiation necrosis.

2. **A.** Before postoperative day 2. Granulation tissue begins to form at approximately 48 hours after surgery; therefore, imaging should be performed before this starts to occur.

3. **A.** Perfusion imaging using contrast can be performed using either gradient echo or spin echo pulse sequences. In dynamic susceptibility contrast perfusion imaging, the intensity decreases in areas of greater contrast concentration as a result of changes in local susceptibility. This differs from dynamic contrast-enhanced MR imaging, in which a T1-weighted sequence detects an increase in intensity proportional to contrast concentration. CT perfusion is performed by rapidly reimaging a volume of brain to acquire time-resolved images, requiring a higher radiation dose to the patient.

4. **C.** Decreased Cho/Cr ratio. Increased Cho/NAA and Cho/Cr ratios are seen in high-grade glioma. Decreased choline is present in radiation necrosis. Elevated lipid/lactate peaks may be seen in both entities.

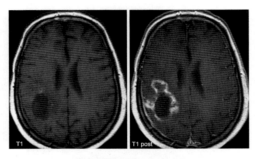

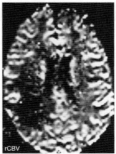

Comment

Post Therapy Magnetic Resonance Imaging

MR imaging is performed to assess for residual neoplasm in patients after brain tumor resection. Findings will determine the need for additional therapy (repeat surgery or the addition of radiation or chemotherapy). Because granulation tissue is often highly vascularized, it can enhance for months after surgery. Typically, granulation tissue develops within the first 3 days after surgery. Therefore, in patients with enhancing tumors before surgical resection, it is especially important to perform postoperative imaging within 48 hours after surgery because granulation tissue is just developing and often does not enhance. The finding of enhancing tissue on these initial postoperative scans should raise concern about residual neoplasm (Figure 132-1). Because T1-weighted hyperintense hemorrhage is usually present in the operative bed after tumor resection, it is important to compare enhanced images with unenhanced T1-weighted images obtained in the same plane as the postcontrast images (see Figure 132-1). Sequential imaging usually distinguishes residual tumor from surgical changes. Postoperative hematoma resolves, and granulation tissue typically decreases in size over time. In contrast, residual tumor grows.

Differentiating Between Radiation Necrosis and Tumor Progression

In patients treated with radiation therapy after surgery, differentiation between radiation necrosis and recurrent high-grade glioma can be challenging. The conventional MR imaging characteristics of recurrent high-grade tumors and radiation necrosis overlap and include edema, mass effect, and contrast enhancement (Figures 132-1 and 132-2). Findings that tend to favor radiation effects over recurrent or progressive neoplasm include conversion from no enhancement to enhancement, new regions of enhancement in areas remote from the primary tumor site, and new periventricular deep white matter enhancement with poorly demarcated margins.

Advanced Techniques

Advanced MR imaging of enhancing regions typically shows low choline and low rCBV in the setting of radiation necrosis. Findings that tend to favor progressive glioma include involvement of the corpus callosum, spread across the midline, and multiple regions of enhancement in the treated bed that have elevated choline and rCBV. In patients treated for high-grade gliomas, it is important to recognize that on a histologic level, microscopic glioma is usually present. In this case of predominant radiation necrosis with low rCBV (Figure 132-3), despite aggressive enhancement that was rapidly progressing over serial examinations, pathologic examination showed less than 5% neoplasm in the enhancing mass.

Reference

Mullins ME, Barest GD, Schaefer PW, et al. Radiation necrosis versus glioma recurrence: conventional MR imaging clues to diagnosis. *Am J Neuroradiol.* 2005;26:1967-1972.

Cross-Reference

Neuroradiology: THE REQUISITES, 4th ed, pp 59, 83-85.

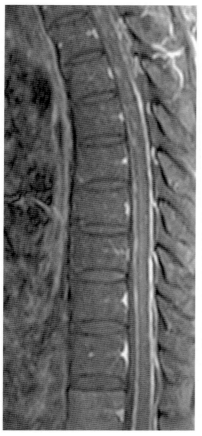

Figure 133-1

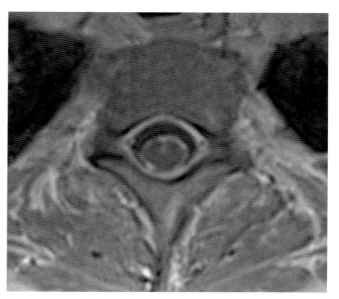

Figure 133-2

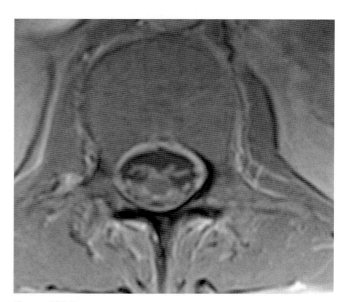

Figure 133-3

HISTORY: A 44-year-old man with a history of a left heel skin lesion removed 5 years ago presents with back pain.

1. What should be *excluded* from the differential diagnosis?
   A. Sarcoid
   B. Tuberculous meningitis
   C. Multiple sclerosis
   D. Leptomeningeal carcinomatosis

2. What cancer has the highest rate of leptomeningeal carcinomatosis?
   A. Lung cancer
   B. Breast cancer
   C. Melanoma
   D. Bladder cancer

3. Where along the spinal axis is leptomeningeal metastasis most likely to be found?
   A. Cervical cord
   B. Thoracic cord
   C. Cauda equina
   D. Thecal sac terminus

4. In the setting of diffuse leptomeningeal involvement, in which of the following processes should a primary intradural mass be localized?
   A. Meningeal melanocytoma
   B. Primary leptomeningeal melanomatosis
   C. Diffuse melanosis
   D. Pigmented meningioma

CASE 133

Leptomeningeal Metastases (Malignant Melanoma)

1. **C.** Multiple sclerosis. Multiple sclerosis does not manifest with leptomeningeal enhancement.

2. **A.** Lung cancer. Small cell lung cancer has the highest rate of spread to the leptomeninges (25%). If including other lung cancer histology, the rate is higher. Breast cancer has a low rate of spread to the leptomeninges (5%); however, because of the high frequency of breast cancer, most patients with leptomeningeal carcinomatosis have breast cancer. Melanoma has the second most common rate of spread to the leptomeninges (23%). Bladder cancer is an uncommon cause of leptomeningeal carcinomatosis.

3. **C.** Cauda equina. The cauda equina is the most common location.

4. **D.** Pigmented meningioma. The pigmented form of meningioma is not considered in the differential diagnosis of diffuse involvement of the subarachnoid space without a primary localized mass. The other disease may have diffuse involvement without a primary or dominant mass.

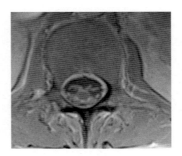

Comment

Background

Diffuse leptomeningeal metastatic disease, or carcinomatosis, has become more common as the longevity of patients with cancer has increased and as techniques for the identification of malignant cells in the cerebrospinal fluid have improved.

Histopathology

Leptomeningeal carcinomatosis occurs with invasion to, and subsequent proliferation of, neoplastic cells in the subarachnoid space, which may cause multifocal or diffuse infiltration of the leptomeninges in a sheetlike fashion along the surface of the spinal cord. This multifocal seeding of the leptomeninges by malignant cells is called leptomeningeal carcinomatosis if the primary is a solid tumor and lymphomatous meningitis or leukemic meningitis if the primary is not a solid tumor. Leptomeningeal metastases may result from hematogenous spread or intrathecal cerebrospinal fluid spread (drop metastases) of malignant cells.

Imaging

Magnetic resonance imaging is the imaging modality of choice and typically demonstrates peripheral linear or nodular enhancement of the cord surface and conus (Figures 133-1 through 133-3). Linear enhancement has been called the "sugarcoating" or "frosting" sign. In addition, thickening and linear or nodular enhancement of the cauda equina roots is often seen (see Figure 133-3).

Management

The therapeutic management of leptomeningeal carcinomatosis includes intrathecal administration of chemotherapy and radiotherapy. Treatment is controversial, and no straightforward guidelines exist in the literature.

References

Chamberlain MC. Leptomeningeal metastasis. *Curr Opin Neurol.* 2009;22(6):665-674.

Gomori JM, Heching N, Siegal T. Leptomeningeal metastases: evaluation by gadolinium enhanced spinal magnetic resonance imaging. *J Neurooncol.* 1998;36(1):55-60.

Holtz AJ. The sugarcoating sign. *Radiology.* 1998;208(1):143-144.

Cross-Reference

Neuroradiology: THE REQUISITES, 4th ed, pp 44, 575-576.

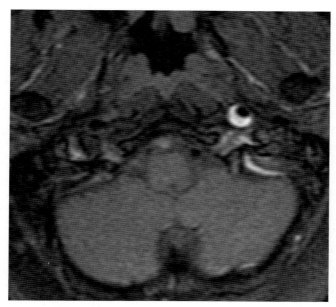

Figure 134-1

HISTORY: A 42-year-old with left neck pain.

1. What is the single best diagnosis in this case?
   A. Left internal carotid artery thrombosis
   B. Left internal carotid artery dissection
   C. Left internal jugular vein thrombosis
   D. Glomus jugulare paraganglioma

2. What is the cause of the crescentic high signal intensity?
   A. Fat
   B. Intraluminal thrombosis
   C. Calcium
   D. Intramural hematoma

3. What is the advantage of acquiring noncontrast fat-suppressed T1-weighted images?
   A. Distinguishes fluid from fat
   B. Distinguishes intramural blood products from perivascular fat
   C. Suppresses mural blood products as well as perivascular fat
   D. Allows for evaluation of intraluminal flow voids

4. In addition to headache, what other clinical presentation is likely?
   A. Seizure
   B. Horner syndrome
   C. Vertigo
   D. Plethora of the head and neck

CASE 134

Internal Carotid Artery Dissection

1. **B.** Left internal carotid artery dissection. There is a dissection of the left internal carotid artery proximal to the skull base characterized by the hyperintense intramural/subintimal thrombus and preservation although narrowing of the hypointense flow void of the vessel lumen.

2. **D.** Intramural hematoma. Intramural hematoma (methemoglobin) causes the high signal intensity around the vessel lumen.

3. **B.** Distinguishes intramural blood products from perivascular fat. Fat suppression allows vascular mural blood products (which remain hyperintense) to be distinguished from perivascular fat (which saturates out).

4. **B.** Horner syndrome. Horner syndrome occurs because of compression of the cervical sympathetic neurons along the carotid adventitia and results in the classic triad of miosis, ptosis, and anhidrosis of the ipsilateral face and neck.

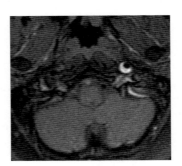

Comment

Imaging

This case illustrates the characteristic appearance of a dissection of the internal carotid artery. Magnetic resonance (MR) imaging shows overall enlargement of the left internal carotid artery, when compared with the right, due to extensive intramural hematoma (methemoglobin) that is hyperintense on unenhanced T1-weighted images (Figure 134-1). The narrowed arterial lumen is still patent because signal void (black blood), consistent with flow, is clearly present. MR imaging combined with MR angiography is sensitive for detecting vascular dissections because it allows evaluation of the vascular lumen (as with angiography), the vessel wall, and the tissues around the vascular structures. An occluded vessel can usually be differentiated from one that is narrowed but patent using a combination of conventional spin echo MR imaging and MR angiography. It is important to acquire phase-contrast MR angiography because, with this sequence, the mural hematoma, which has high signal intensity, is nulled. If only time-of-flight MR angiography is used, mural hematoma may be mistaken for flow because it remains hyperintense on this sequence.

Pathophysiology

Vascular dissections (tears in the intima that allow blood to travel in the arterial wall) can result from trauma or neck manipulation (e.g., as provided by chiropractors) and are more common in patients with underlying vascular dysplasias (fibromuscular dysplasia, Marfan syndrome, Ehlers-Danlos syndrome, and cystic medial necrosis).

Treatment

Treatment in uncomplicated cases usually includes anticoagulation therapy and aspirin. It is important to obtain follow-up MR imaging in these patients to assess for recanalization of the vascular lumen or progressive stenosis. In addition, these patients are at increased risk for the development of pseudoaneurysms, which can be catastrophic if they go undetected and rupture. The most common complication of vascular dissection is thromboembolic disease, which can occur days to weeks after the dissection.

Reference

Ozdoba C, Sturzenegger M, Schroth G. Internal carotid artery dissection: MR imaging features and clinical-radiologic correlation. *Radiology*. 1996;199:191-198.

Cross-Reference

Neuroradiology: THE REQUISITES, 4th ed, pp 173, 505.

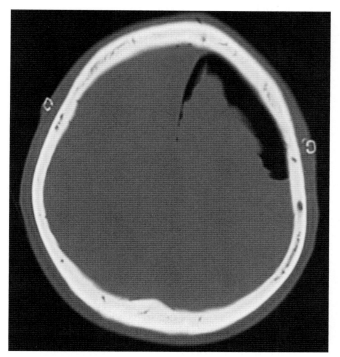

Figure 135-1

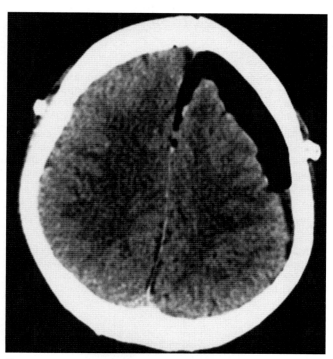

Figure 135-2

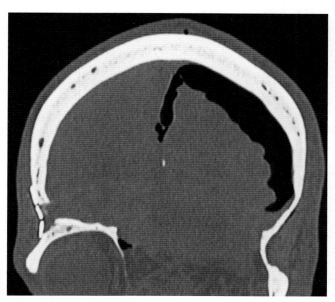

Figure 135-3

HISTORY: A 52-year-old with recent craniofacial surgery and new headache.

1. What is the most critical finding on this postoperative patient?
   A. Extra-axial blood product
   B. Tension pneumocephalus
   C. Acute infarct
   D. Intraparenchymal hemorrhage

2. In what space is the majority of the intracranial air located?
   A. Epidural
   B. Subdural
   C. Subarachnoid
   D. Parenchymal

3. This entity is most commonly described in association with what paranasal sinus tumor?
   A. Fibrous dysplasia
   B. Osteochondroma
   C. Osteoma
   D. Inverted papilloma

4. What is the minimal absorbed dose needed to induce temporary sterility in males?
   A. 0 to 0.20 Gy
   B. 0 to 0.20 mGy
   C. 4 to 5 Gy
   D. Greater than 6 Gy

CASE 135

Tension Pneumocephalus

1. **B.** Tension pneumocephalus. This case demonstrates a perioperative complication of tension pneumocephalus. There is extra-axial air over the anterior left frontal lobe and along the interhemispheric fissure, resulting in mass effect.

2. **B.** Subdural. When fluid (air or blood) insinuates along the interhemispheric fissure, it is almost always subdural. The sulci are compressed rather than enlarged; therefore, the air is not in the subarachnoid space. Epidural air would have a more lentiform configuration.

3. **C.** Osteoma. This entity is most commonly described in association with an osteoma of the frontal sinuses or ethmoid air cells.

4. **A.** 0 to 0.20 Gy. Temporary male infertility occurs at approximately 0.15 Gy absorbed dose. Permanent male sterility occurs at doses above 6 Gy. Females are rendered infertile at doses of approximately 4 to 6 Gy.

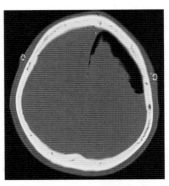

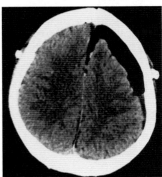

Comment

The term *tension pneumocephalus* describes the situation in which there are neurologic symptoms caused by intracranial air that results in increased intracranial pressure. Symptoms are similar to those of other space-occupying lesions. The most common cause of tension pneumocephalus is trauma resulting in fractures of the frontal sinuses and ethmoid air cells. It can also occur as a result of craniofacial surgery or tumors of the paranasal sinuses (most commonly described with osteomas). In this case, there is evidence of craniofacial surgery (Figure 135-3). The patient's symptoms and the appearance of mass effect upon the left frontal lobe, which is displaced inferiorly and posteriorly by air along the convexity and in the interhemispheric fissure (Figures 135-1 through 135-3), is consistent with tension pneumocephalus. The oddity of this case is that the pneumocephalus is unilateral; bilateral tension pneumocephalus is more commonly found.

Pathogenesis

Tension pneumocephalus can develop when there is communication between the extracranial and intracranial compartments (usually through a bone defect that is accompanied by a dural defect). When the intracranial pressure is lower, such that the ingress of air into the intracranial compartment is favored, tension pneumocephalus can result. The pathogenesis of tension pneumocephalus is ascribed to a ball-valve mechanism. In the presence of a bony defect resulting in communication between the paranasal sinuses and anterior cranial fossa, pressure within the sinuses may be transiently increased with coughing or sneezing. In this situation, air flows from the sinuses into the lower-pressure intracranial compartment until there is equilibration of pressure. Less commonly, a negative intracranial pressure gradient, such as might be seen with a large cerebrospinal fluid leak, can draw air into the cranial compartment.

Diagnosis

The diagnosis of pneumocephalus is readily established with computed tomography (CT), which can detect very small volumes of air (reportedly as small as 0.5 mL). CT also establishes the presence of mass effect and is useful in identifying osseous defects in the cranium.

References

Sprague A, Poulgrain P. Tension pneumocephalus: a case report and literature review. *J Clin Neurosci.* 1999;6:418-424.

Tobey JD, Loevner LA, Yousem DM, Lanza DC. Tension pneumocephalus: a complication of invasive ossifying fibroma of the paranasal sinuses. *AJR Am J Roentgenol.* 1996;166:711-713.

Cross-Reference

Neuroradiology: THE REQUISITES, 4th ed, pp 160, 432.

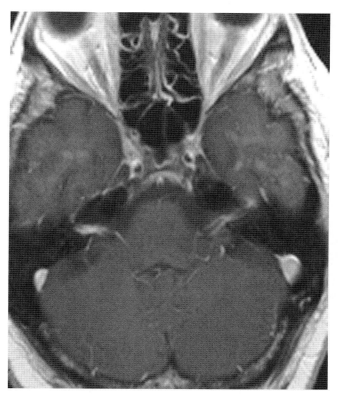

Figure 136-1

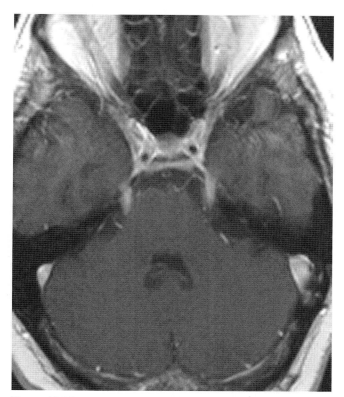

Figure 136-2

HISTORY: A 43-year-old with breast cancer and facial pain.

1. What is the single best diagnosis of this case?
   A. Subarachnoid seeding of malignancy
   B. Dural venous sinus thrombosis
   C. Sarcoidosis
   D. Tuberculosis

2. Blockage of the arachnoid villi can result in what condition?
   A. Normal pressure hydrocephalus
   B. Obstructive communicating hydrocephalus
   C. Pseudotumor cerebri
   D. Venous infarct

3. What is the gold standard for the diagnosis of leptomeningeal metastasis?
   A. Magnetic resonance imaging (MRI) with contrast
   B. Computed tomography (CT) with contrast
   C. Positron emission tomography/computed tomography (PET/CT)
   D. Lumbar puncture

4. Which of the following is the nerve of origin for parasympathetic innervation to the lacrimal gland?
   A. Oculomotor (cranial nerve [CN] III)
   B. Trigeminal (CN V)
   C. Abducens (CN VI)
   D. Facial (CN VII)

CASE 136

Subarachnoid Seeding: Leptomeningeal Carcinomatosis

1. **A.** Subarachnoid seeding of malignancy. There is enhancement of CN V, CN VII, and CN VIII bilaterally. This is the likely diagnosis in a patient with breast cancer. Sarcoidosis and tuberculosis may not infrequently involve the leptomeninges and cranial nerves. There is no evidence of dural venous sinus thrombosis.

2. **B.** Obstructive communicating hydrocephalus. Obstruction of the arachnoid villi results in impaired resorption of cerebrospinal fluid (CSF) resulting in increased CSF volume and hydrocephalus.

3. **D.** Lumbar puncture. Lumbar puncture remains the gold standard for the detection of leptomeningeal malignant dissemination. MRI with contrast is the most sensitive imaging modality for detection of abnormal leptomeningeal enhancement and altered signal.

4. **D.** Facial (CN VII). The facial nerve, particularly the lacrimal nucleus is the origin of the parasympathetic innervation of the lacrimal gland. The neurons synapse at the sphenopalatine ganglion via the pterygoid (vidian) nerve and subsequently join branches of CN V to reach the lacrimal gland, ultimately via the lacrimal nerve.

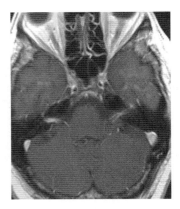

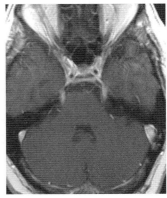

Comment

Incidence and Clinical Presentation

Leptomeningeal carcinomatosis is a relatively uncommon presentation of metastatic disease to the central nervous system in patients with extracranial malignancies. Carcinomatous meningitis is reported in approximately 2% to 3% of patients with such malignancies; however, as treatment for cancer improves and patients live longer, it is likely that the incidence of subarachnoid seeding from systemic malignancies will increase. Patients can present with nonspecific symptoms, including headache and meningeal signs; however, they can also present with cranial neuropathies and symptoms related to obstructive communicating hydrocephalus.

Histology

Histologic examination of leptomeningeal spread typically shows metastatic cellular infiltrates within the subarachnoid space.

Imaging

Contrast-enhanced CT is not sensitive for detecting leptomeningeal spread. Contrast-enhanced MRI is currently the imaging modality of choice for detecting subarachnoid seeding; however, it is not always sensitive. Lumbar puncture to obtain CSF for cytologic evaluation for malignant cells remains the gold standard for diagnosing carcinomatous meningitis; serial punctures may be necessary.

In this case, enhancement can be seen within the internal auditory canals bilaterally, particularly on the right (Figure 136-1). In addition, there is bilateral enhancement of the cisternal portions of CN V (Figure 136-2). In hematologic malignancies, such as leukemia and lymphoma, spread is usually directly to the leptomeninges. In systemic cancers, such as lung and breast carcinoma, although spread can occur directly to the meninges, subarachnoid seeding is often the result of rupture of superficial cerebral metastasis into the subarachnoid space. In patients with carcinomatous meningitis, enhancement may be seen along the perivascular spaces within the brain parenchyma and along the ependymal surface of the ventricles.

Reference

Tsuchiya K, Katase S, Yoshino A, Hachiya J. FLAIR MR imaging for diagnosing intracranial meningeal carcinomatosis. *AJR Am J Roentgenol.* 2001;176:1585-1588.

Cross-Reference

Neuroradiology: THE REQUISITES, 4th ed, pp 47-49.

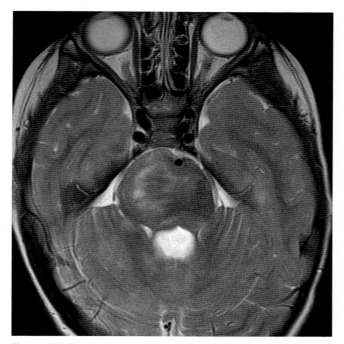

Figure 137-1

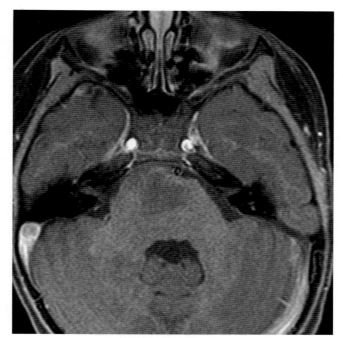

Figure 137-2

HISTORY: A 13-year-old, otherwise healthy, with headache.

1. Considering the imaging findings and the clinical history, what is the single most likely diagnosis of this case?
   A. Low-grade astrocytoma
   B. Glioblastoma
   C. Central pontine myelinolysis
   D. Pontine infarct

2. What part of the brainstem is most commonly affected with this entity?
   A. Cerebral peduncle
   B. Tectal plate
   C. Pons
   D. Medulla

3. What is the most common histologic subtype?
   A. Diffuse fibrillary
   B. Anaplastic
   C. Glioblastoma
   D. Pleomorphic xanthoastrocytoma

4. What is the typical location of a posterior fossa ependymoma?
   A. Cerebellum
   B. Vermis
   C. Fourth ventricle
   D. Medulla

CASE 137

Brainstem Astrocytoma

1. **A.** Low-grade astrocytoma. The differential diagnosis includes astrocytoma; non-neoplastic diseases, such as demyelinating disease (acute disseminated encephalomyelitis), rhombencephalitis, and tuberculosis (more common outside the United States); and lymphoma. Exophytic and enhancing masses can mimic medulloblastoma or ependymoma.

2. **C.** Pons. Overall, 60% to 75% of brainstem astrocytomas are located in the pons.

3. **A.** Diffuse fibrillary. The most common subtype of pontine glioma/astrocytoma is the diffuse fibrillary subtype.

4. **C.** Fourth ventricle. The fourth ventricle is the typical location of a posterior fossa ependymoma.

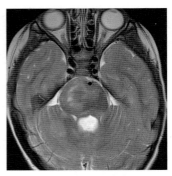

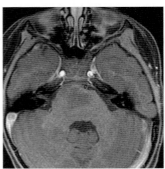

Comment

Case in Point

This case shows the characteristic appearance of a low-grade brainstem astrocytoma, including high signal intensity within the pons on T2-weighted images (Figure 137-1). It also shows marked expansion of the brainstem, most notably the pons but also extending exophytically into the prepontine cistern and around the basilar artery; note effacement of the prepontine cistern and invagination (encasement) of the basilar artery. The enhancement pattern of brainstem gliomas is quite variable, ranging from regions of avid nodular enhancement to minimal or no enhancement, as in this case (Figure 137-2).

Statistics and Disease Progression

Approximately 80% of brainstem gliomas occur during childhood. Brainstem neoplasms are uncommon, accounting for 10% to 15% of central nervous system tumors in children, with a peak age at presentation of younger than 14 years. Most are gliomas, including slow-growing fibrillary or pilocytic astrocytoma, malignant astrocytoma, and glioblastoma. Most tumors are of the diffuse fibrillary subtype; however, more than half of them eventually show regions of anaplastic transformation and have a poor long-term prognosis. These tumors can initially infiltrate the brainstem without tissue destruction, and few deficits may be present, despite extensive disease. Presenting symptoms include cranial nerve deficits, motor or sensory deficits, ataxia, abnormal eye movements, somnolence, and hyperactivity. Hydrocephalus is a late finding, with the exception of tumors arising in immediate proximity to the aqueduct.

Imaging

Magnetic resonance imaging (MRI) is the imaging modality of choice for evaluation of brainstem abnormalities. Its multiplanar capabilities, improved resolution, and relative absence of scanning artifacts commonly present on computed tomography scans have resulted in improved detection of abnormalities in the posterior fossa. In addition, MRI is useful for planning radiation therapy.

Treatment

Because of the infiltrative nature and characteristic location of brainstem astrocytomas, radiation therapy remains the main therapeutic option. In cases in which tumor is exophytic, the exophytic portion can often be resected.

Reference

Young Poussaint T, Yousuf N, Barnes PD, et al. Cervicomedullary astrocytomas of childhood: clinical and imaging follow-up. *Pediatr Radiol.* 1999;29:662-668.

Cross-Reference

Neuroradiology: THE REQUISITES, 4th ed, p 59.

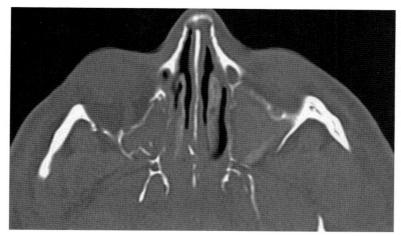

Figure 138-1

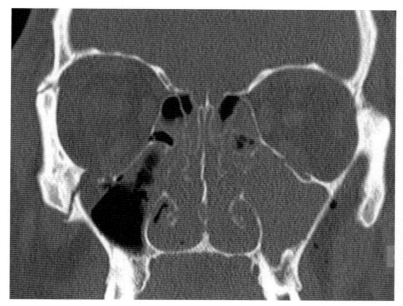

Figure 138-2

HISTORY: The statement "man versus baseball bat" is written on an emergency department requisition, suggesting facial trauma.

1. Which of the following should be included in the differential diagnosis?
   A. Trimalar fracture
   B. Nasoethmoidal strut fracture
   C. Le Fort fracture
   D. Normal

2. What structure or structures are invariably fractured with this fracture pattern/classification?
   A. Maxilla
   B. Pterygoid plates
   C. Orbital floor
   D. Nasal bones

3. In which type(s) of this fracture pattern/classification is the medial orbital wall fractured?
   A. Types I and II
   B. Types II and III
   C. Types I and III
   D. Only type II

4. In which type of this fracture pattern/classification is a nasal bone fractured?
   A. Type I
   B. Type II
   C. Type III
   D. Nasal bone fracture is not specified in this fracture pattern/classification.

CASE 138

Le Fort Fractures

1. **C.** Le Fort fracture. The diagnosis is Le Fort fracture. Le Fort type III fracture on the right side is demonstrated with fractures across lateral and medial orbital walls. Zygomatic attachment fractures are not being demonstrated, so the diagnosis would not include trimalar fractures. In addition, nasoethmoidal strut fractures are not shown.

2. **B.** Pterygoid plates. Pterygoid plates are fractured with Le Fort fractures; they are the sine qua non of Le Fort fractures.

3. **B.** Types II and III. The medial orbital wall is fractured in Le Fort types II and III fractures. Fractures of the maxilla to the medial aspect of the orbit characterize type II, and fractures of the lateral and medial aspects of the orbit characterize type III.

4. **D.** Nasal bone fracture is not specified in this fracture pattern/classification.

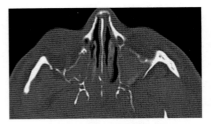

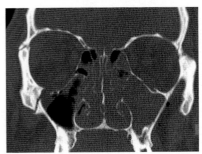

Comment

Associations with Le Fort Fractures

Rhea and Novelline (2005) emphasized that each of the Le Fort fractures is associated with one unique fracture:

- Type I: the anterolateral margin of the nasal fossa
- Type II: the inferior orbital rim
- Type III: zygomatic arch

Le Fort type I fractures predominantly involve the lower maxilla and do not usually involve the orbits, whereas Le Fort type II fractures affect inferior and medial aspects of the orbit (Figures 138-1 and 138-2). Le Fort type I fracture is referred to as the *floating palate fracture* because the fracture crosses from medially at the nasal septum to the maxilla above the teeth and below the zygomaticomaxillary junction and includes the pterygoid plates. This fracture is often bilateral. Le Fort type II fracture is often termed the *pyramidal fracture* because it crosses the body of the maxilla down the midline of the hard palate; through the rim, floor, and medial wall of the orbit; and into the nasal cavity. Le Fort type III fractures, which cross from the lateral to medial aspects of the orbit, are the fracture constellations in which "craniofacial dissociation" may occur; that is, the facial bones inferiorly are relatively disconnected from the skull above them.

Relevant Anatomy

Common to all of these fractures is extension across the pterygoid plates. Trimalar fractures affect the attachments of the zygoma to the maxilla, the frontal bone, and the sphenoid bone. They create a lateral divot out of the side of the face, dissociating the lateral orbit, zygoma, and lateral edge of the maxilla from the rest of the face. It is possible for a patient to have one type of Le Fort fracture on one side and another type of Le Fort fracture on the other side, as well as multiple Le Fort fractures ipsilaterally.

Reference

Rhea JT, Novelline RA. How to simplify the CT diagnosis of Le Fort fractures. *AJR Am J Roentgenol.* 2005;184(5):1700-1705.

Cross-Reference

Neuroradiology: THE REQUISITES, 4th ed, pp 172-173.

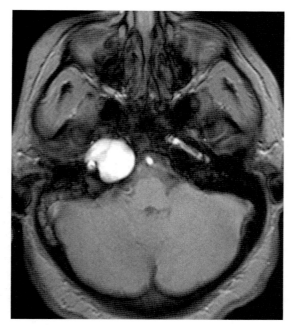

Figure 139-1

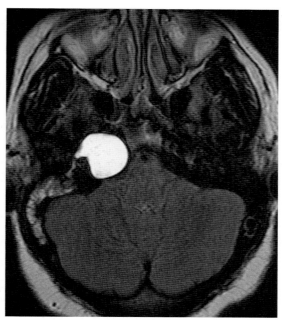

Figure 139-2

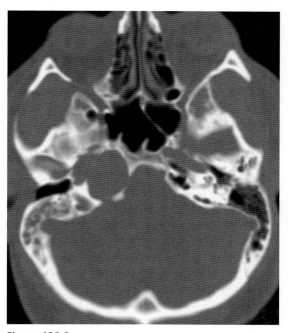

Figure 139-3

HISTORY: A 42-year-old with headache.

1. What is the single best diagnosis in this case?
   A. Cholesterol granuloma
   B. Mucocele
   C. Epidermoid cyst
   D. Schwannoma

2. In what percentage of affected patients is the petrous apex aerated?
   A. 0% to 20%
   B. 21% to 40%
   C. 41% to 60%
   D. More than 60%

3. What is the most likely cause of this lesion?
   A. Posttraumatic
   B. Neoplastic
   C. Recurrent microhemorrhages
   D. Vascular malformation

4. The presence of fluid-fluid levels, especially on T2-weighted images, usually indicates what lesion?
   A. Mucocele
   B. Abscess
   C. Cholesterol granuloma
   D. Epidermoid

CASE 139

Petrous Apex Cholesterol Granuloma

1. **A.** Cholesterol granuloma. This lesion is hyperintense on T1-weighted imaging and T2-weighted imaging and remains hyperintense when fat saturation techniques are used. Fluid-fluid levels are often seen and the lesion is expansile. When a mucocele is bright on T1-weighted imaging (secondary to proteins in the fluid), it usually will not remain as bright on T2-weighted imaging. Epidermoids and schwannomas are not bright on T1-weighted imaging.

2. **B.** 21% to 40%. The petrous apex is aerated in 30% of affected patients. Fatty infiltration is probably just as common.

3. **C.** Recurrent microhemorrhages. Recurrent microhemorrhages resulting from rupture of small blood vessels within the petrous air cells as a result of negative pressure gradients are thought to be the cause of this lesion.

4. **C.** Cholesterol granuloma. These are the most common petrous apex lesions, and fluid-fluid levels are highly characteristic.

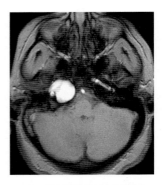

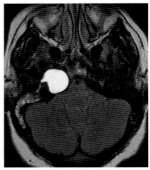

Comment

Cause

Cholesterol granulomas, also known as blue-domed or chocolate cysts, typically arise in the petrous apex. They are believed to be due to chronic obstruction of previously pneumatized petrous air cells, resulting in negative pressure within them. As a result of these negative pressure gradients, there are recurrent microhemorrhages caused by rupture of small blood vessels. A foreign body reaction involving the mucosal lining of the petrous air cells occurs, with giant cell proliferation and a fibroblastic reaction, as well as deposition of cholesterol crystals within the cyst. These are reportedly more common in the setting of chronic otomastoiditis.

Imaging

On computed tomography, these lesions typically have a benign appearance that manifests as an expansile mass lesion with demarcated margins, as in this case involving the right petrous apex (Figure 139-3). Cholesterol granulomas, when large enough, may be multilobular. There is usually thinning of the cortex with large lesions; however, there is no destruction of bone. On magnetic resonance imaging, cholesterol granulomas are hyperintense on all pulse sequences (Figures 139-1 and 139-2). In particular, the marked hyperintensity on unenhanced T1-weighted images (see Figure 139-1) is classic, distinguishing it from many other lesions, and the presence of hemorrhage-fluid levels within these lesions is highly characteristic. Normal fat can occur in the petrous apex and, because it is hyperintense on both T1-weighted and fast spin echo T2-weighted imaging, may be mistaken for a cholesterol granuloma. This error can be avoided by obtaining fat-saturated T1-weighted images in which fat will lose signal but the cholesterol granuloma will remain hyperintense.

Differential Diagnosis

The differential diagnosis of a benign-appearing expansile petrous apex mass includes cholesterol granuloma, mucocele, and epidermoid cyst. Mucoceles are often unilocular and show peripheral enhancement. The signal characteristics of mucoceles vary depending on the protein concentration and viscosity within them, as well as on the cross-linking of glycoproteins. Epidermoid cysts can have a benign appearance, but they can have more concerning radiologic findings, such as bone erosion or destruction. They are typically similar to cerebrospinal fluid on T1-weighted and T2-weighted images, are hyperintense on fluid-attenuated inversion recovery imaging, and show restricted diffusion. Less common and more aggressive "cystic-appearing" masses that can involve the petrous apex include hemorrhagic metastases, plasmacytoma, and multiple myeloma.

References

Chang P, Fagan PA, Atlas MD, Roche J. Imaging destructive lesions of the petrous apex. *Laryngoscope.* 1998;108:599-604.
Palacios E, Valvassori G. Petrous apex lesions: cholesterol granuloma. *Ear Nose Throat J.* 1999;78:234.

Cross-Reference

Neuroradiology: THE REQUISITES, 4th ed, pp 370, 404.

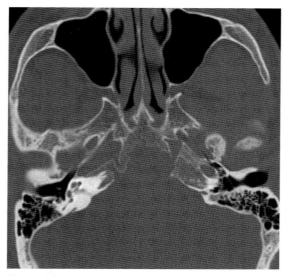

Figure 140-1

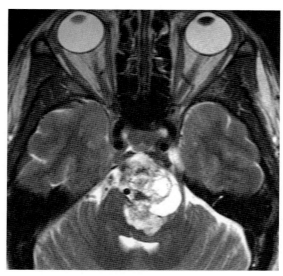

Figure 140-2

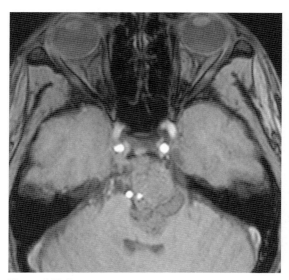

Figure 140-3

HISTORY: A 34-year-old with cranial nerve palsies.

1. This is a tumor arising from a notochord remnant. Where in the body is it most commonly found?
   A. Skull base
   B. Cervical spine
   C. Lumbar spine
   D. Sacrum

2. Which other notochordal remnant lesion occurs intradural along the posterior clivus and is histologically similar to the lesion in this case?
   A. Chondroma
   B. Chondrosarcoma
   C. Osteochondroma
   D. Ecchordosis physaliphora

3. Regarding treatment, which of the following is the most correct statement?
   A. Surgical treatment is often curative.
   B. These tumors are usually resistant to external beam radiation therapy alone.
   C. These tumors are often found malignant on histologic examination, but they often are not aggressive and therefore do not need aggressive therapy.
   D. Treatment for these masses rarely includes surgery because of the surgical morbidities.

4. Which cranial nerve (CN) is most often affected by these masses as located in the case presented?
   A. CN III
   B. CN V
   C. CN VI
   D. CN X

CASE 140

Clival Chordoma

1. **D.** Sacrum. This is a case a clival chordoma, which is the second most common location for this tumor to occur. The sacrum is the most common location.

2. **D.** Ecchordosis physaliphora. This is a histologically similar lesion although there is no infiltration at the tumor margins. These usually are smaller and less aggressive appearing.

3. **B.** These tumors are usually resistant to external beam radiation therapy alone. In fact, surgery, radiation, and chemotherapy are often used together to treat these lesions and proton beam and stereotactic radiation techniques are often used because the tumors are relatively resistant to radiation therapy.

4. **C.** CN VI. As with most skull base lesions that may or may not involve the cavernous sinus, CN VI is often the first nerve affected because of its relatively oblique and long cisternal course and its more medial skull base pathway.

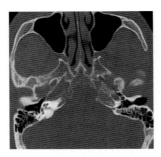

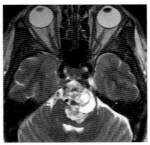

Comment

Chordomas arise in locations where notochordal remnants are found. They occur most commonly in the sacrum (50%), followed by the clivus (35%) and the spine, especially the upper cervical spine (C1-C2, 15%).

Pathophysiology/Histology

Although chordomas are considered benign neoplasms, based on their histologic appearance, they grow quite invasively, particularly at the skull base, where they can invade foramina or the cavernous sinus or extend into the posterior and middle cranial fossa. Like giant cell tumors, chordomas can metastasize in a small percentage of patients.

Imaging

Computed tomography (CT) and magnetic resonance imaging (MRI) play complementary roles in assessing tumors of the base of the skull. On CT, calcification is seen in 50% of cases, and regions of bone erosion or destruction (Figure 140-1) are clearly delineated. Multiplanar MRI allows complete evaluation of the extent of the lesion. On MRI, the signal characteristics of chordomas are variable. These tumors are typically hypointense to isointense to brain on T1-weighted imaging (Figure 140-3) and are normally hyperintense on T2-weighted imaging (Figure 140-2). There may be marked heterogeneity due to cellularity, vascularity, or calcification. Most chordomas enhance, although some predominantly cystic tumors only minimally enhance (not shown). Tumors arising at the C1-C2 region have been associated with less enhancement and more cystic-type changes.

Differential Diagnosis

The differential diagnosis includes chondroid lesions (chondrosarcoma), metastatic disease, multiple myeloma, and lymphoma. The presence of a calcified matrix usually limits the differential diagnosis to chordoma versus chondrosarcoma. In the authors' experiences and as the literature indicates, it may be difficult to distinguish these two entities. Chordomas tend to be midline lesions, whereas chondrosarcomas tend to be more lateral.

Presentation

Clinical symptoms of chordomas and chondrosarcomas may be quite similar at the skull base, including headache and cranial neuropathies (often affecting CN VI). Clinical presentation is usually in the second through fourth decades of life.

Reference

Erdem E, Angtuaco EC, Van Henert R, et al. Comprehensive review of intracranial chordoma. *Radiographics*. 2003;23:995-1009.

Cross-Reference

Neuroradiology: THE REQUISITES, 4th ed, pp 374-376.

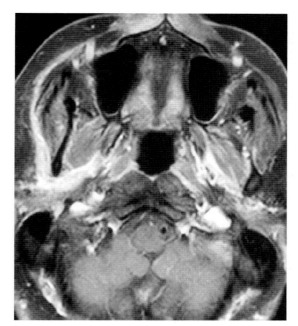

Figure 141-1

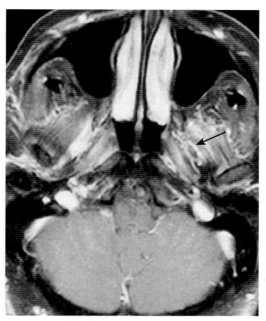

Figure 141-2

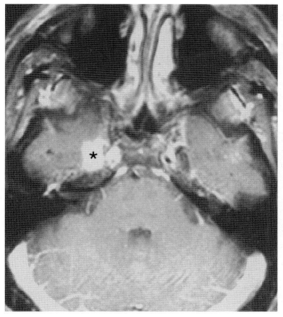

Figure 141-3

HISTORY: A 66-year-old with history of skin cancer removed from right cheek presents with new facial numbness, fasciculations, and mild facial weakness.

1. What is the single best diagnosis of this case?
   A. Perineural spread of tumor
   B. Lymphoma
   C. Perineural spread of infection
   D. Trigeminal neuralgia secondary to neurovascular impingement

2. Aside from cranial nerve (CN) VII, what additional cranial nerve is involved in this case?
   A. III
   B. IV
   C. V
   D. VI

3. What primary tumor of the salivary glands is notorious for its propensity for perineural spread?
   A. Lymphoma
   B. Adenoid cystic carcinoma
   C. Mucinous adenocarcinoma
   D. Warthin tumor

4. What nerve involved in this case provides communication for perineural spread between the facial nerve and the trigeminal nerve?
   A. Lingual nerve
   B. Auriculotemporal nerve
   C. Inferior alveolar nerve
   D. Lateral pterygoid nerve

CASE 141

Perineural Spread of Skin Cancer: Basal Cell Carcinoma

1. **A.** Perineural spread of tumor. The differential diagnosis includes perineural spread of tumor or infection (Lyme disease, herpes zoster), metastatic disease, and lymphoma.

2. **C.** V. Cranial nerves V and VII are involved in this case by perineural spread of basal cell carcinoma. There are multiple places where the nerves are closely or even directly associated in the face.

3. **B.** Adenoid cystic carcinoma. Among patients with adenoid cystic carcinoma, 50% have perineural invasion.

4. **B.** Auriculotemporal nerve. This nerve is a branch of V_3, which splays in the parotid gland joining multiple branches of the facial nerve, CN VII.

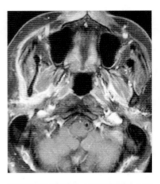

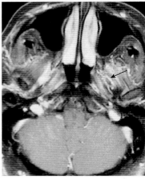

Comment

Findings in This Case

This case illustrates a classic appearance of perineural spread of skin carcinoma (basal cell carcinoma in this patient). The patient, who had previously had a skin cancer removed from his right cheek, presented with new facial numbness, fasciculations, and mild facial weakness. The first image shows prominent enhancement of right CN VII tracking from superficial fibers along the cheek into the parotid gland (Figure 141-1). In addition to CN VII, the parotid gland can also contain branches of the auriculotemporal rami of the third division of CN V. As seen in this case, tumor can spread along branches of the auriculotemporal nerve, through the foramen ovale (*arrow* on the normal left side, Figure 141-2), and into Meckel cave (*asterisk*, Figure 141-3). In Figure 141-3, note the enhancement of the right facial nerve in the temporal bone, including the labyrinthine portion that takes tumor to the fundus of the internal auditory canal.

Pathology

Perineural spread of tumor represents tracking of tumor along nerve sheaths, often discontinuous and remote from the site of the primary neoplasm. It occurs with a spectrum of tumors, including skin cancer (basal cell and desmoplastic melanoma are notorious for this tendency, but squamous cell carcinoma is common and can also have perineural spread); squamous cell carcinoma of the head and neck (in particular, nasopharyngeal cancer); primary salivary neoplasms (most notably, adenoid cystic carcinoma); lymphoma in the periorbital region; and other skull base neoplasms.

Clinical Information

Because perineural spread of tumor might not be symptomatic, the radiologist must always be on the hunt for this in appropriate clinical scenarios. Perineural spread is a poor prognostic indicator. Lesions believed to be resectable for cure may be deemed unresectable. Radiation fields may need to be expanded.

Reference

Ginsberg LE, Eicher SA. Great auricular nerve: anatomy and imaging in a case of perineural tumor spread. *Am J Neuroradiol.* 2000;21: 568-571.

Cross-Reference

Neuroradiology: THE REQUISITES, 4th ed, pp 370-371.

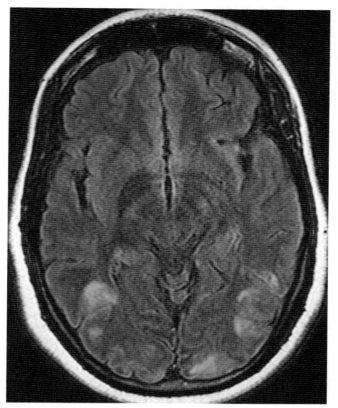

Figure 142-1

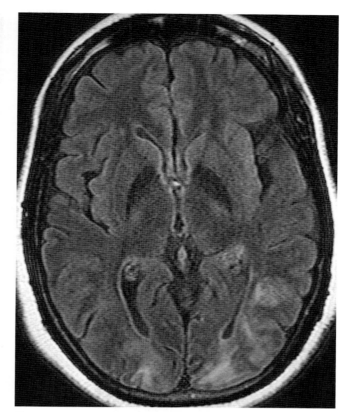

Figure 142-2

HISTORY: A 36-year-old female with postpartum seizures.

1. What is the likely cause of this patient's imaging finding?
   A. Hypertensive encephalopathy
   B. Progressive multifocal leukoencephalopathy
   C. Postviral leukoencephalitis
   D. Infarct

2. There are two major proposed mechanisms. Aside from autonomic dysregulation of the circulation in the posterior fossa, what is the other often accepted mechanism for this process?
   A. Endothelial dysfunction
   B. Venous insufficiency
   C. Venous thrombosis
   D. Proteinemia

3. What areas of the brain are particularly susceptible to the changes of hypertension?
   A. Frontal lobes
   B. Insula cortex
   C. Occipital lobes
   D. Basal ganglia

4. What medication has proven associations with this entity?
   A. Aspirin
   B. Cisplatin
   C. Metoprolol
   D. Erythromycin

CASE 142

Posterior Reversible Encephalopathy Syndrome

1. **A.** Hypertensive encephalopathy. This is a case of hypertensive encephalopathy/posterior reversible encephalopathy syndrome (PRES)/reversible posterior leukoencephalopathy. Control of the patient's hypertension resulted in resolution of the imaging findings and complete clinical recovery.

2. **A.** Endothelial dysfunction. It is thought that microangiopathic hemolysis may result in endothelial damage and, subsequently, cerebral edema.

3. **C.** Occipital lobes. The most commonly affected portions of the brain are the occipital and posterior parietal lobes, but other areas of the brain can be involved, especially when severe.

4. **B.** Cisplatin. Medications implicated in PRES include cisplatin, tacrolimus, cyclosporine, vidarabine, cytarabine, and dimethyl sulfoxide.

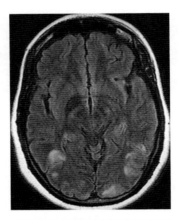

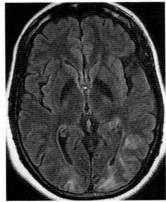

Comment

This case shows many of the typical imaging manifestations of reversible posterior leukoencephalopathy. The images (Figures 142-1 and 142-2) show foci of increased signal intensity within the subcortical white matter (and cortex) that is predominantly in the occipital lobes (see Figure 142-1); however, regions of signal alteration are also present in the parietal lobes.

The imaging findings, in combination with the patient's clinical presentation (elevated blood pressure associated with progressive neurologic symptoms, including change in mental status, headache, blurred vision, seizures, and focal neurologic deficits), facilitate the correct diagnosis to be made. Both the symptoms and the radiologic findings may be reversible with treatment of the elevated blood pressure. In addition to foci of abnormal signal intensity at the gray-white matter interface in the occipital and parietal lobes, the frontal and temporal lobes may be affected, as may the cerebellum and pons. Enhancement in regions of signal abnormality may be observed. Acute hemorrhage may be present, although this is less common.

Cause

One theory is that the normal autoregulatory control of the cerebral vasculature that allows continuous perfusion over a range of blood pressures is exceeded. The posterior circulation is more sensitive to the changes of accelerated hypertension. This may be related to a difference in sympathetic innervation (sparse innervation by sympathetic nerves). This can result in engorgement of the distal cerebral vessels, with hyperperfusion and breakdown of the blood-brain barrier. Signal abnormalities can represent reversible vasogenic edema. Another theory is that microangiopathic hemolysis results in endothelial damage with release of endothelial toxins resulting in localized vasogenic edema.

Medication and Other Treatment Implications

Similar, potentially reversible changes can occur with the use of intravenous drugs, such as cocaine; in patients treated with chemotherapeutic agents (cytosine arabinoside, methotrexate, cisplatin); in patients undergoing radiation therapy; and in patients with eclampsia.

Reference

Casey SO, Sampaio RC, Michel E, Truwit CL. Posterior reversible encephalopathy syndrome: utility of fluid-attenuated inversion recovery MR imaging in the detection of cortical and subcortical lesions. *AJNR Am J Neuroradiol.* 2000;21:1199-1206.

Cross-Reference

Neuroradiology: THE REQUISITES, 4th ed, pp 220-222.

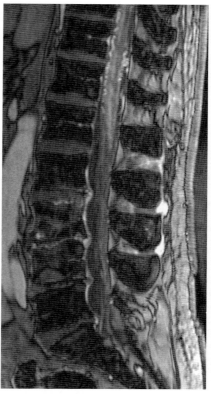

Figure 143-1

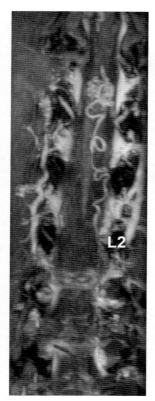

Figure 143-2

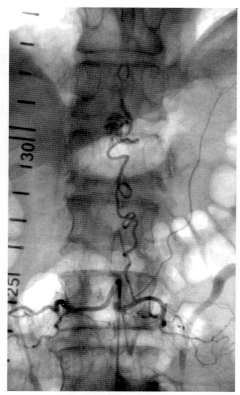

Figure 143-3

HISTORY: This patient presented with progressive numbness in the lower extremities for the past year and recent urinary incontinence.

1. What is the single best diagnosis?
   A. Hemangioblastoma
   B. Leriche syndrome
   C. Dural arteriovenous fistula (DAVF)
   D. Glomus arteriovenous malformation (AVM)

2. Which of the four commonly accepted types of spinal vascular malformation is the most likely in this patient?
   A. Type I
   B. Type II
   C. Type III
   D. Type IV

3. Which of the following patients best fits the demographic for the lesion in this case?
   A. 50-year-old woman
   B. 20-year-old woman
   C. 12-year-old boy
   D. 60-year-old man

4. What is the most common location of spinal DAVF along the spinal axis?
   A. High cervical spine (at level of the foramen magnum)
   B. Lower cervical spine (below C2 and above T1)
   C. Thoracolumbar region
   D. Sacral spine

CASE 143

Dural Arteriovenous Fistula (L2)

1. **C.** Dural arteriovenous fistula (DAVF). The findings of dilated early filling intradural veins on magnetic resonance angiography (MRA) and on spinal angiography are essentially diagnostic for spinal DAVF. No mass lesion is noted. Hemangioblastoma would have a discrete lesion and likely have a dilated anterior spinal artery. Leriche syndrome, or occlusion of the infrarenal abdominal aorta, can result in hypertrophy of the anterior spinal artery but would not have venous hypertrophy. An intramedullary AVM would have a hypertrophied anterior spinal artery and an intramedullary nidus (which is not seen in this case).

2. **A.** Type I. Type I (DAVF) is the most common.

3. **D.** 60-year-old male. DAVF typically occurs in men 50 to 70 years old.

4. **C.** Thoracolumbar region. More than 80% of all DAVFs are located between T6 and L2.

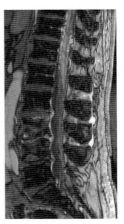

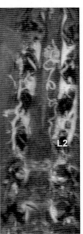

Comment

Background

Spinal DAVF is the most commonly encountered spinal vascular malformation; however, it is still an underdiagnosed entity. Because presenting clinical symptoms are nonspecific, the neuroradiologist is often the first to raise the possibility of this diagnosis. Patients typically present with progressive myelopathy.

Pathophysiology and Classification

Spinal DAVF is presumed to be an acquired disease, although the exact cause is unknown. A commonly accepted classification scheme for spinal vascular malformations is that of Anson and Spetzler, in which the four types of spinal AVM are described. Type I is DAVF, which is subclassified into types IA (single feeding artery) and IB (multiple feeding arteries). The nidus is located within or on the dura mater of the proximal nerve root sleeve in the neural foramen.

Imaging

Spinal DAVF may occur anywhere from the level of the foramen magnum to the sacrum; identification of the arteriovenous shunt location may be difficult and challenging, especially in cases in which cord edema is extensive. The noninvasive evaluation of the shunt location is extremely helpful to guide invasive conventional angiography. Contrast-enhanced spinal MRA (Figures 143-1 and 143-2) has contributed greatly to diagnosing and demonstrating the level of the fistula and helps avoid unnecessary superselective injections of all possible arterial feeders. Two methods may be used: standard three-dimensional time-of-flight (TOF) technique and dynamic bolus injected contrast-enhanced MRA. Although the three-dimensional TOF technique offers good spatial resolution, only normal (large) veins are depicted, whereas dynamic contrast-enhanced MRA allows the differentiation of normal spinal cord arteries and veins. MRA shows increased tortuosity, length, and size of the intradural vessels (see Figure 143-1). The fistula level is diagnosed by following the dominant and often tortuous draining medullary vein to the foraminal level (see Figure 143-2). Selective spinal angiography (Figure 143-3) is necessary to confirm the diagnosis and fistula level.

Management

Treatment consists of interruption of the draining medullary vein, either surgically or by superselective endovascular embolization with a liquid embolic agent. Careful angiographic evaluation is required before treatment of this lesion to identify the artery of Adamkiewicz and confirm that it is not supplied by the same segmental artery as the fistula to prevent cord infarction.

References

Anson JA, Spetzler RF. Spinal dural arteriovenous malformations. In: Awad IA, Barrow DL, eds. *Dural Arteriovenous Malformations*. Park Ridge, IL: American Association of Neurological Surgeons; 1993:175-191.

Bowen BC, Fraser K, Kochan JP, et al. Spinal dural arteriovenous fistulas: evaluation with magnetic resonance angiography. *AJNR Am J Neuroradiol*. 1995;16(10):2029-2043.

Krings T, Geibprasert S. Spinal dural arteriovenous fistulas. *AJNR Am J Neuroradiol*. 2009;30(4):639-648.

Saraf-Lavi E, Bowen BC, Quencer RM, et al. Detection of spinal dural arteriovenous fistulae with MRI and contrast-enhanced MR angiography: sensitivity, specificity, and prediction of vertebral level. *AJNR Am J Neuroradiol*. 2002;23(5):858-867.

Cross-Reference

Neuroradiology: THE REQUISITES, 4th ed, pp 147-149.

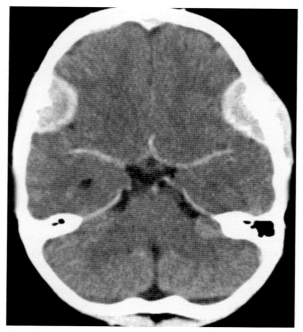

Figure 144-1

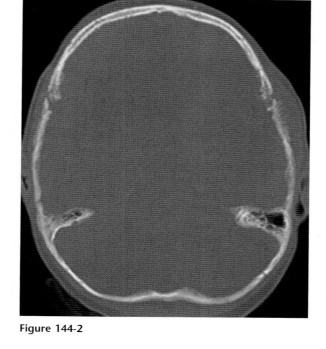

Figure 144-2

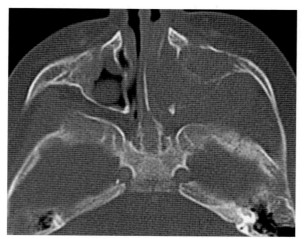

Figure 144-3

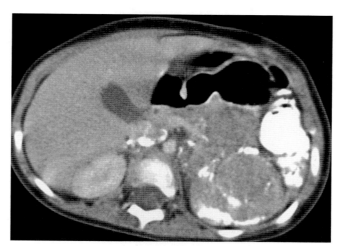

Figure 144-4

HISTORY: A 1-year-old boy who presented to the emergency department because his parents felt "bumps" on his head.

1. What is the single best diagnosis of this case?
   A. Neuroblastoma
   B. Chondrosarcoma
   C. Wilms tumor
   D. Osteosarcoma

2. What type of nuclear medicine scan is most specific for neuroendocrine tumors in children?
   A. Three-phase bone scan
   B. Iodine-123–labeled metaiodobenzylguanidine (I-123-MIBG) scan
   C. Indium-labeled white blood cell scan
   D. Positron emission tomography/computed tomography (PET/CT)

3. What are the approximate physical half-lives of I-131 and I-123, respectively?
   A. 8 hours and 13 hours
   B. 8 days and 13 days
   C. 8 days and 13 hours
   D. 13 hours and 12 hours

4. What is the critical organ for I-123-MIBG?
   A. Thyroid
   B. Urinary bladder
   C. Bone
   D. Liver

CASE 144

Neuroblastoma: Metastases to the Cranium

1. **A.** Neuroblastoma. There is a calcified left suprarenal mass arising from the adrenal gland, and there are also aggressive bone lesions with soft tissue components involving the calvarium, skull base, and face.

2. **B.** Iodine-123–labeled metaiodobenzylguanidine (I-123-MIBG) scan. I-131-MIBG and I-123-MIBG scans are used in the routine staging of this entity.

3. **C.** 8 days and 13 hours. The physical half-life of I-131 is approximately 8 days, and the physical half-life of I-123 is approximately 13 hours.

4. **D.** Liver. The critical organ is the organ that is most susceptible to the radiation damage and the first organ to receive the maximal dose for a given radiotracer/pharmaceutical. In the case of I-123-MIBG, this organ is the liver.

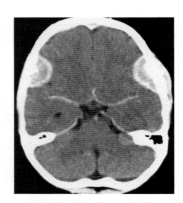

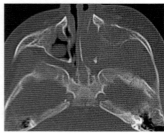

Comment

Neuroblastoma is the most common extracranial pediatric solid tumor and the most common neoplasm in infancy. The majority of cases occur in children by the age of 5 years. These neoplasms arise from precursors of the sympathetic nervous plexus. The primary site is usually the adrenal gland, but these tumors can arise in paraspinal locations anywhere from the neck through the pelvis. High urinary catecholamine levels are present in more than 90% of cases. The embryonal type of this neoplasm often encases vascular structures and usually manifests with metastatic disease (bone, lymph nodes, liver).

Prognosis

Defining the extent of disease requires CT (Figures 144-1 through 144-4) or MRI, bone scan, MIBG scan, bone marrow tests, and urine catecholamine measurements. The natural history is variable, but it is largely predictable from the clinical and biologic features. The biologic features distinguish low-risk (90% survival) from high-risk (30% survival) cases. Some patients with a favorable clinical profile (localized tumor) are likely to have fatal metastatic disease because of the biologic features of the tumor, whereas other patients with widespread disease are likely to survive because of good biologic markers of the tumor.

Presentation

Patients usually present with symptoms attributable to the local effects of the primary or metastatic tumor. Ecchymotic orbital proptosis ("raccoon eyes") results from metastatic involvement of the periorbital bones and soft tissue (spread to the skull is common). This 1-year-old boy was brought to the emergency room because his parents felt "bumps" on his head. A small subset of patients, approximately 2%, present with a paraneoplastic syndrome that can include watery diarrhea or opsoclonus-myoclonus-ataxia syndrome. The diarrhea mimics intestinal malabsorption and results from vasoactive intestinal peptide production by tumor cells that resolves after tumor resection.

Reference

Kushner BH. Neuroblastoma: a disease requiring a multitude of imaging studies. *J Nucl Med.* 2004;45:1172-1188.

Cross-Reference

Neuroradiology: THE REQUISITES, 4th ed, p 342.

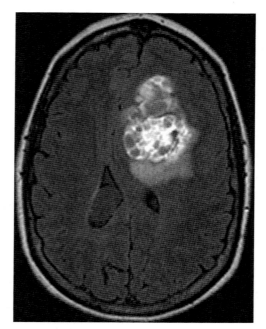

Figure 145-1

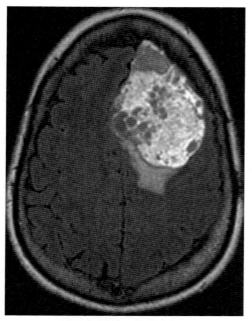

Figure 145-2

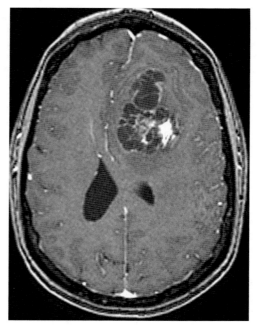

Figure 145-3

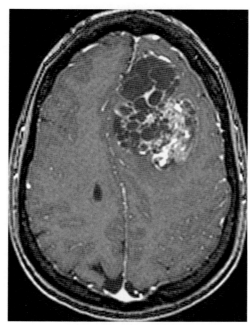

Figure 145-4

HISTORY: A 44-year-old with headache.

1. Assuming this mass is not malignant and primarily extra-axial, what is the single most likely diagnosis?
   A. Meningioma
   B. Epidermoid cyst
   C. Teratoma
   D. Abscess

2. What percentage of these masses are cystic?
   A. Less than 2%
   B. 2% to 10%
   C. 11% to 15%
   D. 16% to 25%

3. What is the most common site of these masses?
   A. Planum sphenoidale
   B. Cerebellopontine angle
   C. Cerebral convexity
   D. Along the tentorium cerebelli

4. Which tumor would most likely cause cystic intracranial metastases?
   A. Squamous cell carcinoma of the larynx
   B. Adenocarcinoma of the colon
   C. Hodgkin lymphoma
   D. Osteosarcoma of the femur

CASE 145

Cystic Meningioma

1. **A.** Meningioma. The most common benign intracranial extra-axial mass is a meningioma. The cystic subtype is uncommon and can be confused with metastatic disease or gliomas. These usually have solid enhancing components and may have more aggressive features.

2. **B.** 2% to 10%. The percentage of meningiomas that are cystic is between 2% and 5%, with some series reporting as high as 10%.

3. **C.** Cerebral convexity. Most of these lesions occur along the cerebral convexities or the sphenoid wing.

4. **B.** Adenocarcinoma of the colon. When metastatic, adenocarcinomas tend to result in cystic metastatic foci in the brain. Squamous cell carcinoma metastasis may have necrosis if large but are generally more solid than cystic. Lymphoma and osteosarcoma, if metastatic, would be solid, but even this less commonly occurs.

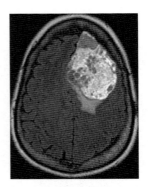

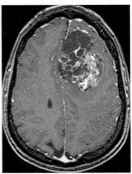

Comment

Cystic meningiomas are uncommon tumors, representing approximately 2% to 5% of meningiomas (some series report up to 10%), and they can be confused with metastatic or glial tumors with cystic components. Cystic meningiomas typically occur at the cerebral convexity or along the greater wing of the sphenoid. In rare cases, they have been found in the ventricles and suprasellar cistern.

Subtypes

Cystic meningiomas may be morphologically divided into three major types: cystic areas contained within the tumor; cystic areas at the periphery of the tumor, but within the tumor margins (as in this case, Figures 145-1 through 145-4); and cystic areas peripheral to the tumor, lying on, or occasionally within, the adjacent brain. There is still debate about the cause of the cyst wall.

Risk of Malignancy

The majority of cystic meningiomas are histopathologically meningothelial. Cellular atypia and sometimes malignant features are seen in a higher percentage of these cystic variants (compared with the garden variety meningioma); therefore, multiple intraoperative biopsies and frozen sections are recommended.

Imaging

Magnetic resonance imaging (MRI) shows the extra-axial location of these tumors and their cystic components. MRI with contrast enhancement (see Figures 145-3 and 145-4) can distinguish cyst walls containing tumor cells (these cyst walls enhance) from cyst walls containing gliotic tissue without tumor invasion (these cyst walls typically do not enhance). There is no clear correlation between cyst signal intensity and cyst content. MRI findings correlate well with the surgical appearance and pathologic results, and these findings allow the preoperative diagnosis of cystic meningioma.

Treatment

Division of this entity into three types of cysts aids the neurosurgeon, who must decide whether total resection is feasible. To obtain total resection and reduce the risk of recurrence, the surgeon must ensure that the plane of resection is between the thin enhancing membrane of the tumor cyst and the adjacent arachnoid. In cases in which the cyst is intra-axial or trapped cerebrospinal fluid, the cyst wall adjacent to or within the brain parenchyma usually is not included in the resection.

Reference

Wasenko JJ, Hochhauser L, Stopa EG, Winfield JA. Cystic meningiomas: MR characteristics and surgical correlations. *Am J Neuroradiol.* 1994;15:1959-1965.

Cross-Reference

Neuroradiology: THE REQUISITES, 4th ed, p 41.

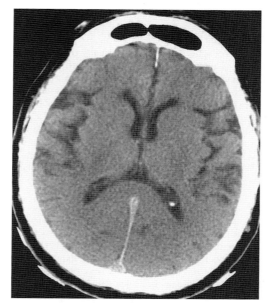

Figure 146-1 Patient A.

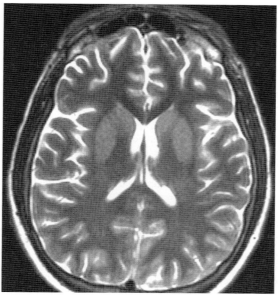

Figure 146-2 Patient A.

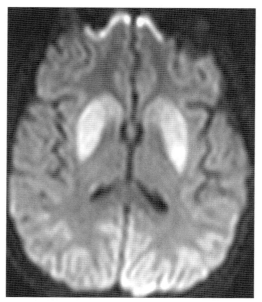

Figure 146-3 Patient A.

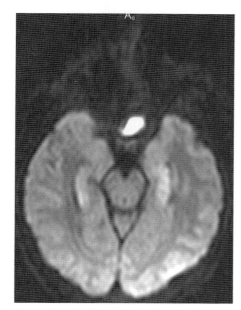

Figure 146-4 Patient B.

HISTORY: A 23-year-old with prolonged hypotension after a motor vehicle collision.

1. What is the single most likely diagnosis of this case?
   A. Methanol toxicity
   B. Anoxic brain injury
   C. Metastatic disease
   D. Diffuse axonal injury

2. Of the choices provided, an angiogram may likely show which of the following?
   A. Beaded middle cerebral artery branches
   B. Absence of contrast in the anterior circulation
   C. Prominent lenticulostriate vessels
   D. Multiple aneurysms

3. What is the most common cause of hypoxic-ischemic injury in a 60-year-old person?
   A. Respiratory arrest
   B. Cardiac arrest
   C. Trauma
   D. Seizures

4. What is the watershed territory in fetuses and newborns?
   A. Anterior frontal and frontal-parietal cortices
   B. Subcortical white matter
   C. Deep periventricular white matter
   D. Posterior fossa

CASE 146

Global Anoxic Brain Injury

1. **B.** Anoxic brain injury. In this case of a patient with sustained hypotension following a motor vehicle collision, the findings are most compatible with hypoxic-ischemic encephalopathy (HIE).

2. **B.** Absence of contrast in the anterior circulation. In cases of HIE, the diffuse cerebral edema and increased intracranial pressure may overcome cerebral perfusion pressure and result in brain death.

3. **B.** Cardiac arrest. Cardiac arrest is the most likely cause for HIE in a 60-year-old person.

4. **C.** Deep periventricular white matter. The watershed territory in fetuses and newborns is the deep periventricular white matter. As a result, radiologic and pathologic manifestations of global hypoxic-ischemic injury are present within the deep white matter and result in periventricular leukomalacia.

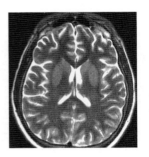

Comment

Pathophysiology

Global hypoxic-ischemic injury is typically related to decreased perfusion; less commonly, it may be related to a disturbance in blood oxygenation. Postanoxic encephalopathy typically occurs after a period in which a diffuse episode of cerebral hypoperfusion has occurred. The patient may have a lucid interval but then, over a 1- to 2-week period, undergo a precipitous decline that can even result in death. In this scenario, the pathologic changes are most pronounced in the white matter, where there is demyelination and sometimes necrosis. Carbon monoxide poisoning can produce a similar clinical course and radiologic appearance.

Imaging

In the acute setting of global hypoxic-ischemic injury, unenhanced computed tomography can show global loss of gray-white matter differentiation, diffuse gray matter hypodensity, and sulcal effacement (Figure 146-1). On magnetic resonance imaging, T2-weighted hyperintensity may be seen in the watershed territories and/or in the basal ganglia (Figure 146-2). The hippocampus and basal ganglia are particularly susceptible to anoxic injury (Figures 146-1 through 146-4). In laminar necrosis, T2-weighted hyperintensity may be seen globally throughout the cortex. Imaging in the subacute phase can demonstrate cortical hemorrhage in the setting of laminar necrosis, which is commonly of high signal intensity on unenhanced T1-weighted images. In the subacute to chronic stages, hypointensity in the cortex and on gradient echo images may be noted.

Reference

Dettmers C, Solymosi L, Hartmann A, et al. Confirmation of CT criteria to distinguish pathophysiologic subtypes of cerebral infarction. *AJNR Am J Neuroradiol.* 1997;18:335-342.

Cross-Reference

Neuroradiology: THE REQUISITES, 4th ed, pp 117, 308.

Challenge

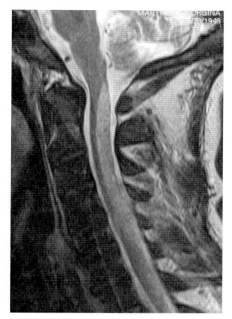

Figure 147-1

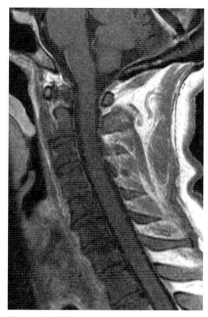

Figure 147-2

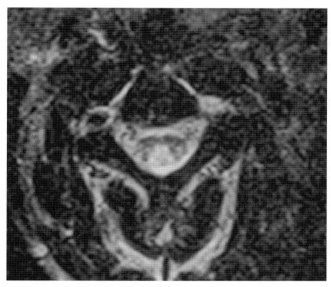

Figure 147-3

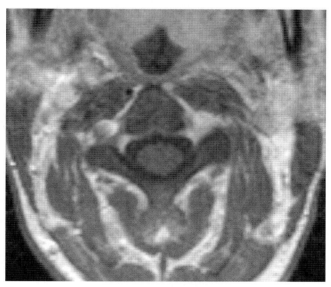

Figure 147-4

HISTORY: A 57-year-old woman presents with difficulty walking and bilateral upper extremity weakness for several weeks, 3 months status post partial gastrectomy.

1. Considering both imaging and clinical presentation, what is the single best diagnosis?
   A. Multiple sclerosis
   B. Wallerian degeneration
   C. Spinal dural arteriovenous fistula
   D. Subacute combined degeneration

2. Which of the following conditions is *not* associated with vitamin B_{12} deficiency?
   A. Acquired immunodeficiency syndrome (AIDS)
   B. Alcoholism
   C. Multiple sclerosis
   D. Metformin therapy

3. What commonly used anesthetic agent has been implicated in vitamin B_{12} deficiency?
   A. Propofol
   B. Amobarbital
   C. Nitrous oxide
   D. Ketamine

4. Which imaging finding is *least* likely to be seen with subacute combined degeneration?
   A. High signal intensity on T2-weighted images in the posterior columns
   B. Contrast enhancement
   C. Expansion of the spinal cord
   D. Low signal intensity on T1-weighted images in the posterior columns

CASE 147

Subacute Combined Degeneration

1. **D.** Subacute combined degeneration (SCD). A high-intensity signal in the dorsal columns is typically seen in SCD. Although multiple sclerosis involves the dorsal columns, the exquisite symmetry of the signal abnormality confined to the dorsal columns over several vertebral segments, as in this case, would be unlikely. There is no volume loss to suggest Wallerian degeneration, and the patient's history does not suggest a causative injury. Spinal dural arteriovenous fistula may manifest with cord signal changes; however, no abnormal intradural vessels are seen to suggest that.

2. **C.** Multiple sclerosis. The symptoms of vitamin B_{12} deficiency often mimic symptoms of multiple sclerosis; however, there is no association between the two. In recent years, an increasing prevalence of vitamin B_{12} deficiency has been reported in patients who tested positive for human immunodeficiency virus (HIV), especially patients with AIDS. Alcohol abuse can lead to gastritis and damage to the lining of the intestines, both of which can interfere with vitamin B_{12} absorption. There is a high prevalence of vitamin B_{12} deficiency in patients with type 2 diabetes mellitus on metformin therapy.

3. **C.** Nitrous oxide. In individuals with borderline vitamin B_{12} serum levels, SCD may be promoted by nitrous oxide anesthesia during surgery. Nitrous oxide enhances the oxidation of vitamin B_{12}. There is no association between the other medications listed and SCD.

4. **D.** Low signal intensity on T1-weighted images in the posterior columns. High T2 signal in the posterior columns with or without enhancement and with or without expansion of the cord is seen in SCD. Low T1 signal in the posterior columns is not characteristic.

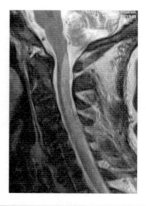

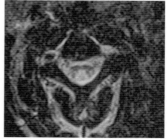

Comment

Background

SCD is the manifestation of vitamin B_{12} deficiency in the spinal cord. The cause of vitamin B_{12} (cyanocobalamin) deficiency can be divided into three main categories: (1) inadequate intake (e.g., vegetarians); (2) malabsorption (e.g., pernicious anemia, gastrectomy, intestinal infections, Crohn disease, tropical sprue); and (3) other conditions (e.g., nitrous oxide anesthesia, transcobalamin II deficiency). The most common cause of vitamin B_{12} deficiency in the United States is pernicious anemia.

Histopathology

Histopathologic studies demonstrate degeneration of myelin sheaths and axonal loss in the posterior, lateral, and sometimes anterior columns.

Imaging

On sagittal images, T2-weighted images reveal increased signal intensity of variable length in the posterior columns (Figure 147-1). On transverse images, the signal abnormality appears as an inverted "V" (Figure 147-3). This configuration reflects greater involvement of the lateral than the medial portions of the dorsal columns and corresponds to relative sparing of proprioceptive sensation in the lower extremities clinically. Lesions typically occur in the thoracic and cervical cord, most often exceeding several vertebral bodies in length. The hyperintensity may or may not be associated with postcontrast enhancement on T1-weighted images (Figures 147-2 and 147-4). Cord enlargement has been observed in some cases. Restricted diffusion in the posterior columns has also been described. Lateral column hyperintensity is uncommon, even in cases with histologic and clinical evidence of lateral column involvement.

Management

Therapy with vitamin B_{12} results in partial to full recovery, depending on the duration and extent of neurodegeneration. Vitamin B_{12} supplements must be taken throughout life to prevent symptoms from recurring.

References

Ravina B, Loevner LA, Bank W. MR findings in subacute combined degeneration of the spinal cord: a case of reversible cervical myelopathy. *AJR Am J Roentgenol.* 2000;174(3):863-865.

Renard D, Dutray A, Remy A, et al. Subacute combined degeneration of the spinal cord caused by nitrous oxide anaesthesia. *Neurol Sci.* 2009;30(1):75-76.

Tian C. Hyperintense signal on spinal cord diffusion-weighted imaging in a patient with subacute combined degeneration. *Neurol India.* 2011;59(3):429-431.

Cross-Reference

Neuroradiology: THE REQUISITES, 4th ed, pp 563-564.

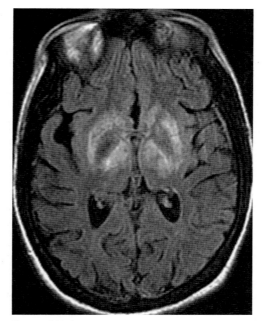

Figure 148-1

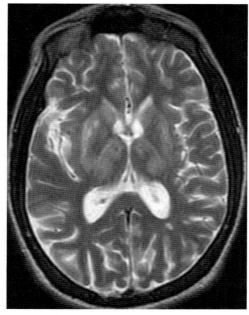

Figure 148-2

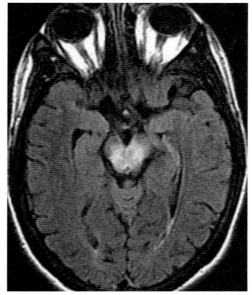

Figure 148-3

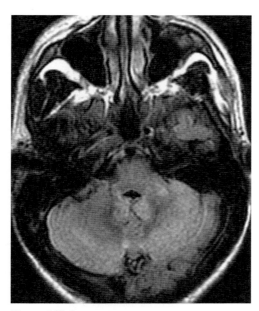

Figure 148-4

HISTORY: Tremors.

1. Which group of differential diagnoses is most correct for T1 hyperintensity in the basal ganglia?
   A. Acute infarct, lymphoma
   B. Creutzfeldt-Jakob disease, methanol toxicity
   C. Extrapontine myelinolysis, Leigh disease
   D. Wilson disease, neurofibromatosis type 1

2. What neurodegenerative disease is caused by loss of dopaminergic neurons?
   A. Dementia with Lewy bodies
   B. Alzheimer disease
   C. Progressive supranuclear palsy
   D. Parkinson disease

3. What is the inheritance pattern of Wilson disease?
   A. Autosomal recessive
   B. Autosomal dominant
   C. Sporadic
   D. X-linked

4. What mineral deposition has been postulated to be contributory to the cause for abnormal signal in the globus pallidus with hepatic encephalopathy?
   A. Copper
   B. Manganese
   C. Magnesium
   D. Iron

CASE 148

Wilson Disease

1. **D.** Wilson disease, neurofibromatosis type 1. Both of these are causes of hyperintense T1 signal on magnetic resonance imaging (MRI) in the basal ganglia. Acute infarct, lymphoma, Creutzfeldt-Jakob disease, methanol toxicity, extrapontine myelinolysis, and Leigh disease all cause hypointense signal on T1-weighted images.

2. **D.** Parkinson disease. Primary Parkinson disease is characterized by loss of dopaminergic receptors. Dementia with Lewy bodies is from accumulation of Lewy bodies resulting in volume loss that spares the hippocampi. Alzheimer disease is extracellular B-amyloid plaque deposition with intracellular accumulation of neurofibrillary tangles resulting in atrophy in the temporal and parietal lobes. Progressive supranuclear palsy is from abnormal accumulation of phosphorylated tau protein within the brain, causing postural instability and dementia.

3. **A.** Autosomal recessive. Wilson disease is inherited in an autosomal recessive pattern affecting chromosome 13.

4. **B.** Manganese. It is most accepted that manganese accumulation in the globus pallidus results in the signal abnormality. In hepatic failure, manganese bypasses normal detoxification.

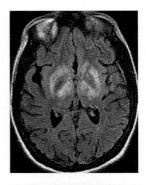

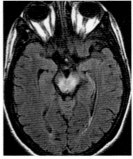

Comment

Cause

Wilson disease (hepatolenticular degeneration) is an autosomal recessive hereditary disease that results from abnormal metabolism of copper caused by deficiency of its carrier protein, ceruloplasmin. As a result, there is extensive abnormal deposition of copper in multiple organ systems (most pronounced in the liver and brain). Although neurologic symptoms may be directly related to copper deposition within the brain parenchyma, they may also be a manifestation of hepatic encephalopathy caused by liver failure.

Clinical

Neurologic signs and symptoms may include a pseudoparkinsonian-like syndrome, with rigidity, gait disturbance, and difficulty with fine motor skills. Dysarthria and progressive cognitive and psychiatric disturbances may also be present. Symptoms usually begin at 10 to 20 years of age but sometimes do not begin until the age of 30 years and beyond. Presentation before 5 years of age is rare, even though the biochemical defect is present at birth. The diagnosis is made by laboratory analysis in which there are elevated copper levels within the urine as well as low serum ceruloplasmin levels. Treatment of Wilson disease is with D-penicillamine (chelation therapy).

Imaging

On MRI, the most common finding may be atrophy (Figures 148-1 through 148-4). Regions of abnormal T2 hyperintensity involve the deep gray matter of the basal ganglia and the thalami, as well as the white matter (see Figure 148-2). In particular, the putamen of the lentiform nucleus and the caudate are involved (see Figure 148-2). In addition to signal abnormality, atrophy of the caudate nuclei may be present. Regions of T2 hyperintensity have also been noted in the basal ganglia and have been attributed either to the paramagnetic effects of copper or possibly to associated iron deposition. Abnormalities on MRI may also be present in the brainstem and in the white matter of the cerebellum, as in this case (see Figures 148-3 and 148-4).

References

Akhan O, Akpinar E, Oto A, et al. Unusual findings in Wilson's disease. *Eur Radiol.* 2002;12(suppl 3):S66-S69.

van Wassenaer-van Hall HN, van den Heuvel AG, Algra A, Hoogenrad TU, Mali WP. Wilson's disease: findings at MR imaging and CT of the brain with clinical correlation. *Radiology.* 1996;198:531-536.

Cross-Reference

Neuroradiology: THE REQUISITES, 4th ed, pp 250-252.

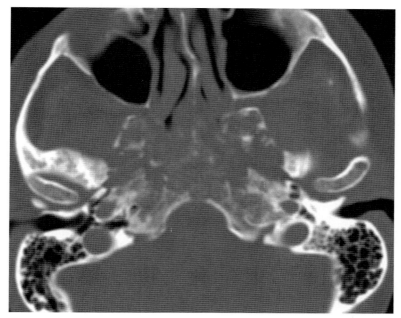

Figure 149-1

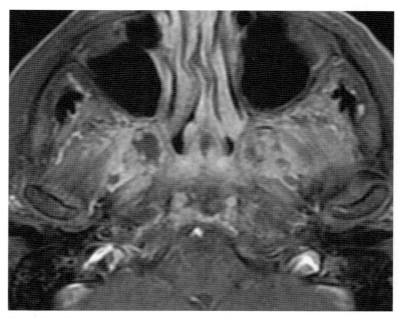

Figure 149-2

HISTORY: A patient with previously treated cancer had a severe headache.

1. Which of the following is the single best diagnosis?
   A. Myeloma
   B. Chordoma
   C. Fibrous dysplasia
   D. Radiation necrosis

2. Which of the following is the tumor for which treatment most commonly causes radiation necrosis of the skull base?
   A. Sinonasal cancer
   B. Nasopharyngeal carcinoma
   C. Glioblastoma
   D. Retinoblastoma

3. Which of the following is the strongest risk factor for nasopharyngeal carcinoma?
   A. Smoking
   B. Human papillomavirus
   C. Epstein-Barr virus
   D. Alcohol

4. What is the first line of therapy for nasopharyngeal cancer?
   A. Surgery
   B. Chemoradiation
   C. Brachytherapy
   D. Laser

CASE 149

Radiation Necrosis

1. **D.** Radiation necrosis. Radiation necrosis may destroy bone, and nasopharyngeal carcinoma can grow through bone. The pattern of destruction and location are not correct for myeloma or chordoma.

2. **B.** Nasopharyngeal carcinoma. Nasopharyngeal carcinoma is the tumor for which treatment most commonly causes radiation necrosis of the skull base. There may also be radiation changes and/or necrosis in the temporal lobes. The retinoblastoma gene may also cause sarcomas. Sinonasal cancer and glioblastoma very rarely erode the clivus.

3. **C.** Epstein-Barr virus. The Epstein-Barr virus is the strongest risk factor for nasopharyngeal carcinoma, along with Southeast Asian ancestry. Smoking and alcohol (wine, in particular) cause a slight risk.

4. **B.** Chemoradiation. Chemoradiation is first line of therapy for nasopharyngeal cancer. Brachytherapy is sometimes used for recurrence.

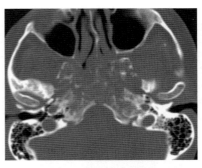

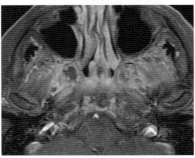

Comment

Differential Diagnosis

The permeative and diffuse pattern of destruction of the skull base and surrounding tissues, including the adjacent musculature, is typical of radiation necrosis (Figures 149-1 and 149-2). The other possible diagnosis is malignant otitis externa with *Pseudomonas* infection, osteomyelitis, and myositis. There really is very little mass in this case; it is more a destructive tissue-limited process and hence suggestive of radiation necrosis.

Treatment of Nasopharyngeal Carcinoma

For nasopharyngeal carcinoma, radiation therapy is often the primary mode of ablation. Recurrence or residual disease may be treated with second-line treatment regimens such as brachytherapy, inasmuch as surgery is not an option. Chemotherapy is often used concomitantly. After multiple treatments, the risk of radiation necrosis increases. Intensity-modulated radiotherapy with doses of up to 70 Gy for recurrent nasopharyngeal carcinoma leads to temporal lobe necrosis in 6% to 19% of patients. Osteoradionecrosis occurs in 10% of cases of successfully treated nasopharyngeal carcinoma; if pharyngeal mucosa necrosis is evident endoscopically, the rate of osteoradionecrosis is as high as 56%.

Imaging Findings

If this bone destruction pattern is accompanied by white matter changes bilaterally and symmetrically in the temporal lobes or, worse, by areas of peripheral enhancement in the temporal lobes with extreme vasogenic edema, radiation injury to the brain has probably occurred as well. These features suggest this diagnosis, as opposed to nasopharyngeal carcinoma, which could also aggressively destroy the skull base or grow intracranially, or both. Usually the intracranial growth is via skull base foramina or the cavernous sinus.

Reference

Chen MY, Mai HQ, Sun R, et al. Clinical findings and imaging features of 67 nasopharyngeal carcinoma patients with postradiation nasopharyngeal necrosis. *Chin J Cancer.* 2013;32(10):533-538.

Cross-Reference

Neuroradiology: THE REQUISITES, 4th ed, pp 83-85.

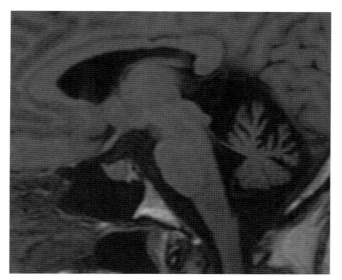

Figure 150-1

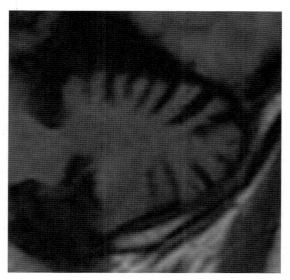

Figure 150-2

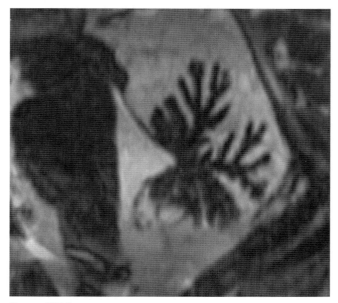

Figure 150-3

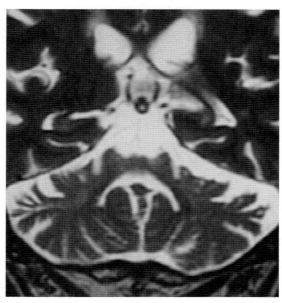

Figure 150-4

HISTORY: A patient presents with ataxia and nystagmus.

1. Which of the following is a cause of cerebellar atrophy?
   A. Alcohol abuse
   B. Chiari type I malformation
   C. Arachnoid cyst
   D. Posterior fossa pilocytic astrocytoma

2. What is the most common clinical presentation in olivopontocerebellar degeneration (OPCD)?
   A. Ataxia
   B. Muscle spasms
   C. Tremor
   D. Nystagmus

3. Which structure is spared from atrophy in OPCD?
   A. Pons
   B. Middle cerebellar peduncle
   C. Dentate nuclei
   D. Substantia nigra

4. Where does the loss in myelin and gliosis begin in OPCD?
   A. Cerebellum
   B. Pons
   C. Middle cerebellar peduncle
   D. Inferior olives

CASE 150

Olivopontocerebellar Degeneration

1. **A.** Alcohol abuse. Excessive chronic alcohol use results in cerebral and cerebellar atrophy. Chiari type I malformation may result in gliosis and encephalomalacia of the cerebellar tonsils but not global atrophy. Mass lesions such as an arachnoid cyst or tumor do not cause an atrophic appearance.

2. **A.** Ataxia. The most common presentation of OPCD is ataxia. Muscle spasms, tremor, and nystagmus occur but not more commonly than ataxia.

3. **C.** Dentate nuclei. The dentate nuclei do not atrophy in OPCD. There is or may be volume loss in the pons, middle cerebellar peduncles, and the substantia nigra.

4. **B.** Pons. Degeneration begins in the pons and progresses along the pontocerebellar tracts through the middle cerebellar peduncle into the cerebellum.

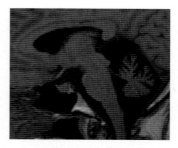

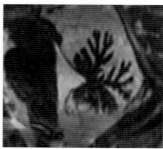

Comment

Epidemiology/Etiology

OPCD may be transmitted through autosomal dominant inheritance or may occur sporadically. Although the onset of symptoms in OPCD may span several decades, two peaks of presentation are noted. Sporadic cases are more common and tend to affect middle-aged adults, whereas familial cases usually occur earlier in young adulthood. The cause of sporadic olivopontocerebellar atrophy is unknown, but the disease is progressive.

Clinical

The main clinical presentation is truncal ataxia, first involving the legs and then the arms. Patients may also have nystagmus, dysarthria, and tremors. Parkinsonian features may develop, accompanied by mild dementia and ophthalmoplegia, pyramidal tract signs, and autonomic disturbance.

Pathology

Pathologically, there is loss of myelin and gliosis of the ponto-cerebellar pathways, beginning in the pontine nuclei and progressing into the cerebellum (the hemispheres and, to a lesser degree, the vermis), with neuronal loss of the cerebellar cortex. OPCD is characterized by atrophy of the cerebellum, pons, medullary olives, and other brainstem structures.

Imaging

Advanced quantitative assessment using magnetic resonance imaging (MRI) has greatly enhanced the ability to evaluate the degenerative processes of the brain including those diseases affecting the cerebellum, brainstem, and spinal cord. On MRI, atrophy of the involved structures (pons, middle cerebellar peduncles, inferior olives, and cerebellum) is evident (Figures 150-1 through 150-4). In addition, there may be mild hyperintensity on T2-weighted images of the involved structures in OPCD.

Reference

Matsusue E, Fujii S, Kanasaki Y, et al. Cerebellar lesions in multiple system atrophy: postmortem MR imaging–pathologic correlations. *AJNR Am J Neuroradiol.* 2009;30:1725-1730.

Cross-Reference

Neuroradiology: THE REQUISITES, 4th ed, pp 255-256.

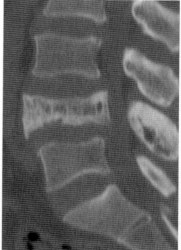

Figure 151-1

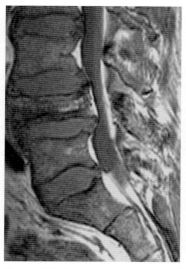

Figure 151-2

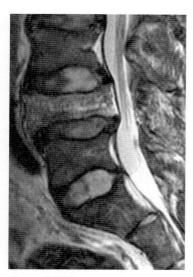

Figure 151-3

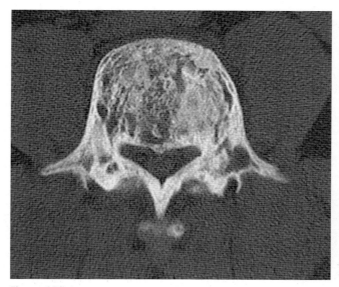

Figure 151-4

HISTORY: A 63-year-old man presents with lower back pain.

1. What is the single best diagnosis?
   A. Paget disease
   B. Lymphoma
   C. Fibrous dysplasia
   D. Osteoblastic metastasis

2. What is the most common spinal complication of this disease?
   A. Spondylolysis
   B. Synovial cyst
   C. Pathologic fracture
   D. Sarcomatous transformation

3. Which of the following statements regarding this disease is *true?*
   A. Thinning of the cortex is often seen.
   B. Associated soft tissue mass is common.
   C. The disease has five phases.
   D. PET/CT is more accurate than bone scintigraphy in the imaging of Paget disease.

4. What is an *uncommon* radiologic finding of uncomplicated disease in this entity?
   A. Bone enlargement
   B. Cortical thickening
   C. Cortical destruction
   D. Disorganized trabecular thickening

CASE 151

Paget Disease in the Lumbar Spine

1. **A.** Paget disease. This is the most likely diagnosis. Lymphoma tends to have a more uniform increase in bone density and is unlikely to cause vertebral expansion. Monostotic involvement in Paget disease may be mistaken for fibrous dysplasia. The absence of a "ground-glass" appearance, seen with fibrous dysplasia, and the presence of cortical thickening suggest Paget disease. Osteoblastic metastasis, commonly from carcinoma of the breast or prostate, may be difficult to differentiate from Paget disease. The key to the diagnosis is the appearance of the spinous process, which shows cortical thickening and enlargement (Figure 151-2).

2. **C.** Pathologic fracture. Pathologic fracture occurs during the early osteolytic phase of Paget disease. Spondylolysis is due to pagetoid involvement of the pars interarticularis with insufficiency fracture; however, it is not the most common complication. Synovial cyst is not a complication of Paget disease. Sarcomatous transformation is a rare complication.

3. **D.** PET/CT is more accurate than bone scintigraphy in the imaging of Paget disease. PET/CT has superior spatial resolution and offers more accurate quantification of bone activity. Thickening of the cortex is a hallmark of the disease. Associated soft tissue is uncommon and, if present, would suggest sarcomatous transformation. The disease has lytic, mixed, and blastic phases.

4. **C.** Cortical destruction. Bone enlargement, cortical thickening, and disorganized trabecular thickening are common findings in Paget disease. Cortical destruction would suggest sarcomatous transformation, which is uncommon.

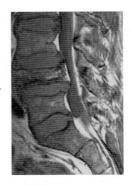

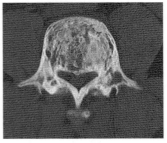

Comment

Background

Paget disease is one of the most common metabolically active bone diseases, second in prevalence only to osteoporosis. The overall prevalence of Paget disease is 3% to 3.7%, and it increases with age. The spine is the second most commonly affected site after the pelvis. Common complications include osseous weakening (with secondary deformity and fracture), spinal stenosis from enlargement of the affected vertebral body or neural arch or both, facet arthropathy, neurologic compromise, and sarcomatous transformation.

Histopathology

Paget disease is characterized by a disturbance in bone modeling and remodeling caused by an increase in osteoblastic and osteoclastic activity. The disease is polyostotic in 66% of cases.

Imaging

Radiography is typically used for diagnostic purposes and may be indicated to evaluate for fracture. Common CT findings of uncomplicated Paget disease include bone enlargement, disorganized trabecular thickening, and cortical thickening (Figures 151-1 and 151-4). The magnetic resonance imaging (MRI) signal intensity pattern is variable. In the lytic (early, active) phase, the marrow space is heterogeneous in signal on T1-weighted and T2-weighted images. In the mixed (intermediate) phase, there is preservation of marrow fat signal (Figures 151-2 and 151-3). Speckled enhancement is found on images after contrast agent administration. The mixed phase is the most commonly seen. In the blastic (late, inactive) phase, low signal intensity is usually found on all sequences; this corresponds to bony sclerosis. All MRI sequences must be carefully examined to exclude sarcomatous transformation.

Management

Patients presenting with neurogenic pain secondary to cord compression by expanded pagetic bone respond well to medical treatment with calcitonin and bisphosphonates. Because of the increased risk of malignancy, patients with Paget disease should be monitored indefinitely. Chemotherapy, radiation, or both may be used to treat neoplasms that arise from pagetic bone.

References

Dell'Atti C, Cassar-Pullicino VN, Lalam RK, et al. The spine in Paget's disease. *Skeletal Radiol.* 2007;36(7):609-626.

Smith SE, Murphey MD, Motamedi K, et al. From the archives of the AFIP. Radiologic spectrum of Paget disease of bone and its complications with pathologic correlation. *Radiographics.* 2002;22(5):1191-1216.

Cross-Reference

Neuroradiology: THE REQUISITES, 4th ed, p 584.

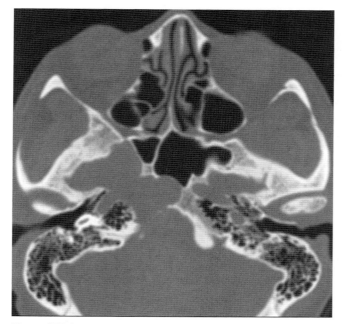

Figure 152-1

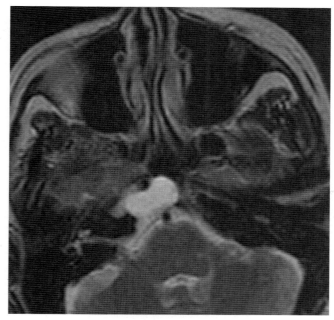

Figure 152-2

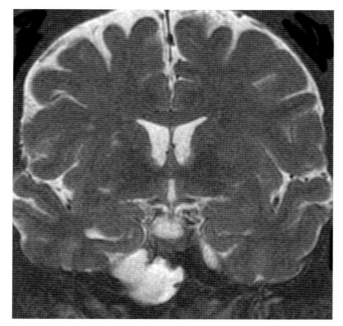

Figure 152-3

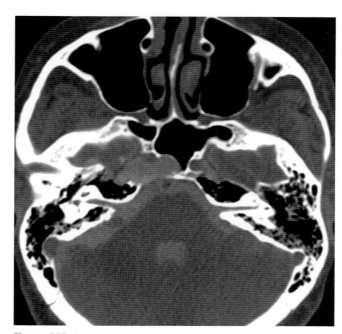

Figure 152-4

HISTORY: A patient presents with headache.

1. What is the single best diagnosis in this case?
   A. Epidermoid
   B. Cholesterol granuloma
   C. Mucocele
   D. Meningocele

2. What lesion in the petrous apex is most commonly differentiated from other T2 hyperintense lesions by presence of restricted diffusivity?
   A. Epidermoid
   B. Cholesterol granuloma
   C. Mucocele
   D. Meningocele

3. What is the characteristic location for meningoencephalocele with Chiari type III malformation?
   A. Orbital
   B. Frontal
   C. Occipital
   D. Lumbosacral

4. Which of the following can be seen with intracranial hypertension?
   A. Meningoceles
   B. Reduction in perioptic subarachnoid spaces
   C. Cerebral edema
   D. Enlarged cortical veins

CASE 152

Meningocele of the Skull Base (Petrous Apex)

1. **D.** Meningocele. There is a well-defined lesion contiguous with cerebrospinal fluid (CSF), following CSF signal on magnetic resonance imaging, and showing contrast-laden CSF on the cisternogram.

2. **A.** Epidermoid. Also called a cholesteatoma when in the temporal bone, these lesions demonstrate restricted diffusion, which allows differentiation from other T2 hyperintense lesions.

3. **D.** Occipital. In Chiari type III malformation, there is an occipital meningoencephalocele.

4. **A.** Meningoceles. Intracranial hypertension is associated with meningoceles, arachnoid pits, distended perioptic subarachnoid spaces, and diminished venous spaces. Cerebral edema is not typically seen in intracranial hypertension.

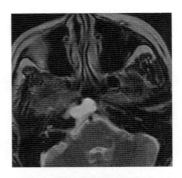

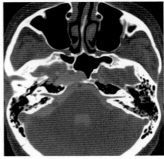

Comment

Imaging

This case shows a well-demarcated, chronic-appearing lesion of the right petrous apex (Figures 152-1 through 152-4) consistent with a cephalocele, more specifically a meningocele, as no brain parenchyma is herniating to consider it a meningoencephalocele. There is expansion, smooth cortical bone thinning without bone destruction, and cortication medially, suggesting a long-standing process (see Figures 152-1 and 152-4). The lesion is isointense to CSF on T2-weighted images (see Figures 152-2 and 152-3); on the coronal T2-weighted image, it is difficult to determine whether this lesion is separate from, or an extension of, Meckel cave into the osseous base of the skull (see Figure 152-3). Computed tomography (CT) cisternography (instillation of contrast material into the thecal sac by lumbar puncture, followed by CT imaging after tilting of the patient so that the contrast agent spreads through the subarachnoid spaces in the head) confirms that the petrous apex lesion communicates with the CSF spaces (see Figure 152-4).

Differential Diagnosis of Petrous Apex Lesions

The differential diagnosis of a benign-appearing, expansile petrous apex mass includes cholesterol granuloma, mucocele, epidermoid, meningocele, and, occasionally, aneurysm of the internal carotid artery. Mucoceles are frequently unilocular and show peripheral enhancement. The signal characteristics of mucoceles vary depending on the protein concentration and viscosity. Epidermoid cysts may have a benign appearance, or they can have more concerning radiologic findings, such as bone erosion or destruction. They typically appear similar to CSF on T1-weighted and T2-weighted images, hyperintense on fluid-attenuated inversion recovery (FLAIR) imaging, and show restricted diffusion. Cholesterol granulomas, when large, may be multilocular. There is usually thinning of the cortex with large lesions without bone destruction. Cholesterol granulomas are often hyperintense on all pulse sequences. In particular, the marked hyperintensity on unenhanced T1-weighted images distinguishes these from many other lesions, and the presence of hemorrhage-fluid levels within these lesions is highly characteristic.

Reference

Silver RI, Moonis G, Schlosser RJ, et al. Radiographic signs of elevated intracranial pressure in idiopathic CSF leaks: a possible presentation of idiopathic intracranial hypertension. *Am J Rhinol.* 2007; 21:257-261.

Cross-Reference

Neuroradiology: THE REQUISITES, 4th ed, p 374.

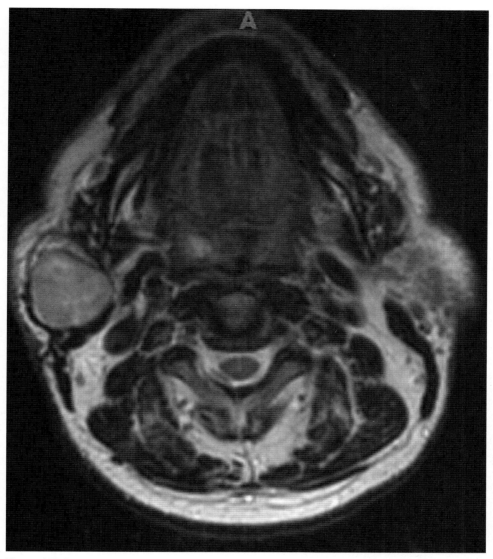

Figure 153-1

HISTORY: A 70-year-old male patient has a complaint of right ear swelling, and a palpable mass was present.

1. Which of the following should be *excluded* from the differential diagnosis?
   A. Warthin tumor
   B. First branchial cleft cyst
   C. Pleomorphic adenoma
   D. Myoepithelioma

2. What is the most common location for this lesion in the head and neck?
   A. Palate minor salivary glands
   B. Submandibular glands
   C. Lacrimal glands
   D. Parotid glands

3. Which of the following best describes the features of Warthin tumor?
   A. It occurs primarily in older men; it occurs in the tail of the parotid gland.
   B. It occurs primarily in middle-aged women; it occurs in the superficial lobe of the parotid gland.
   C. It occurs primarily in older men; it occurs in the deep lobe of the parotid gland.
   D. It occurs primarily in young men; it occurs in the deep lobe of the parotid gland.

4. Why are Warthin tumors electively removed at the patient's option?
   A. On resection, the rate of facial nerve paralysis is high, and so surgeons are reluctant to remove them.
   B. They respond very well to chemotherapy and radiation therapy.
   C. They seed the operative bed.
   D. They have no malignant potential.

CASE 153

Parotid Myoepithelioma

1. **B.** First branchial cleft cyst. Because of the location, the diagnosis is most likely a Warthin tumor. The diagnosis should also include pleomorphic adenoma because it is the most common parotid mass. The actual pathologic diagnosis was myoepithelioma. The T2-weighted image suggests a solid mass, and so a first branchial cleft cyst should not be considered.

2. **D.** Parotid glands. The parotid gland is the primary site of occurrence of most reported tumors (40% to 50%), followed by the minor salivary glands as the second most preferred site (of which the palate is the most common location; 20%). The submandibular gland accounts for 10% of the tumors.

3. **A.** It occurs primarily in older men; it occurs in the tail of the parotid gland. Warthin tumors are often seen in older men. They are seen in the tail of the parotid gland near the angle of the mandible.

4. **D.** They have no malignant potential. Warthin tumors have no malignant potential, so their removal is the patient's choice.

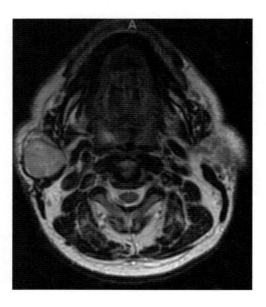

Comment

Features of a Warthin Tumor

Although this case histologically proved to be a myoepithelioma, it had the classical features of a Warthin tumor:

- It occurred in a man.
- The man was older.
- The lesion was in the tail of the parotid gland.
- It appeared heterogeneous on T2-weighted images, with darker areas in it (Figure 153-1).

Features of Myoepitheliomas

Myoepitheliomas are varieties of monomorphic adenomas characterized by a variable course. The parotid glands are the locations in 45% of the cases; however, in all salivary glands, pleomorphic adenomas are the most common benign salivary tumors. Monomorphic adenoma masses usually are well defined and enhance avidly. However, there are malignant varieties of salivary gland myoepithelial tumors, and 39% have aggressive features.

Site of Parotid Tumors

With regard to sites of tumors, the most common tumor of the superficial and deep lobes of the parotid gland is the pleomorphic adenoma. The tail of the parotid gland near the angle of the mandible is the only location where Warthin tumor predominates.

Reference

Khademi B, Kazemi T, Bayat A, Bahranifard H, Daneshbod Y, Mohammadianpanah M. Salivary gland myoepithelial neoplasms: a clinical and cytopathologic study of 15 cases and review of the literature. *Acta Cytol.* 2010;54(6):1111-1117.

Cross-Reference

Neuroradiology: THE REQUISITES, 4th ed, p 490.

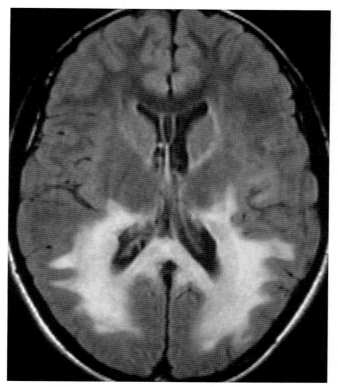

Figure 154-1

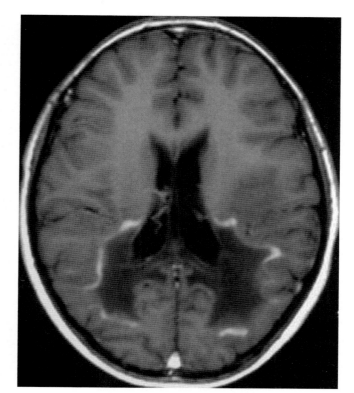

Figure 154-2

HISTORY: A 6-year-old male presents with seizures and behavioral difficulties.

1. What is the diagnosis?
   A. Adrenoleukodystrophy
   B. Metachromatic leukodystrophy
   C. Alexander disease
   D. Canavan disease

2. What is the most common dysmyelinating disease?
   A. Adrenoleukodystrophy
   B. Canavan disease
   C. Metachromatic leukodystrophy
   D. Alexander disease

3. What is the deficiency in adrenoleukodystrophy?
   A. Arylsulfatase A
   B. N-acetylaspartoacylase
   C. Lysosomal β-galactocerebrosidase
   D. Peroxysomal acyl coenzyme A (acyl-CoA) synthetase

4. What is the deficiency in Canavan disease?
   A. Arylsulfatase A
   B. N-acetylaspartoacylase
   C. Lysosomal β-galactocerebrosidase
   D. Peroxysomal acyl-CoA synthetase

CASE 154

Adrenoleukodystrophy

1. **A.** Adrenoleukodystrophy. In this case, abnormal signal is localized to the parietal and occipital lobes. There is usually symmetric diffuse T2 hyperintense signal throughout all white matter, with sparing of the subcortical U-fibers in metachromatic leukodystrophy. In Alexander disease, there is usually symmetric abnormal signal involving predominately the frontal lobes, which can eventually spread posteriorly. In Canavan disease, there is symmetric abnormal signal involving all white matter, including the subcortical U-fibers.

2. **C.** Metachromatic leukodystrophy. Metachromatic leukodystrophy is the most common dysmyelinating disease.

3. **D.** Peroxysomal acyl-CoA synthetase. This enzyme is necessary for the β oxidation of very long-chain fatty acids.

4. **B.** *N*-acetylaspartoacylase. This enzyme deficiency in Canavan disease results in toxic accumulation of *N*-acetylaspartate in the brain as evidenced on magnetic resonance spectroscopy.

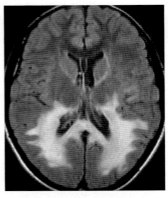

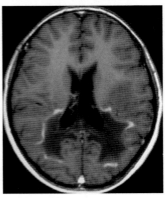

Comment

Clinical

Adrenoleukodystrophy is an X-linked or autosomal recessive disorder that is related to a single enzyme deficiency (acyl-CoA synthetase) within intracellular peroxisomes. This enzyme is necessary for β oxidation in the breakdown of very long-chain fatty acids that accumulate in erythrocytes, plasma, and fibroblasts in the central nervous system white matter and adrenal cortex. Boys typically present between ages 4 and 10 years. The clinical presentation may include behavioral disturbance, visual symptoms, hearing loss, seizures, and, eventually, spastic quadriparesis. Patients often present with adrenal insufficiency (Addison disease), which may occur before or after the development of neurologic symptoms.

Imaging

As in other demyelinating and dysmyelinating disorders, magnetic resonance imaging (MRI) is the imaging modality of choice for the detection of white matter disease, being far superior to computed tomography. In adrenoleukodystrophy, the most common pattern of white matter disease is bilaterally symmetric abnormalities within the parietal and occipital white matter, extending across the splenium of the corpus callosum (Figures 154-1 and 154-2). The disease may continue to progress anteriorly to involve the frontal and temporal lobes. The region of active demyelination, usually along the anterior margin, may show contrast enhancement (see Figure 154-2). Less typical presentations include predominantly frontal lobe involvement or holohemispheric involvement. Adrenoleukodystrophy also involves the cerebellum, spinal cord, and peripheral nervous system. Findings on MRI correlate well with the patient's neuropsychiatric assessment.

Reference

Rajanayagam V, Balthazor M, Shapiro EG, et al. Proton MR spectroscopy and neuropsychological testing in adrenoleukodystrophy. *AJNR Am J Neuroradiol.* 1997;18:1909-1914.

Cross-Reference

Neuroradiology: THE REQUISITES, 4th ed, pp 225-226.

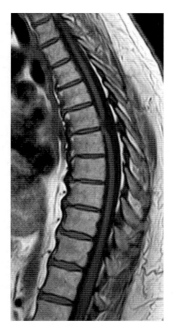

Figure 155-1

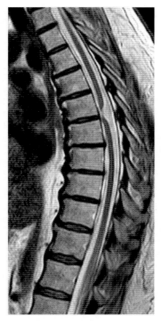

Figure 155-2

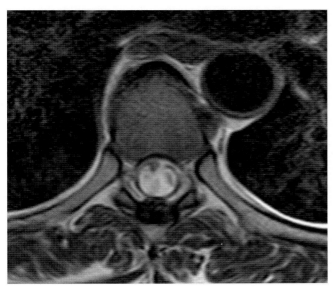

Figure 155-3

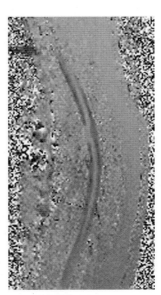

Figure 155-4

HISTORY: A 55-year-old woman presents with a history of progressive paraparesis and rapidly progressive myelopathy.

1. What is the single best diagnosis?
   A. Spinal cord herniation
   B. Arachnoid cyst
   C. Diastematomyelia
   D. Dermoid cyst

2. Where does this most often occur?
   A. C2-C6
   B. C7-T3
   C. T4-T7
   D. T8-T12

3. What finding is common to patients with this entity?
   A. Scalloping of the vertebral body
   B. Focal cord atrophy
   C. Dural tear at the level of an intervertebral disc
   D. Schmorl node

4. Which of the following imaging features has been described in patients with spinal cord herniation?
   A. Fluid sign
   B. Nuclear trail sign
   C. Mercedes-Benz sign
   D. Empty sac sign

CASE 155

Idiopathic Spinal Cord Herniation

1. **A.** Spinal cord herniation. The findings in this case are typical of spinal cord herniation. A dorsal arachnoid cyst may cause mass effect and ventral displacement of the cord. The signal within the lesion is slightly hyperintense compared with the cerebrospinal fluid signal, and thin margins visible at the superior and inferior ends of the lesion are suggestive of a cyst. There is no evidence of split cord on the axial images. Dermoid cyst may manifest as an intramedullary cystic lesion; however, no defined lesion is present in this case.

2. **C.** T4-T7. Idiopathic spinal cord herniations most commonly occur in the mid-thoracic spine between the T4 and the T7 levels.

3. **C.** Dural tear at the level of an intervertebral disc. A dural tear is a characteristic finding in all cases of spinal cord herniation. Scalloping of the vertebral bodies, focal spinal cord atrophy, and signal abnormality in the spinal cord can be seen but are variably present.

4. **B.** Nuclear trail sign. Nuclear trail sign has been described in association with spinal cord herniation. Fluid sign has been described with benign vertebral body fractures. Mercedes-Benz sign has been described as pathognomonic of epidural lipomatosis involving the lumbar spine. Empty sac sign has been described in arachnoiditis.

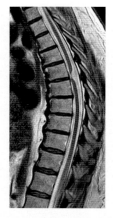

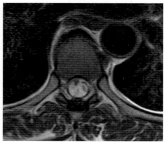

Comment

Background and Clinical Findings

Idiopathic thoracic spinal cord herniation, in contrast to spinal cord herniation with a known traumatic or postoperative origin, is an uncommon cause of thoracic myelopathy in which the anterior portion of the spinal cord herniates or prolapses through a defect in the ventral dura. Brown-Séquard syndrome is the most frequently reported clinical feature. Early manifestations include numbness and decreased temperature sensation in the legs, gait disturbances, pain, and incontinence. Symptoms often worsen over time, but timely diagnosis and treatment may allow the reversal of neurologic deficits.

Pathophysiology

The pathophysiology of this condition is unclear. Some authors suggest that it is initiated by incidental or unnoticed trauma to the anterior surface of the thoracic dura by disc protrusions or osteophytes. Subsequent herniation of spinal cord tissue through a dural defect results from the action of cerebrospinal fluid pulsation and mechanical factors, which lead to progressive myelopathy.

Imaging

Radiologic imaging is the main method for diagnosing idiopathic spinal cord herniation. On sagittal magnetic resonance imaging (MRI), an acute, anterior kink of the thoracic spinal cord is observed with an enlargement of the dorsal subarachnoid space (Figures 155-1 and 155-2). Cord deviation is generally limited to one or two thoracic spine segments. The dural defect occurs in the thoracic spine, most commonly between the levels of the T4 and T7 vertebrae (Figure 155-3). Associated cord atrophy and high T2 signal intensity may be observed within the thoracic cord. Scalloping of the vertebral body also may be seen occasionally. Imaging features of spinal cord herniation generally include a dural tear through which a portion of the cord protrudes. Cerebrospinal fluid flows freely through the defect, causing increased turbulence in the fluid just dorsal to the site of herniation. The observation of this feature and the demonstration of uninterrupted flow on phase contrast cine MRI may allow the differentiation of spinal cord herniation from an arachnoid cyst (Figure 155-4). The nuclear trail sign, a linear area of hyperdensity on computed tomography at the endplate, related to herniation of the disc nucleus, has been described although this is often seen with disc herniation of the thoracic spine without dural tears or spinal cord herniation.

Management

The best treatment option is surgical reduction, especially in the case of progressive clinical deterioration. Patients whose symptoms are less severe may be eligible for less invasive therapy and monitoring.

References

Brus-Ramer M, Dillon WP. Idiopathic thoracic spinal cord herniation: retrospective analysis supporting a mechanism of diskogenic dural injury and subsequent tamponade. *AJNR Am J Neuroradiol.* 2012; 33(1):52-56.

Parmar H, Park P, Brahma B, et al. Imaging of idiopathic spinal cord herniation. *Radiographics.* 2008;28(2):511-518.

Prada F, Saladino A, Giombini S, et al. Spinal cord herniation: management and outcome in a series of 12 consecutive patients and review of the literature. *Acta Neurochir.* 2012;154(4):723-730.

Cross-Reference

Neuroradiology: THE REQUISITES, 4th ed, p 567.

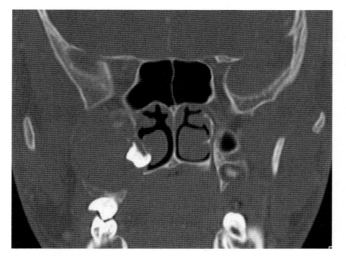

Figure 156-1

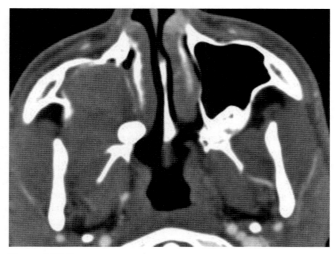

Figure 156-2

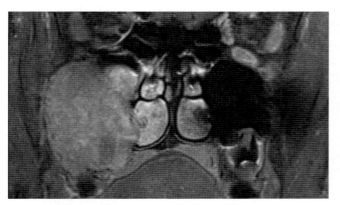

Figure 156-3

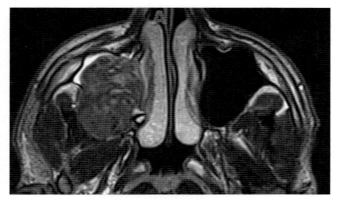

Figure 156-4

HISTORY: A child with sinus congestion is being evaluated before endoscopic surgery.

1. What is the single best diagnosis?
   A. Odontogenic cyst
   B. Metastasis
   C. Keratogenic odontogenic tumor
   D. Juvenile ossifying fibroma

2. How often are ameloblastomas in the mandible, as opposed to the maxilla?
   A. They occur more often in the mandible by a ratio of 4:1.
   B. They occur more often in the mandible by a ratio of 2:1.
   C. They occur more often in the maxilla by a ratio of 2:1.
   D. They occur more often in the maxilla by a ratio of 4:1.

3. What percentage of ameloblastomas are associated with an unerupted tooth or dentigerous cyst?
   A. 0% to 25%
   B. 26% to 50%
   C. 51% to 75%
   D. 76% to 100%

4. What imaging features are characteristic of giant cell reparative granulomas of the maxilla?
   A. Neoplastic tissue that is associated with onion skinning
   B. Cystic degeneration and aneurysmal bone cyst features
   C. Unilocular lesion without enhancement
   D. Osteoid production and hemorrhagic components

CASE 156

Juvenile Ossifying Fibroma

1. **D.** Juvenile ossifying fibroma. Juvenile ossifying fibroma could account for the dark signal on T2-weighted images. An odontogenic lesion that enhances on magnetic resonance imaging (MRI) may be an ameloblastoma. In view of the dark T2-weighted signal, this is probably not a cyst. The solid enhancement also indicates that this is probably not an odontogenic keratocyst (keratogenic odontogenic tumor).

2. **A.** They occur more often in the mandible by a ratio of 4:1. Ameloblastomas occur more often in the mandible by a ratio of 4:1. Nonetheless, they are common primary odontogenic neoplasms of the maxilla as well.

3. **A.** 0% to 25%. Ameloblastomas are associated with an unerupted tooth or dentigerous cyst in 20% of cases. However, they have solid components and therefore should not be confused with odontogenic cysts.

4. **D.** Osteoid production and hemorrhagic components. Osteoid production and hemorrhagic components are characteristic of giant cell reparative granulomas of the maxilla. These are common lesions of the maxilla and mandible.

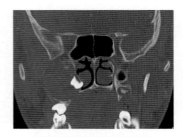

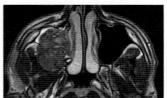

Comment

Imaging Findings

This lesion is unique in that it produces such dark signal on T2-weighted images and enhances in a solid manner (Figures 156-1 through 156-4). That characteristic is unusual for all dental lesions, but it can be seen with juvenile ossifying fibromas. These lesions typically are located in the mandible (10%) and maxilla (80% to 90%), arising from the periodontal ligament, and develop in the first two decades of life. They may be aggressive lesions that infiltrate bone widely. They have a high rate of recurrence and differ from conventional ossifying fibromas by their rapid growth cycle. Usually their edges are surrounded by a thin bone shell, and they may have internal calcifications.

Differential Diagnosis

The differential diagnosis includes the desmoplastic variety of ameloblastomas. These are lesions dominated by their fibrous content and hence produce a dark signal on T2-weighted images. Most ameloblastomas produce a higher signal on T2-weighted images and have a cystic component. Ameloblastomas are tumors that occur more often in the mandible than in the maxilla by a 4:1 ratio. They may be unilocular (37.5%) or multilocular (62.5%); the latter have a high rate of recurrence (60% to 80%). In 20% of cases, they may be associated with an unerupted tooth and/or a dentigerous cyst.

Types of Odontogenic Tumors

Odontomas are more common dental tumors than ameloblastomas. With the reclassification of odontogenic keratocysts as neoplasms referred to as *keratocystic odontogenic tumors*, ameloblastomas are the third most common odontogenic tumors. The amount of solid versus cystic tissue in ameloblastomas is usually more than in karatocystic odontogenic tumors. Giant cell reparative granulomas are nonneoplastic lesions that occur in the maxillomandibular region, as well as in the extremities. They occur more often in women than in men, and 80% are found in patients younger than 30 years. They are often partially cystic and have hemorrhagic elements. Myxomas, also included in the differential diagnosis, characteristically appear bright on T2-weighted MRI and usually have only a peripheral rim of enhancement.

References

Asaumi J, Hisatomi M, Yanagi Y, et al. Assessment of ameloblastomas using MRI and dynamic contrast-enhanced MRI. *Eur J Radiol.* 2005;56(1):25-30.

Keles B, Duran M, Uyar Y, Azimov A, Demirkan A, Esen HH. Juvenile ossifying fibroma of the mandible: a case report. *J Oral Maxillofac Res.* 2010;1(2):e5.

Cross-Reference

Neuroradiology: THE REQUISITES, 4th ed, pp 342-343.

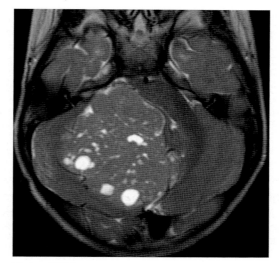

Figure 157-1

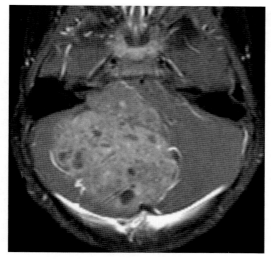

Figure 157-2

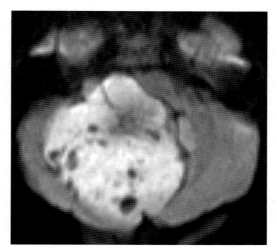

Figure 157-3

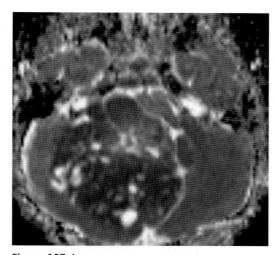

Figure 157-4

HISTORY: A patient presents with headache.

1. What is the single best diagnosis?
   A. Medulloblastoma
   B. Desmoplastic infantile ganglioglioma
   C. Juvenile pilocytic astrocytoma
   D. Ependymoma

2. From where in the posterior fossa do these tumors characteristically originate when presenting in adults?
   A. Vermis
   B. Cerebellar hemisphere
   C. Fourth ventricle
   D. Leptomeninges

3. What causes these tumors to be high density on unenhanced computed tomography (CT) scans?
   A. Hemorrhage
   B. Calcifications
   C. Hypercellularity
   D. Hypervascularity

4. What percentage of patients with this tumor present with subarachnoid seeding?
   A. 0% to 20%
   B. 21% to 40%
   C. 41% to 60%
   D. 61% to 80%

CASE 157

Medulloblastoma

1. **A.** Medulloblastoma. There is a mass in the posterior fossa in a pediatric male patient that demonstrates restricted diffusion and enhancement. It compresses rather than fills the fourth ventricle. Juvenile pilocytic astrocytoma tends to not show restricted diffusion, and ependymomas arise within the ventricle. Desmoplastic infantile gangliogliomas are typically supratentorial lesions.

2. **B.** Cerebellar hemisphere. In children, medulloblastomas arise from the superior medullary velum, whereas in adults, these usually present as a lateral cerebellar mass.

3. **C.** Hypercellularity. Medulloblastomas typically have dense cellularity causing hyperattenuation on unenhanced CT scans and diffusion restriction on diffusion-weighted imaging.

4. **B.** 21% to 40%. Approximately 30% to 40% of patients with medulloblastoma will present with subarachnoid seeding.

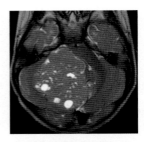

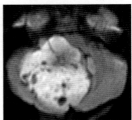

Comment

Medulloblastomas account for up to one third of all pediatric posterior fossa tumors. They occur more commonly in boys than in girls (approximately 3 : 1) and arise from the superior medullary velum of the fourth ventricle from primitive neuroectoderm. In children, medulloblastomas are typically midline masses associated with the inferior vermis, but occasionally they may manifest as a lateral cerebellar hemispheric mass, as in this case. Subarachnoid seeding of the leptomeninges is very common at presentation (reported in 30% to 40% of cases in some series); patients should have a screening contrast-enhanced magnetic resonance imaging (MRI) study of the spine to exclude this type of spread.

Imaging and the Differential Diagnosis

On unenhanced CT, medulloblastomas are typically hyperdense relative to brain parenchyma because of their dense cellularity. They are demarcated masses, and calcification, cystic change, or hemorrhage may be present in 10% to 20% of lesions. On MRI, the signal characteristics of medulloblastomas vary considerably on T2-weighted imaging, depending on the presence of hemorrhage and the degree of cellularity. Most medulloblastomas show avid but heterogeneous contrast enhancement (Figure 157-2). Typically, medulloblastomas efface the fourth ventricle and manifest with hydrocephalus (Figures 157-1 and 157-4).

Accurate preoperative diagnosis is important in pediatric cerebellar tumors because this may affect the surgical approach. Diffusion MRI allows assessment of microscopic water diffusion within tissues; with neoplasms, this diffusion seems to be primarily based on cellularity. Increasing cellularity leads to increased signal intensity on diffusion imaging and hypointensity on corresponding apparent diffusion coefficient (ADC) maps. Studies have suggested that diffusion imaging and ADC values may be useful in helping to distinguish among histologic types of pediatric brain tumors. Juvenile pilocytic astrocytomas have shown high ADC values and ratios. In contrast, medulloblastomas that characteristically are cellular have shown restricted diffusion, as in this case, with high signal intensity on diffusion images (Figure 157-3) and hypointensity on ADC maps (see Figure 157-4). The cellularity of ependymomas is between that of astrocytomas and that of medulloblastomas. On ADC maps, pilocytic astrocytomas are most often hyperintense, medulloblastomas are hypointense, and ependymomas fall somewhere in between.

Reference

Rumboldt Z, Camacho DLA, Lake D, et al. Apparent diffusion coefficients for differentiation of cerebellar tumors in children. *AJNR Am J Neuroradiol.* 2006;27:1362-1369.

Cross-Reference

Neuroradiology: THE REQUISITES, 4th ed, pp 62-65.

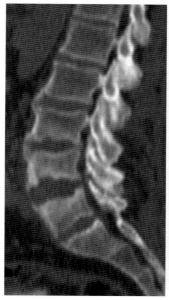

Figure 158-1

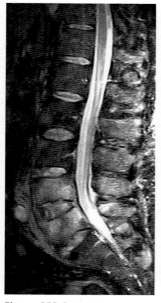

Figure 158-2

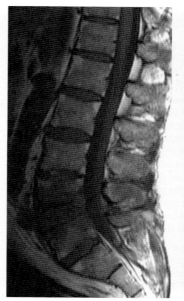

Figure 158-3

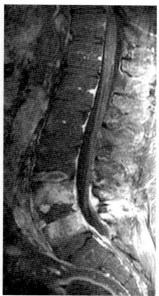

Figure 158-4

HISTORY: A 47-year-old man presents with a history of increasing back pain for the past 3 years.

1. Considering the history and imaging findings, what is the single best diagnosis?
   A. Pyogenic discitis-osteomyelitis
   B. Ankylosing spondylitis
   C. Modic type I degenerative changes
   D. Metastatic disease

2. Which of the following is an imaging feature of an Andersson lesion?
   A. Disc space widening
   B. Preservation of vertebral endplates
   C. Sclerosis of adjacent bone
   D. Large prevertebral fluid collection

3. Which of the following statements regarding Romanus lesions is *true*?
   A. Romanus lesions are focal destructive areas at the center of the discovertebral junction.
   B. Romanus lesions have been described as rugger jerseys on radiographs.
   C. Magnetic resonance imaging (MRI) is less sensitive than radiography in detecting early Romanus lesions.
   D. MRI has an important role in assessment of treatment response.

4. Identification of anticyclic citrullinated peptide (anti-CCP) antibodies is most useful to diagnose which arthritis?
   A. Ankylosing spondylitis
   B. Rheumatoid arthritis
   C. Reactive arthritis
   D. Calcium pyrophosphate deposition disease (pseudogout)

CASE 158

Ankylosing Spondylitis Discovertebral (Andersson) Lesions

1. **B.** Ankylosing spondylitis. The insidious onset and findings of the MRI "corner" sign would make ankylosing spondylitis the most likely diagnosis. Discitis osteomyelitis may manifest with similar signal abnormality and enhancement in the disc space and endplates. Modic type I degenerative changes would not be expected to involve the entire vertebral body, as seen in this case. There is no bony cortical destruction to suggest metastatic disease. In addition, the disc space is not usually involved with metastatic disease. Involvement of multiple contiguous vertebral segments with relative preservation of the disc space is typically seen with tuberculous spondylitis, although this was not an answer option.

2. **C.** Sclerosis of adjacent bone. Sclerosis of bone adjacent to the endplate changes is a feature of an Andersson lesion. Disc space narrowing may be seen. Destruction of the endplate is a feature. A prevertebral fluid collection would suggest infection and is not associated with Andersson lesions.

3. **D.** MRI has an important role in assessment of treatment response. Clinical improvement has been shown to correlate with a reduction in the acute spinal changes documented by MRI. MRI is more sensitive than radiography in detecting early lesions. These destructive changes are seen in the corners of the vertebral body. Reactive sclerosis at the edges of the vertebral endplates when the erosions heal has been described as "shiny corners" on radiographs.

4. **B.** Rheumatoid arthritis. Anti-CCP antibodies are potentially important markers for diagnosis and prognosis in rheumatoid arthritis. Anti-CCP antibody detection is as sensitive as, and more specific than, immunoglobulin M (IgM) rheumatoid factor (RF) in early and fully established disease.

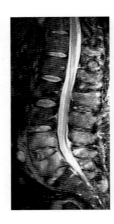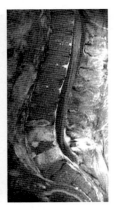

Comment

Background

A known complication of ankylosing spondylitis is the development of discovertebral lesions of the spine, known as Andersson lesions (also referred to as spondylodiscitis, aseptic discitis, and pseudarthrosis). The exact cause of these lesions is unknown; however, they are characterized by inflammation and stress fractures with the resulting development of pseudarthrosis.

Histopathology

On pathology, nonspecific reactive changes are found with the intervertebral disc, which is replaced by hypovascular fibrous tissue with endplate destruction extending into the subchondral bone. Mild inflammatory changes may also be present.

Imaging

A computed tomography scan of an Andersson lesion shows irregular discovertebral osteolysis with surrounding reactive sclerosis (Figure 158-1), which may mimic infection. Fractures of the posterior elements or nonfusion of the facet joints may also be seen. MRI shows increased short tau inversion recovery (STIR) signal (Figure 158-2) and decreased T1-weighted signal (Figure 158-3) of the disc space and surrounding vertebral bodies with corresponding enhancement (Figure 158-4). Contrast-enhanced fat suppression imaging allows better differentiation between fat and enhanced lesions (see Figure 158-4). Spinal canal stenosis may be seen resulting from hypertrophic ligamentum flavum and facet joints and from hypertrophic callus formation of the anterior and posterior elements of the Andersson lesion. An additional significant feature of ankylosing spondylitis is the MRI "corner" sign (see Figure 158-3), which represents enthesitis at the site of attachment of the anulus fibrosus to the vertebral endplate. These marginal erosions of the anterior vertebral corners, first described by Romanus, are related to inflammation of the anterior anulus fibrosus in patients with an Andersson lesion. In the healing phase, the erosions are enclosed by a rim of sclerosis, which later results in the formation of syndesmophytes and eventually in a complete ankylosed spinal segment.

Management

Initial treatment is conservative with nonsteroidal antiinflammatory drugs, intensive physical therapy, or tumor necrosis factor-α inhibitors. Surgical instrumentation and fusion is considered the principal management in symptomatic Andersson lesions that fail to resolve after conservative treatment.

References

Bron JL, de Vries MK, Snieders MN, et al. Discovertebral (Andersson) lesions of the spine in ankylosing spondylitis revisited. *Clin Rheumatol.* 2009;28(8):883-892.

Kim NR, Choi JY, Hong SH, et al. "MR corner sign": value for predicting presence of ankylosing spondylitis. *AJR Am J Roentgenol.* 2008;191(1):124-128.

Cross-Reference

Neuroradiology: THE REQUISITES, 4th ed, pp 550, 552.

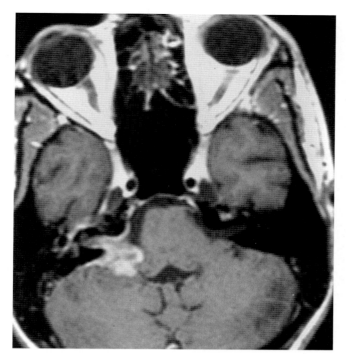

Figure 159-1

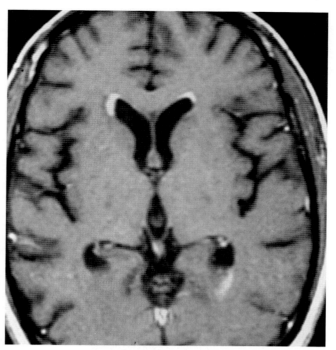

Figure 159-2

HISTORY: Sensorineural hearing loss and vertigo.

1. What is the most common human immunodeficiency virus (HIV)–associated opportunistic infection of the central nervous system?
   A. Cytomegalovirus (CMV)
   B. Toxoplasmosis
   C. Cryptococcosis
   D. Tuberculosis

2. What is the most common cause of ependymal enhancement in a patient with acquired immunodeficiency syndrome (AIDS)?
   A. CMV
   B. Toxoplasmosis
   C. Lymphoma
   D. Cryptococcosis

3. In a patient with recent serologic conversion to HIV positivity, what is the most likely cause for meningitis?
   A. CMV
   B. Toxoplasmosis
   C. HIV
   D. Tuberculosis

4. In a healthy population, what is the risk of congenital infection of CMV secondary to reactivation of latent maternal infection?
   A. Less than 1%
   B. 2% to 5%
   C. 6% to 10%
   D. Greater than 10%

CASE 159

Cytomegalovirus Meningitis and Ependymitis in a Patient with AIDS

1. **C.** Cryptococcosis. Cryptococcal meningitis is the most common HIV-associated central nervous system infection. It affects 5% to 10% of all HIV-positive patients.

2. **C.** Lymphoma. The most common cause for ependymal enhancement in patients with AIDS is lymphoma.

3. **C.** HIV. HIV is the most common cause for meningitis in a patient with recent seroconversion and normal CD4 count.

4. **B.** 2% to 5%. Reactivation of CMV has a 3.4% risk, whereas primary infection poses a 30% to 50% risk.

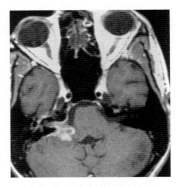

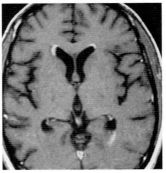

Comment

CMV is present in the latent form in the majority of the U.S. population. Reactivation usually results in a subclinical or mild flulike syndrome. In immunocompromised patients, reactivation can result in disseminated infection, usually involving the respiratory and gastrointestinal tracts; however, in rare cases, it can infect the nervous system. In the central nervous system, CMV may cause meningoencephalitis (Figure 159-1) and ependymitis (Figure 159-2). Symptoms may be acute or chronic, developing over months. Patients may have fever, altered mental status, and progressive cognitive decline. Patients may also present with cranial neuropathies (as in this case). CMV polymerase chain reaction in the cerebrospinal fluid is sensitive and specific for the diagnosis of AIDS-related CMV infection of the central nervous system. However, conventional cerebrospinal fluid findings and neuroimaging may not adequately assess the severity of central nervous system CMV disease, as demonstrated at autopsy.

Imaging

Magnetic resonance imaging is the diagnostic study of choice in assessing immunocompromised patients suspected of having central nervous system infection. Imaging may show atrophy; high signal intensity in the periventricular white matter, typically not associated with significant mass effect; and retinitis, frequently seen in the AIDS population, in patients with CMV infection. Although patients with central nervous system infection may also have ependymal and subependymal (see Figure 159-2) involvement, associated imaging findings often are not present. When present, T2-weighted signal abnormality and enhancement along the ependyma (see Figure 159-2) are valuable in establishing this diagnosis.

Currently, the most common cause of ependymal enhancement in the setting of AIDS is lymphoma.

References

Boska MD, Mosley RL, Nawab M, et al. Advances in neuroimaging for HIV-1 associated neurological dysfunction: clues to diagnosis, pathogenesis and therapeutic monitoring. *Curr HIV Res.* 2004;2: 61-68.

Vinters HV, Kwok MK, Ho HW, et al. Cytomegalovirus in the nervous system of patients with the acquired immune deficiency syndrome. *Brain.* 1989;112:245-268.

Cross-Reference

Neuroradiology: THE REQUISITES, 4th ed, pp 182, 188-192.

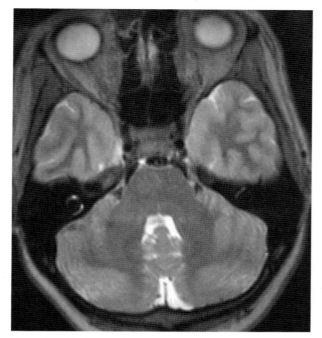

Figure 160-1 Patient A.

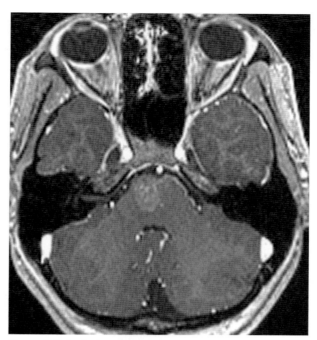

Figure 160-2 Patient A.

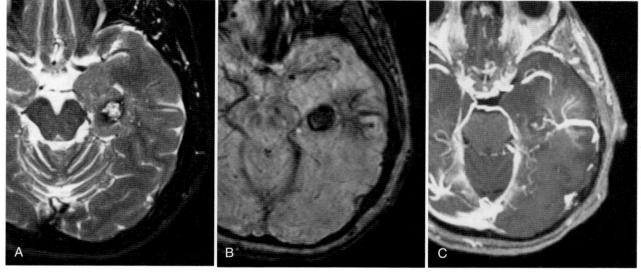

Figure 160-3 Patient B.

HISTORY: Patient A suffers from chronic headaches and is otherwise healthy. Patient B has seizures.

1. What is the diagnosis for Patient A?
   A. Capillary telangiectasia
   B. Cavernous malformation
   C. Subacute infarct
   D. Pontine glioma

2. What lesion is classically considered a high-flow vascular malformation?
   A. Capillary telangiectasia
   B. Developmental venous anomaly
   C. Cavernous malformation
   D. Arteriovenous malformation

3. What are the lesions present in Patient B?
   A. Thrombosed venous varix and arteriovenous malformation
   B. Parenchymal hematoma and dural arteriovenous fistula
   C. Capillary telangiectasia and developmental venous anomaly
   D. Developmental venous anomaly and cavernous malformation

4. What is the incidence rate of cavernomas being associated with developmental venous anomalies?
   A. Less than 2%
   B. 2% to 3%
   C. 4% to 5%
   D. More than 5%

CASE 160

Capillary Telangiectasia of the Brainstem, Cavernous Malformation, and Developmental Venous Anomaly

1. **A.** Capillary telangiectasia. The lesion within the pons in Patient A is a capillary telangiectasia as demonstrated by minimal signal abnormality on T2-weighted imaging (Figure 160-1) and feathery or smudgy enhancement without mass effect (Figure 160-2).

2. **D.** Arteriovenous malformation. Intracranial vascular malformations can be classified as low or high flow. Arteriovenous malformations are high-flow lesions.

3. **D.** Developmental venous anomaly (DVA) and cavernous malformation. The venous structure is a DVA. The focus of susceptibility and well-defined hemosiderin staining is compatible with a cavernous malformation.

4. **B.** 2% to 3%. The incidence of cavernous malformation occurring in a patient with a DVA is between 2% and 3%.

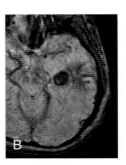

Comment

Capillary Telangiectasia (Patient A, Figures 160-1 and 160-2)

Capillary telangiectasias represent a cluster of abnormally dilated capillaries with intervening normal brain tissue. They usually are clinically silent lesions that are detected incidentally. On angiography, they are most often occult. The images for Patient A illustrate the typical appearance of a capillary telangiectasia on magnetic resonance imaging (MRI): T2-weighted images show little or no signal abnormality (Figure 160-1), and a poorly demarcated region of "feathery" contrast enhancement (Figure 160-2) is identified. Gradient echo images would show hypointensity in the lesion. Capillary telangiectasias may coexist with other vascular malformations, including cavernomas and DVAs.

Developmental Venous Anomalies (Patient B, Figure 160-3, B and C)

DVAs are typically incidental vascular malformations that represent an aberration in venous drainage. Within the venous network is intervening normal brain tissue, and no arterial elements are associated with these lesions. DVAs are composed of a tuft of enlarged venous channels that drain into a common venous trunk, best seen on Figure 160-3, C, which subsequently drains into the deep or superficial venous system. DVAs typically are clinically silent, although they may be associated with intracranial hemorrhage. There is usually no significant signal abnormality in the adjacent brain parenchyma. On angiography, the arterial and capillary phases are normal, and there may be opacification of the DVA during the venous phase.

Cavernous Malformation (Cavernoma) (Patient B, Figures 160-3, A and B)

In the absence of edema, acute hemorrhage within the cavernous malformation is unlikely. The differentiation of a cavernous malformation from a hemorrhagic neoplasm on MRI occasionally can be difficult in the face of acute hemorrhage, particularly in the presence of edema and mass effect. Several imaging features may help to distinguish these two lesions. Findings favoring a cavernous malformation include focal heterogeneous high signal intensity, representing methemoglobin; a complete hypointense peripheral ring, representing hemosiderin, as in the case of Patient B (see Figures 160-3, A and B); and the absence of enhancing solid tissue (see Figure 160-3, C). When all else fails, follow-up imaging may be performed to assess for the expected evolution of hemorrhage. Cavernous malformations may be present in 5% of the population. Cavernous malformations occur less frequently in the infratentorial compartment. The most common brainstem location is the pons. Many are incidental and asymptomatic, although symptoms may be related to acute hemorrhage or location.

References

Barr RM, Dillon WP, Wilson CB. Slow-flow vascular malformations of the pons: capillary telangiectasias? *AJNR Am J Neuroradiol.* 1996;17:71-78.

Lee C, Pennington MA, Kenney CM. MR evaluation of developmental venous anomalies: medullary venous anatomy of venous angiomas. *AJNR Am J Neuroradiol.* 1996;17:61-70.

Porter RW, Detwiler PW, Spetzler RF, et al. Cavernous malformations of the brainstem: experience with 100 patients. *J Neurosurg.* 1999;90:50-58.

Zausinger S, Yousry I, Brueckmann H, et al. Cavernous malformations of the brainstem: three-dimensional-constructive interference in steady-state magnetic resonance imaging for improvement of surgical approach and clinical results. *Neurosurgery.* 2006;58:322-330.

Cross-Reference

Neuroradiology: THE REQUISITES, 4th ed, pp 145-146.

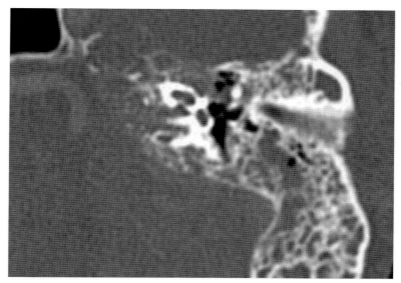

Figure 161-1

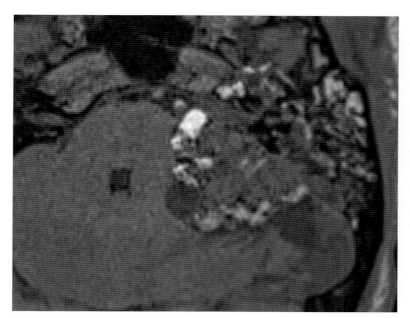

Figure 161-2

HISTORY: A patient has left-sided hearing loss after nephrectomy for renal cell carcinoma.

1. Aside from a metastatic lesion, following nephrectomy for renal cell carcinoma in this patient, what hypervascular lesion should be considered specific to this location?
   A. Chondrosarcoma
   B. Chordoma
   C. Schwannoma
   D. Endolymphatic sac tumor

2. With what syndrome are these tumors associated?
   A. Neurofibromatosis 1 (NF1)
   B. Tuberous sclerosis complex (TSC)
   C. Gorlin syndrome
   D. Von Hippel–Lindau (VHL)

3. What is the characteristic magnetic resonance imaging feature of this lesion that distinguishes it from glomus tumors?
   A. Flow voids
   B. Enhancement
   C. Hyperintensity on T1-weighted images
   D. Hyperintensity on T2-weighted images

4. What percentage of these lesions has a syndrome-associated presentation?
   A. Less than 10%
   B. 11% to 25%
   C. 26% to 50%
   D. More than 50%

CASE 161

Endolymphatic Sac Tumor

1. **D.** Endolymphatic sac tumor. A hypervascular lesion may represent renal cell carcinoma metastasis or endolymphatic sac tumor (ELST). Renal cell carcinoma metastasis is also destructive. The location best characterizes ELST. The lesion could also be a paraganglioma, although such tumors have a predilection for the jugular foramen. Chondrosarcomas and chordomas are not hypervascular, and chordomas are not found in this location. Schwannomas are not typically destructive lesions.

2. **D.** Von Hippel–Lindau (VHL). VHL disease is associated with hemangioblastomas and ELSTs.

3. **C.** Hyperintensity on T1-weighted images. Hyperintensity on T1-weighted images distinguishes ELST from glomus tumors. Both have flow voids, enhance vividly, and have a speckled appearance on T2-weighted images from flow voids.

4. **B.** 11% to 25%. Twenty percent of ELSTs are associated with VHL disease. Of patients with VHL disease, 11% have an ELST.

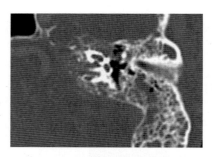

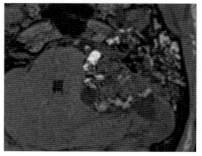

Comment

Imaging Findings

ELSTs arise in the temporal bone along the plane of the endolymphatic sac and vestibular aqueduct. They are oriented obliquely and are destructive-looking lesions that may have finely calcified matrix, which may explain their characteristic hyperintense appearance on T1-weighted images (Figures 161-1 and 161-2). They are associated with VHL disease in approximately 20% of cases, and 11% of patients with VHL disease have an ELST. In the presence of a renal cell carcinoma, metastases to the temporal bone should also be considered because both would be hypervascular. ELSTs are bilateral in 33% of patients with VHL disease.

Clinical Findings

The most common clinical finding is hearing loss in the third decade of life, which may be the presenting symptom of VHL disease. Tinnitus and vertigo may plague affected patients as well. The hearing loss is sensorineural, and its onset may be progressive or sudden.

Reference

Manski TJ, Heffner DK, Glenn GM, et al. Endolymphatic sac tumors. A source of morbid hearing loss in von Hippel–Lindau disease. *JAMA.* 1997;277(18):1461-1466.

Cross-Reference

Neuroradiology: THE REQUISITES, 4th ed, pp 405-406.

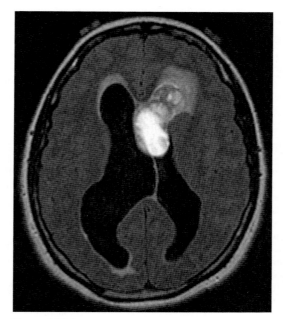

Figure 162-1

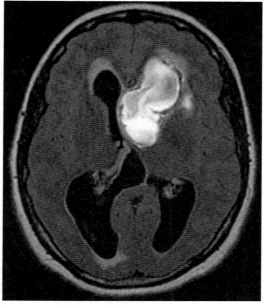

Figure 162-2

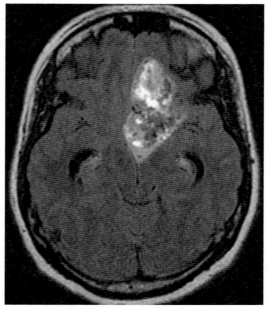

Figure 162-3

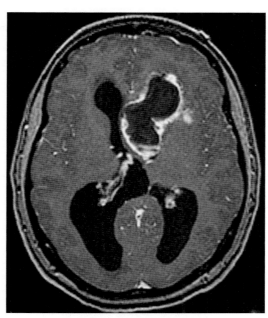

Figure 162-4

HISTORY: A 30-year-old patient presents with headache.

1. What is the most likely diagnosis?
   A. Subependymal giant cell tumor
   B. Central neurocytoma
   C. Choroid plexus papilloma
   D. Germinoma

2. This tumor is histologically similar to what other tumor, which can be differentiated by the presence of a mutation of chromosome 19?
   A. Anaplastic astrocytoma
   B. Glioblastoma
   C. Oligodendroglioma
   D. Ependymoma

3. At what age are these tumors most frequently diagnosed?
   A. 0 to 19 years
   B. 20 to 40 years
   C. 41 to 60 years
   D. 61 to 80 years

4. What is the normal volume per day of cerebrospinal fluid (CSF) production in a healthy adult?
   A. 100 to 300 mL
   B. 500 to 700 mL
   C. 800 to 1000 mL
   D. 1200 to 1500 mL

CASE 162

Central Neurocytoma

1. **B.** Central neurocytoma. This lesion arises from near the foramen of Monro and extends into the lateral ventricle. There is irregular peripheral enhancement and heterogenous signal on T2 fluid-attenuated inversion recovery (FLAIR) imaging. It results in obstructive hydrocephalus and is distinct from the choroid plexus. Subependymal giant cell tumors occur in patients with tuberous sclerosis. There is no evidence of subependymal nodularity. Germinomas commonly arise in the pineal region or the suprasellar region and not in the ventricle.

2. **C.** Oligodendroglioma. Central neurocytoma and oligodendroglioma appear similar histologically. Central neurocytomas test positive for synaptophysin and oligodendrogliomas are differentiated from other tumors by the presence a mutation involving chromosomes 1 and 19 (1p19q deletion).

3. **B.** 20 to 40 years. The mean age of presentation is approximately 29 years.

4. **B.** 500 to 700 mL. The ventricular system and thecal sac contain approximately 150 to 250 mL of CSF. The rate of production is approximately 0.4 to 0.7 mL/min. The best answer is therefore 500 to 700 mL/day, which must be resorbed by arachnoid granulations.

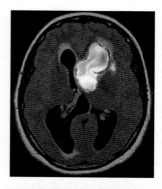

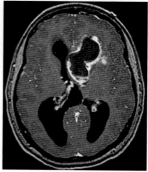

Comment

Presentation

Central neurocytomas are benign neuroepithelial neoplasms that occur in young and middle-aged adults. Patients may be asymptomatic or may present with headache and signs of increased intracranial pressure, frequently because of hydrocephalus, as in this case (Figure 162-1).

Pathologic and Imaging Characteristics

Central neurocytomas typically have a homogeneous cell population with neuronal differentiation. Central neurocytomas arise most commonly within the body of the lateral ventricle (less frequently, the third ventricle), adjacent to the septum pellucidum and foramen of Monro (Figure 162-3). They have a characteristic attachment to the superolateral ventricular wall. Most are confined to the ventricles, although occasionally parenchymal extension may occur, as in this case, where there is growth into the frontal lobe (Figure 162-4). These features may help to distinguish neurocytomas from other intraventricular tumors, such as astrocytoma, giant cell astrocytoma, ependymoma, intraventricular oligodendroglioma, and meningioma.

Importance of Accurate Diagnosis

Preoperative diagnosis of central neurocytoma may help in planning therapy because this tumor has a better prognosis than other intraventricular tumors arising in this area. On imaging and conventional pathologic evaluation (light microscopy), central neurocytomas are frequently indistinguishable from oligodendrogliomas. The distinction between these two neoplasms is important because central neurocytomas have a more benign course, and treatment may differ. Although neurocytomas have a favorable prognosis, malignant variants and recurrences may, in rare cases, occur.

Additional Imaging Characteristics

On computed tomography and magnetic resonance imaging (MRI), neurocytomas typically are heterogeneous masses that contain multiple cysts. They are well demarcated, with smooth, lobulated margins and moderate vascularity. Most neurocytomas have calcifications. On MRI, the more solid component of these tumors tends to follow the signal characteristics of gray matter. Signal voids may be related to calcification or tumor vascularity. Contrast enhancement is variable, ranging from none to moderate (Figure 162-2).

References

Cooper JA. Central neurocytoma. *Radiographics.* 2002;22:1472.

Shin JH, Lee HK, Khang SK, et al. Neuronal tumors of the central nervous system: radiologic findings and pathologic correlation. *Radiographics.* 2002;22:1177-1189.

Cross-Reference

Neuroradiology: THE REQUISITES, 4th ed, pp 52-54.

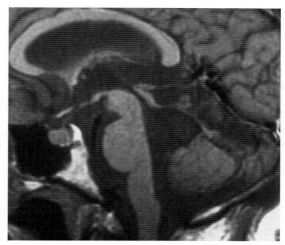

Figure 163-1

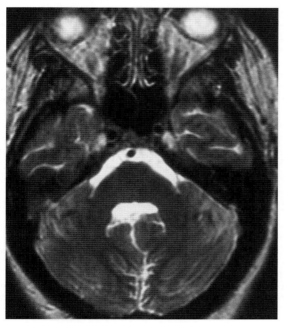

Figure 163-2

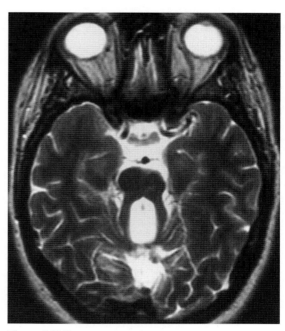

Figure 163-3

HISTORY: A patient presents with developmental delay and abnormal ocular movements.

1. What is the correct diagnosis?
   A. Chiari malformation type II
   B. Dandy-Walker malformation
   C. Mega cisterna magna
   D. Joubert syndrome

2. What is the most common inheritance pattern for this entity?
   A. X-linked dominant
   B. Autosomal recessive
   C. Autosomal dominant
   D. X-linked recessive

3. What is a mandatory imaging characteristic to diagnose this entity?
   A. Dysgenesis of the corpus callosum
   B. Cortical dysplasia
   C. Molar tooth sign
   D. Rhombencephalosynapsis

4. What is one of the necessary characteristics of rhombencephalosynapsis?
   A. Colpocephaly
   B. Vermian agenesis and continuity of the cerebellar hemispheres
   C. Corpus callosum dysgenesis
   D. Intact septum pellucidum

CASE 163

Joubert Syndrome

1. **D.** Joubert syndrome. The correct diagnosis is arrived upon by identification of the two mandatory findings, vermian hypoplasia and the molar tooth sign, the second of which is pathognomonic for Joubert syndrome.

2. **B.** Autosomal recessive. Multiple genes have been identified and associated with Joubert syndrome. Mutations in all these genes are inherited with an autosomal-recessive pattern. Only mutations within the *OFD1* gene are inherited with an X-linked recessive pattern.

3. **C.** Molar tooth sign. The molar tooth sign and vermian hypoplasia are mandatory imaging characteristics of Joubert syndrome.

4. **B.** Vermian agenesis and continuity of the cerebellar hemispheres. This finding is diagnostic for rhombencephalosynapsis and is best seen on posterior coronal magnetic resonance (MR) images.

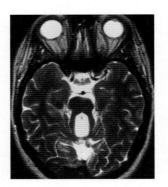

Comment

Many classifications of developmental anomalies of the posterior fossa have been proposed in the literature. A simple classification scheme based on the neuroimaging pattern divides these diseases into (1) predominantly cerebellar, (2) cerebellar and brainstem, (3) predominantly brainstem, and (4) predominantly midbrain anomalies. Predominantly cerebellar anomalies include the Dandy-Walker malformation, other cystic malformations of the posterior fossa, and rhombencephalosynapsis. Dandy-Walker malformation and rhombencephalosynapsis affect primarily the cerebellar vermis. Other anomalies may globally involve the cerebellum or affect only one cerebellar hemisphere. Anomalies involving both the cerebellum and the brainstem are Joubert syndrome or the group of pontocerebellar hypoplasias. Predominant brainstem abnormalities are rare and include, for example, pontine tegmental cap dysplasia.

A consistent abnormality in Joubert syndrome is aplasia or hypoplasia and dysplasia of the vermis (Figures 163-1 and 163-2). The molar tooth sign is pathognomonic for Joubert syndrome and is characterized by elongated, thickened, and horizontally oriented superior cerebellar peduncles and a deepened interpeduncular fossa. In addition, about 30% of the patients have abnormalities of the brainstem, such as dysplasia of the tectum and midbrain or interpeduncular heterotopia. Supratentorial abnormalities are present in about 30% of the patients and can include dysgenesis of the corpus callosum, encephaloceles, and disorders of cortical migration. Diffusion tensor imaging showed absence of the decussation of the superior cerebellar peduncles and corticospinal tracts. Mutations in the majority of the genes associated with Joubert syndrome are inherited with an autosomal recessive pattern.

MR imaging in these patients shows a characteristic appearance. Specifically, sagittal images show hypoplasia and dysplasia of the cerebellar vermis and enlargement of the fourth ventricle with displacement of the fastigium (see Figure 163-1). Axial images, in particular, show an enlarged fourth ventricle with a "bat-wing" shape and the molar tooth sign (Figures 163-2 and 163-3).

References

Bosemani T, Orman G, Boltshauser E, Tekes A, Huisman TA, Poretti A. Congenital abnormalities of the posterior fossa. *Radiographics*. 2015;35:200-220.

Poretti A, Huisman TA, Scheer I, Boltshauser E. Joubert syndrome and related disorders: spectrum of neuroimaging findings in 75 patients. *AJNR Am J Neuroradiol*. 2011;32:1459-1463.

Poretti A, Vitiello G, Hennekam RC, et al. Delineation and diagnostic criteria of oral-facial-digital syndrome type VI. *Orphanet J Rare Dis*. 2012;7:4.

Romani M, Micalizzi A, Valente EM. Joubert syndrome: congenital cerebellar ataxia with the molar tooth. *Lancet Neurol*. 2013;12:894-905.

Cross-Reference

Neuroradiology: THE REQUISITES, 4th ed, pp 282-283.

The editor would like to acknowledge Dr. Andrea Poretti's contribution to this case.

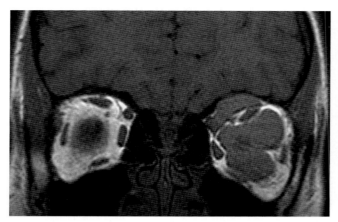

Figure 164-1

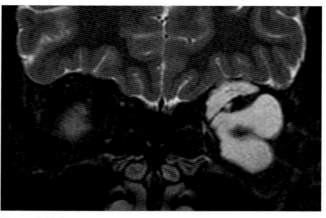

Figure 164-2

HISTORY: A patient presents with a left orbital mass that is palpable during coughing.

1. What is the best diagnosis in this case?
   A. Hemangioma
   B. Lymphatic malformation
   C. Mucocele
   D. Schwannoma

2. What is the most common orbital mass in an adult?
   A. Lymphoma
   B. Vascular malformation
   C. Meningioma
   D. Orbital pseudotumor

3. Which of the following statements about the lesion in this case is correct?
   A. These lesions are often treated with radiation therapy.
   B. Sclerotherapy is a commonly used minimally invasive treatment option.
   C. These lesions rarely extend into different compartments or through fascial planes.
   D. These are neoplastic lesions and grow unless treated.

4. Which of the following statements regarding extraoccular muscle innervation and function is correct?
   A. The lateral rectus muscle is innervated by the third cranial nerve.
   B. The superior oblique and superior rectus muscle share common motor innervation and function.
   C. The inferior oblique muscle is innervated by the sixth cranial nerve.
   D. The superior oblique muscle and the inferior rectus act to inferiorly direct the eye from a neutral position.

CASE 164

Orbital Lymphatic Malformation

1. **B.** Lymphatic malformation. The lesion is homogeneous, has low signal intensity on T1-weighted images and high signal intensity on T2-weighted images, and involves the intraconal and extraconal left orbit, insinuating around the optic nerve/sheath complex.

2. **B.** Vascular malformation. The most common orbital mass is a vascular malformation, more specifically a venous malformation.

3. **B.** Sclerotherapy is a commonly used minimally invasive treatment option. Other treatment options are surgery and medical management.

4. **D.** The superior oblique muscle and the inferior rectus act to inferiorly direct the eye from a neutral position. The lateral rectus is innervated by the sixth cranial nerve. The superior oblique is innervated by the fourth cranial nerve. Each of the other extraoccular muscles is innervated by the third cranial nerve. The torsional force of the superior oblique muscle apposes the rotation imposed upon by the inferior rectus in inferior gaze. This allows for direct downward motion of the eye.

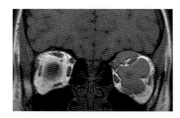

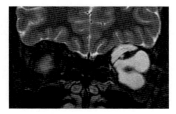

Comment

Evolving Knowledge

The knowledge regarding etiology, pathophysiology, histology, and treatment of vascular lesions has been continuously expanding. Over decades, there have been multiple revisions and reclassifications, resulting in some confusion among pathologists, radiologists, clinicians, and patients.

Classification

The newest and most widely accepted classification system approved by the General Assembly of the International Society for the Study of Vascular Anomalies (ISSVA) can be found at issva.org/classification.

In keeping with the 2014 classification, this lesion in the left orbit is best characterized as a lymphatic malformation. These are non-neoplastic lesions further subclassified into micro, macro, or mixed cystic lymphatic malformations or additional subtypes that may be associated with other diseases. The lesion demonstrated is a macrocystic subtype. As in this case, these lesions are generally iso-intense to muscle on T1-weighted imaging (Figure 164-1), and when macrocystic, homogeneously hyperintense on T2-weighted imaging (Figure 164-2). Fluid levels may be seen, especially in mixed types. These lesions tend to be trans-spacial. The septations, if present, tend to enhance so when the cysts are small, such as in microcystic lymphatic malformations, more solid enhancement can be perceived.

Vascular malformations can be pure capillary, lymphatic, or venous. They may be mixed histologically and may have high or low flow. High-flow vascular malformations include arteriovenous malformations and arteriovenous fistulas.

Furthermore, appropriate use of nomenclature is necessary to avoid confusion with regard to non-neoplastic and neoplastic vascular lesions. Vascular tumors include benign congenital hemangiomas and malignant vascular tumors such as angiosarcomas.

It is discouraged to use words ending in the suffix *-oma*, which implies neoplasm, when describing non-neoplastic vascular lesions such as a lymphatic malformation.

Treatment

Treatment options include surgical removal, chemical ablation/sclerosis, and medical therapy.

References

Bilaniuk LT. Orbital vascular lesions: role of imaging. *Radiol Clin North Am*. 1999;37:169-183.

ISSVA Classification of Vascular Anomalies. Little Rock, AR: International Society for the Study of Vascular Anomalies; 2014.

Kazim M, Kennerdell JS, Rothfus W, Marquardt M. Orbital lymphangioma: correlation of magnetic resonance images and intraoperative findings. *Ophthalmology*. 1992;99:1588-1594.

Cross-Reference

Neuroradiology: THE REQUISITES, 4th ed, p 332.

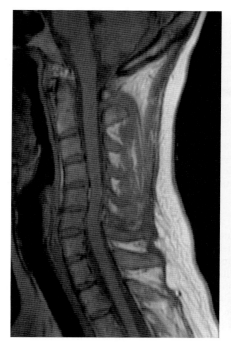

Figure 165-1

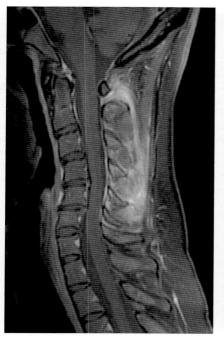

Figure 165-2

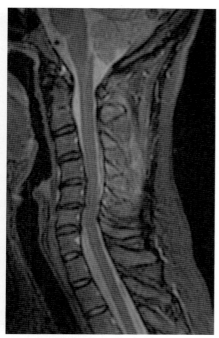

Figure 165-3

HISTORY: A 60-year-old woman reports a several-week history of severe neck and shoulder pain and morning stiffness. X-rays of the axial and appendicular skeleton are negative.

1. What is the single best diagnosis?
   A. Psoriasis
   B. Rheumatoid arthritis
   C. Polymyalgia rheumatica
   D. Fibromyalgia

2. Which imaging modality is the *least* useful in the detection of this disease?
   A. Radiography
   B. Magnetic resonance imaging (MRI)
   C. Ultrasound
   D. Positron emission tomography (PET) and PET/computed tomography (PET/CT)

3. Which of the following statements regarding patients with this disease and interspinous bursitis is true?
   A. The most commonly affected region is C1-C4.
   B. The most commonly affected region is L2-L4.
   C. Bacterial cultures are often positive for surface pathogens.
   D. Moderate to severe cervical or lumbar interspinous bursitis in the absence of other articular changes might be helpful to support the diagnosis.

4. Which of the following statements in reference to the imaging diagnosis of this disease is the *least* accurate?
   A. Imaging allows appreciation of the multifaceted nature of the disease.
   B. Imaging patterns of inflammation are helpful in the diagnosis and differential diagnosis of the disease.
   C. It is unnecessary to differentiate this disease from giant cell arteritis on clinical examination and imaging.
   D. In patients with late-onset rheumatoid arthritis and polymyalgia-like symptoms, MRI can be helpful in the differentiation from this disease.

CASE 165

Cervical Interspinous Bursitis in Polymyalgia Rheumatica

1. **C.** Polymyalgia rheumatica (PMR). PMR is a good possibility given the patient's clinical presentation; the findings of interspinous bursitis on MRI; and negative x-rays. There is no spinal syndesmophytes, sacroiliitis, or peripheral arthropathy to suggest psoriasis. Although rheumatoid arthritis may produce inflammation of synovial tissue and bursae, selective involvement of the cervical interspinous bursa without erosive arthritis at C1-C2 is unlikely. Fibromyalgia is not an inflammatory condition; rather, it is caused by abnormal sensory processing in the central nervous system. No characteristic imaging findings for fibromyalgia are known.

2. **A.** Radiography. There are no characteristic changes on plain films; however, they may be useful to rule out other rheumatologic conditions mimicking symptoms of PMR. MRI shows areas of active inflammation secondary to bursitis, tenosynovitis, and tendinitis. Although less sensitive than MRI, ultrasound may show changes characteristic of bursitis in the shoulders and hips, shoulder synovitis, and biceps tenosynovitis. Although not specific, PET and PET/CT are highly sensitive in the detection of areas of PMR inflammation, particularly in the interspinous bursa of the cervical spine, lumbar spine, shoulders, and sternoclavicular joints.

3. **D.** Moderate to severe cervical or lumbar interspinous bursitis in the absence of other articular changes might be helpful to support the diagnosis. MRI evidence of bursitis affecting the cervical or lumbar spine might be useful in discriminating PMR from the subgroup of late-onset spondyloarthropathies that have PMR manifestations. The cervical interspinous bursae most often affected are C5, C6, and C7. PMR affecting upper lumbar vertebra interspinous bursae is unusual. This is not an infection and the cultures would not grow.

4. **C.** It is unnecessary to differentiate this disease from giant cell arteritis on clinical examination and imaging. The discovery of coexisting vasculitis could help tailor treatment. Imaging allows identification of areas of synovitis, bursitis, tenosynovitis, and vasculitis. The classic extraarticular synovial inflammatory process related to PMR in middle-aged and older patients is easy to recognize on imaging. MRI may be helpful by demonstrating subtle erosions in joints affected with late-onset rheumatoid arthritis, which are not characteristics of PMR.

Comment

Background

PMR is a common condition of unknown cause that affects older adults. Whites are affected more than other ethnic groups. PMR is twice as common in women. Median age at diagnosis is 72 years. PMR is characterized clinically by proximal myalgia of the shoulders and hip girdles with accompanying morning stiffness that lasts more than 1 hour. PMR is known to cause synovitis, bursitis, and tenosynovitis around joints such as shoulders, hips, and knees and inflammation of interspinous bursa at the cervical and lumbar spine. Approximately 20% of patients with PMR develop giant cell arteritis, and 40% of patients with giant cell arteritis have associated PMR.

Imaging

Imaging studies and the patient's clinical presentation are helpful in distinguishing PMR from other rheumatologic conditions. Radiographs reveal either normal joints or evidence of osteoarthritis. Ultrasound may show changes characteristic of bursitis in the shoulders and hips, shoulder synovitis, and biceps tenosynovitis. MRI is excellent in showing areas of active inflammation secondary to bursitis, tenosynovitis, and tendinitis in the shoulders (subacromial and subdeltoid bursitis and glenohumeral joint synovitis are found in most patients), cervical spine interspinous bursae, and trochanters (trochanteric bursitis) (Figures 165-1 through 165-3).

Management

Corticosteroids are considered the treatment of choice. A rapid response to low-dose corticosteroids is considered pathognomonic. Prognosis for patients is excellent, although exacerbations may occur if corticosteroids are tapered too soon or too rapidly.

References

Paroli M, Garlaschi G, Silvestri E, et al. Magnetic resonance imaging in the differential diagnosis between polymyalgia rheumatica and elderly onset rheumatoid arthritis. *Clin Rheumatol*. 2006;25(3): 402-403.

Salvarani C, Barozzi L, Cantini F, et al. Cervical interspinous bursitis in active polymyalgia rheumatica. *Ann Rheum Dis*. 2008;67(6): 758-761.

Salvarani C, Cantini F, Hunder GG. Polymyalgia rheumatica and giant-cell arteritis. *Lancet*. 2008;372(9634):234-245.

Cross-Reference

Neuroradiology: THE REQUISITES, 4th ed, pp 119, 549.

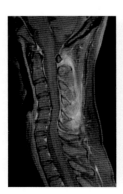
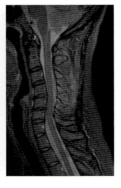

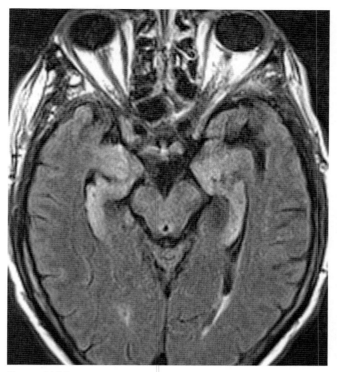

Figure 166-1

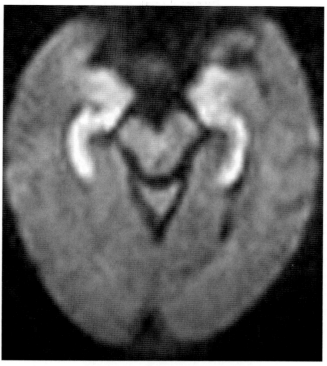

Figure 166-2

HISTORY: A patient presents with altered mental status and disorientation.

1. What is the appropriate treatment for the presumptive diagnosis?
   A. Supportive care
   B. Antiviral medications
   C. Antiretroviral medications
   D. Chemotherapy

2. What percentage of the population would test positive for human herpesvirus 6 (HHV-6)?
   A. 0% to 25%
   B. 26% to 50%
   C. 51% to 75%
   D. 76% to 100%

3. What primary tumors are most commonly associated with paraneoplastic limbic encephalitis?
   A. Testicular germ cell
   B. Renal cell
   C. Thyroid
   D. Prostate

4. What is the earliest and most common finding for herpes encephalitis in the temporal lobe?
   A. Diffusion restriction
   B. Hemorrhage
   C. Enhancement
   D. Vasogenic edema

CASE 166

Herpes Encephalopathy—Human Herpesvirus 6 Infection after Organ Transplantation

1. **B.** Antiviral medications. The presumptive diagnosis and diagnosis of exclusion is viral encephalitis, most commonly caused by the herpesvirus. These findings may be present in cases of limbic encephalitis, but the delay in the initiation of antiviral treatment for the work-up of a potential malignancy would be detrimental to the patient. Supportive care alone would be negligent, and herpesvirus is not a retrovirus.

2. **D.** 76% to 100%. Population studies have shown 90% or more of patients have been infected with HHV-6.

3. **A.** Testicular germ cell. Small cell carcinoma of the lung, testicular germ cell, thymic, ovarian, breast, hematologic, and gastrointestinal malignancies all have been associated with paraneoplastic encephalitis.

4. **D.** Vasogenic edema. Vasogenic edema precedes hemorrhage, enhancement, and cytotoxic edema in herpes encephalitis.

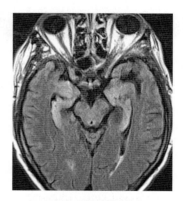

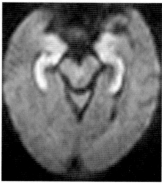

Comment

Etiology and Pathophysiology

HHV-6 is a double-stranded DNA virus. More than 90% of the general population is seropositive for HHV-6. It is excreted by the salivary glands and may be passed to infants from their mothers. HHV-6 has a strong affinity for the central nervous system and has been detected by polymerase chain reaction in one third of normal brain specimens; this suggests that the brain might be a latent viral site. HHV-6 encephalopathy has been reported in immunocompromised patients, especially patients who have undergone hematopoietic stem cell or solid-organ transplantation (lung and liver). Infection has typically been identified within 4 weeks of transplantation. The pathogenesis is considered to be reactivation of the recipient's latent HHV-6 infection and not infection from the donor. Immunocompromised patients are at risk for a spectrum of disease processes that may affect the central nervous system, and their symptoms are frequently nonspecific. Common neurologic symptoms in HHV-6 infection include disorientation, confusion, and short-term memory loss. Coma, hypopnea, and seizures have been reported.

Imaging

Early magnetic resonance imaging (MRI) findings, as in this case, include high signal intensity on fluid-attenuated inversion recovery (Figure 166-1), T2-weighted, and diffusion-weighted (Figure 166-2) images of the mesial temporal lobe structures (hippocampus and amygdala). The diffusion-weighted abnormality (see Figure 166-2) is accompanied by hypointensity (low values) on apparent diffusion coefficient maps. Enhancement usually is not present.

Treatment

In transplantation, acyclovir is routinely administered to prevent reactivation of herpesviruses. Acyclovir is not effective against HHV-6, however, because it lacks virus-specific thymidine kinase. Ganciclovir and foscarnet can be effective against HHV-6, but serious side effects, including myelosuppression and nephrotoxicity, may occur. These drugs are not usually given prophylactically. Early diagnosis is crucial to prevent serious neurologic sequelae. Mesial temporal involvement seen on MRI in a transplant recipient receiving preventive treatment with acyclovir is highly suggestive of HHV-6–associated encephalopathy.

Reference

Noguchi T, Mihara F, Yoshiura T, et al. MR imaging of human herpesvirus-6 encephalopathy after hematopoietic stem cell transplantation in adults. *AJNR Am J Neuroradiol.* 2006;27:2191-2195.

Cross-Reference

Neuroradiology: THE REQUISITES, 4th ed, pp 185, 220.

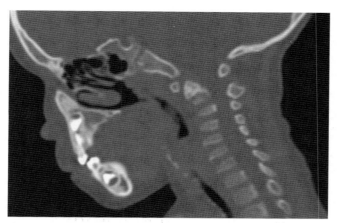

Figure 167-1

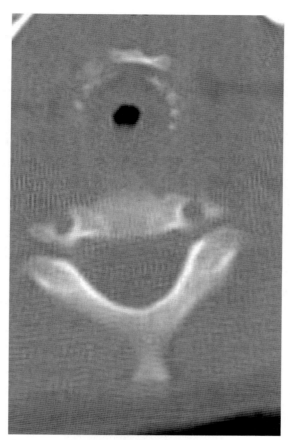

Figure 167-2

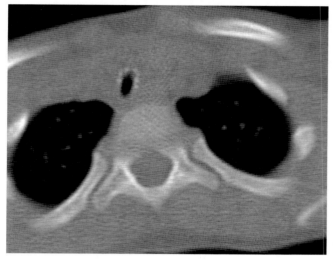

Figure 167-3

HISTORY: A patient presents with dwarfism.

1. Which of the following is the single best diagnosis?
   A. Chondrodysplasia punctata
   B. Chondroectodermal dysplasia
   C. Enchondromatosis
   D. Campomelic dysplasia

2. Which of the following statements is true?
   A. Chondroectodermal dysplasia occurs in Amish populations and is associated with wormian bones in the skull.
   B. Chondroectodermal dysplasia occurs in Ashkenazi Jewish populations and is associated with stenosis at the foramen magnum.
   C. Chondroectodermal dysplasia occurs sporadically and is associated with subependymal nodules and astrocytomas.
   D. Chondroectodermal dysplasia occurs in Southeast Asian populations and is associated with craniosynostosis of the skull.

3. Patients with chondrodysplasia punctata have which of the following characteristics?
   A. High incidence of cleft palate
   B. High incidence of enchondromas
   C. Normal life expectancy
   D. Normal height

4. What is the rate of sarcomatous transformation in Ollier disease?
   A. 0% to 20%
   B. 21% to 40%
   C. 41% to 60%
   D. 61% to 80%

CASE 167

Chondrodysplasia Punctata

1. **A.** Chondrodysplasia punctata. The correct diagnosis is chondrodysplasia punctata. Chondroectodermal dysplasia does not cause tracheal punctate hyperdensities. No enchondromas are shown. Campomelic dysplasia may be associated with laryngotracheomalacia but not punctate hyperdensities either.

2. **A.** Chondroectodermal dysplasia occurs in Amish populations and is associated with wormian bones in the skull. Chondroectodermal dysplasia, also known as Ellis–van Creveld syndrome, is also associated with high rates of polydactyly, congenital heart defects, and short limbs.

3. **A.** High incidence of cleft palate. The characteristics of chondrodysplasia punctata include a high incidence of cleft palate, multiple stippled epiphyses, foci of hyperdensity in respiratory cartilage (on imaging), and dwarfism.

4. **B.** 21% to 40%. The rate of sarcomatous transformation in Ollier disease is 21% to 40%. As expected, these tumors are typically chondrosarcomas.

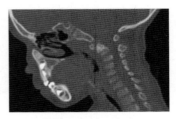

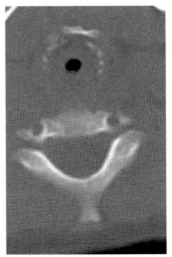

Comment

Features of Chondrodysplasia Punctata

Chondrodysplasia punctata is also known as *congenital stippled epiphyseal syndrome,* and it is typically associated with rhizomelic dwarfism, although there are non-rhizomelic forms. It is most commonly an autosomal recessive disorder accompanied by congenital heart defects, cleft palate, distal phalangeal hypoplasia, midface hypoplasia, mental retardation, and death before the age of 2 years. On imaging, multiple punctate hyperdensities are visible in the epiphyses of the extremities and axial skeleton; moreover, these same fine calcifications are also visible in the trachea and bronchi (Figures 167-1 through 167-3). Clefts in the vertebral bodies are also characteristic. The most common manifestation of the disorder is cataract, occurring in more than 70% of cases, and ichthyosis is also prevalent. Tracheal stenosis, as in this case, is another reported complication of the disease. Flat facies, well demonstrated in the sagittal reconstruction (Figure 167-1), is another feature of the disorder.

Laboratory Manifestations of Chondrodysplasia Punctata

A defect in the *PEX7* gene, which encodes the receptor for a subset of peroxisomal matrix enzymes affecting vitamin K–dependent arylsulfatase, is associated with chondrodysplasia punctata and has been mapped to chromosome 6. Levels of red cell plasmalogens are depressed, but phytanic acid progressively accumulates.

Reference

Mundinger GS, Weiss C, Fishman EK. Severe tracheobronchial stenosis and cervical vertebral subluxation in X-linked recessive chondrodysplasia punctata. *Pediatr Radiol.* 2009;39(6):625-628.

Cross-Reference

Neuroradiology: THE REQUISITES, 4th ed, pp 306-307.

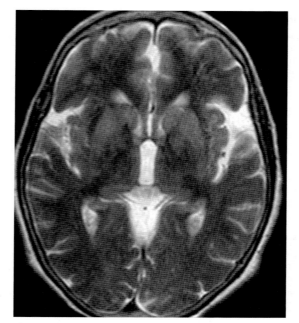

Figure 168-1

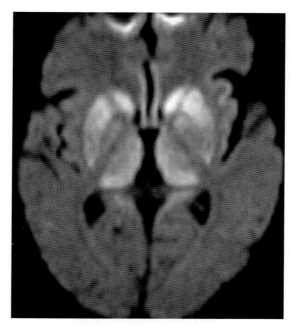

Figure 168-2

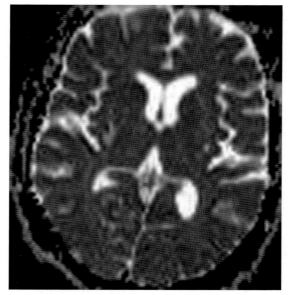

Figure 168-3

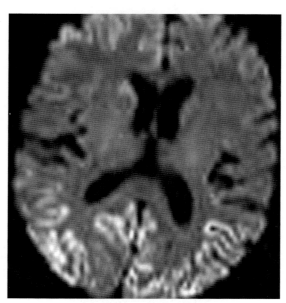

Figure 168-4

HISTORY: Dementia.

1. Which of the following could cause symmetric diffusion restriction in the basal ganglia?
   A. Artery of Heubner infarct
   B. Fahr disease
   C. Wilson disease
   D. Encephalitis

2. Which of the following is the most common finding on computed tomography (CT) in patients with Creutzfeldt-Jakob disease (CJD)?
   A. Edema in the basal ganglia
   B. Cortical atrophy
   C. Intracranial hemorrhage
   D. No abnormality is usually present on CT

3. How is CJD most commonly transmitted?
   A. Liver transplant
   B. Maternal/perinatal
   C. Blood transfusion
   D. Consumption of meat from infected animals

4. Where is an abnormal T2 signal and/or restricted diffusion seen most frequently in CJD aside from the basal ganglia?
   A. Paramedian cortices
   B. Cranial nerves
   C. Substantia nigra
   D. Pons

CASE 168

Creutzfeldt-Jakob Disease

1. **D.** Encephalitis. Encephalitis commonly affects the basal ganglia and often results in symmetric signal abnormality in the basal ganglia. Artery of Heubner infarct would cause asymmetric restricted diffusion in the caudate nucleus. Fahr disease and Wilson disease are associated with signal abnormality in the basal ganglia but not restricted diffusion.

2. **D.** No abnormality is usually present on CT. Most commonly there is no abnormality on CT, but when there is abnormality on CT, it is most commonly cortical atrophy.

3. **D.** Consumption of meat from infected animals. CJD is transmitted by corneal transplant, cerebral electrode implantation, eating infected meat, and cannibalism.

4. **A.** Paramedian cortices. Signal changes in the cortices may be more frequent than those changes typically described in the basal ganglia.

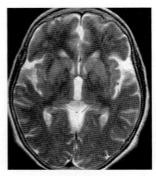

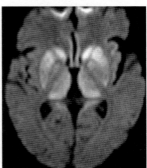

Comment

CJD is rare and is caused by a prion agent composed of protease-resistant protein that affects the central nervous system and results in rapid, progressive neurodegeneration. Approximately 1 in every 1 million persons worldwide is infected.

Clinical

The most common clinical presentation is that of rapidly progressive dementia. Other neurologic symptoms include upper motor neuron signs, ataxia, myoclonus, and sensory deficits. The characteristic diagnostic triad of progressive dementia, myoclonic jerks, and periodic sharp-wave electroencephalographic activity is present in approximately 75% of cases. Prognosis is poor, with death usually occurring within 1 year from the onset of symptoms.

Histopathology

Histologic evaluation shows neuronal degeneration and gliosis in the gray matter, especially the cortex, but also in the deep gray matter of the corpus striatum and thalami, as in this case. Spongiform changes are characteristic. Inflammatory changes are usually not present.

Associated Diseases

The disease is best known in association with mad cow disease (bovine spongiform encephalopathy) in the United Kingdom; however, there have been scattered sporadic cases described with corneal transplantation as well as with implantation of cerebral electrodes. A less known prion infection called chronic wasting disease is found in deer and elk in North America.

Imaging

CT may show no abnormality; however, atrophy (most commonly cortical) is the next most common presentation. On magnetic resonance imaging, in addition to cortical atrophy, T2-weighted hyperintensity in the deep gray matter, especially the caudate and putamen nuclei, but also the thalami, is observed (Figure 168-1). Lesions typically are bilateral and are not associated with enhancement or significant mass effect. In addition, abnormalities involving the gray and white matter have been noted within the cerebral hemispheres. Several reported cases of sporadic CJD have shown increased signal intensity in the basal ganglia or cerebral cortex on diffusion-weighted images (reduced diffusion), as in this case (Figures 168-2 through 168-4). Ribbon-like areas of hyperintensity in the cerebral cortex on diffusion-weighted images (see Figure 168-4) have also corresponded to the localization of periodic sharp-wave complexes on electroencephalogram.

References

Hori M, Ishigame K, Aoki S, Araki T. Creutzfeldt-Jacob disease shown by line scan diffusion-weighted imaging. *AJR Am J Roentgenol.* 2003;180:1481-1482.

Mao-Drayer Y, Braff SP, Nagle KJ, Pendlebury W, Penar PL, Shapiro RE. Emerging patterns of diffusion-weighted MR imaging in Creutzfeldt-Jakob disease: case report and review of the literature. *AJNR Am J Neuroradiol.* 2002;23:550-556.

Cross-Reference

Neuroradiology: THE REQUISITES, 4th ed, p 243.

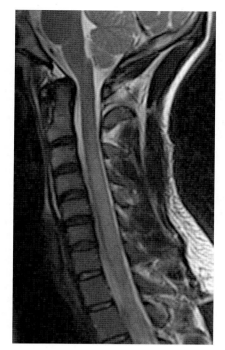

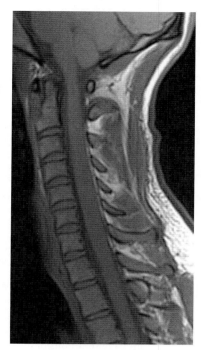

Figure 169-1

Figure 169-2

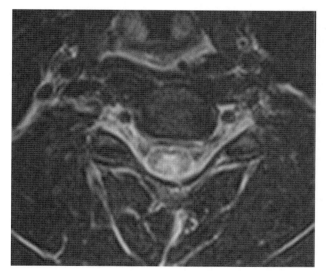

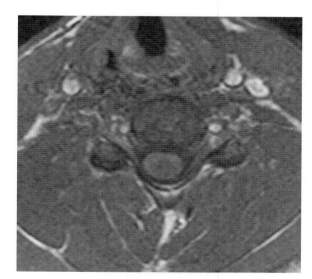

Figure 169-3

Figure 169-4

HISTORY: A 23-year-old male complains of headache after his first multitank SCUBA expedition.

1. What is the single best diagnosis?
   A. Astrocytoma
   B. Decompression sickness
   C. Multiple sclerosis
   D. Carbon monoxide poisoning

2. What is the most frequently affected organ system in this entity?
   A. Musculoskeletal
   B. Neurologic
   C. Cutaneous
   D. Pulmonary

3. Which of the following magnetic resonance imaging (MRI) patterns would be *unlikely* in this disease?
   A. Focal involvement of the gray and white matter
   B. Long segment involvement of the gray and white matter
   C. Isolated white matter involvement
   D. Isolated gray matter involvement

4. Which of the following statements regarding this disease is true?
   A. Negative MRI findings exclude it.
   B. Improvement in MRI findings correlates with clinical improvement.
   C. The diagnosis of the disease is clinical, and the patient's transfer to a hyperbaric oxygen treatment center should not be delayed.
   D. MRI has high sensitivity in detecting spinal lesions.

CASE 169

Caisson Disease (Decompression Sickness)

1. **B.** Decompression sickness (DCS; also called Caisson disease). Involvement of both gray matter and dorsal white matter is typical of decompression injury. There is relatively mild cord expansion to the degree of cord involvement suggesting a demyelinating, inflammatory, or vascular cause. The signal abnormality involving multiple contiguous levels would be unusual in multiple sclerosis. Carbon monoxide poisoning typically affects the basal ganglia and white matter of the brain and does not affect the spinal cord.

2. **A.** Musculoskeletal. DCS is most frequently observed in the appendicular joints. Musculoskeletal symptoms are present in 60% to 70% of all DCS cases. Neurologic symptoms are present in 10% to 15% of DCS cases with headache and visual disturbances being the most common symptom. Skin manifestations are present in about 10% to 15% of cases. Pulmonary DCS ("the chokes") is very rare in divers and has been observed much less frequently in aviators since the introduction of oxygen prebreathing protocols.

3. **D.** Isolated gray matter involvement. Isolated gray matter involvement is highly unusual, and other possible causes for the patient's symptoms should be considered. Focal involvement of the gray and white matter may be seen. Long segment involvement of gray and white matter may be seen and is predictive of poor outcome. Isolated white matter involvement may be seen.

4. **C.** The diagnosis of the disease is clinical, and the patient's transfer to a hyperbaric oxygen treatment center should not be delayed. The decision to pursue hyperbaric oxygen therapy is based on clinical findings and should not be guided by MRI findings. MRI has low sensitivity in DCS; therefore, MRI findings do not exclude DCS. Improvement in MRI findings does not correlate with clinical improvement.

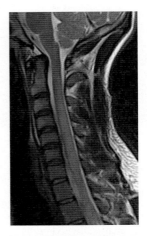

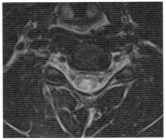

Comment

Background

DCS, also known as Caisson disease, is a clinical syndrome caused by rapid reduction in pressure during ascent from depth that can lead to spinal cord infarction. DCS is classified into two types based on clinical symptoms. Type I includes joint pain, skin rash, or localized edema. Type II has more serious complications and is subdivided into four subtypes according to the organ affected (central nervous system, spinal cord, inner ear, and lungs). Spinal cord involvement may occur in 50% of patients with type II DCS.

Pathophysiology

Ascending too quickly causes the dissolved nitrogen from compressed air that accumulates in blood and tissues to return to its gas form causing bubble formation. The pathophysiology of cord injury is not completely understood. Three possible mechanisms have been proposed: (1) venous infarction resulting from bubble formation in epidural veins, causing clotting and leading to obstruction; (2) autochthonous bubble formation where gas bubbles form space-occupying lesions within the myelin of the spinal cord, especially in the lateral and posterior columns affected secondary to high fat content; and (3) arterial gas embolization, which is considered to be a less frequent cause.

Imaging

Patchy increased T2-weighted signal changes affecting multiple levels (Figures 169-1 and 169-2) and mixed venous and arterial patterns with signal changes involving the dorsal column white matter and the gray matter (Figures 169-3 and 169-4) are typically found.

Management

Initial treatment is with 100% oxygen until hyperbaric oxygen therapy can be provided.

References

Hennedige T, Chow W, Ng YY, et al. MRI in spinal cord decompression sickness. *J Med Imaging Radiat Oncol.* 2012;56(3):282-288.

Kei PL, Choong CT, Young T, et al. Decompression sickness: MRI of the spinal cord. *J Neuroimaging.* 2007;17(4):378-380.

Yoshiyama M, Asamoto S, Kobayashi N, et al. Spinal cord decompression sickness associated with scuba diving: correlation of immediate and delayed magnetic resonance imaging findings with severity of neurologic impairment—a report on 3 cases. *Surg Neurol.* 2007;67(3):283-287.

Cross-Reference

Neuroradiology: THE REQUISITES, 4th ed, p 588.

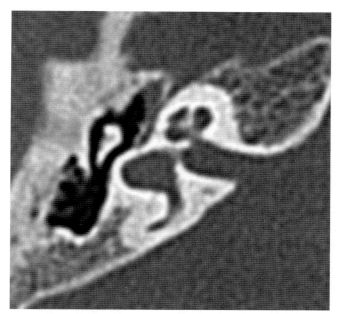

Figure 170-1

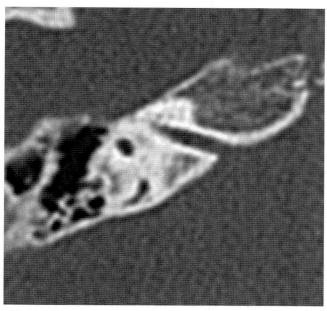

Figure 170-2

HISTORY: These scans show the temporal bones of two children with hearing loss since birth who have the same diagnosis.

1. Which of the following is the single best diagnosis?
   A. Malignant otitis externa
   B. Mondini malformation
   C. Down syndrome
   D. Labyrinthitis ossificans

2. Which part of the temporal bone is most malformed in Down syndrome?
   A. Squamosal
   B. Inner ear
   C. Middle ear
   D. External ear

3. What is the most common external ear finding in Down syndrome?
   A. External auditory canal (EAC) stenosis
   B. EAC atresia
   C. Osteoma
   D. Epidermoid

4. What is the most common inner ear abnormality in Down syndrome?
   A. Malformed bone islands of the lateral semicircular canal
   B. Cochlear aperture stenosis
   C. Internal auditory canal (IAC) narrowing
   D. Mondini malformation

CASE 170

Inner Ear in Down Syndrome

1. **C.** Down syndrome. The inner ear abnormalities (malformed bone island of the semicircular canal and IAC stenosis) indicate Down syndrome as the diagnosis. There is no erosion of the EAC, which would indicate malignant otitis externa. In addition, there is no evidence of incomplete partition, which would indicate Mondini malformation. Finally, there is no bone replacement of the inner ear structures, which would indicate labyrinthitis ossificans.

2. **D.** External ear. The external ear is the part most commonly malformed in Down syndrome.

3. **A.** External auditory canal (EAC) stenosis. EAC stenosis is the most common external ear finding in Down syndrome. This occurs in 40% to 50% of cases. EAC atresia is less common than stenosis. Osteoma and epidermoid are uncommon in this patient population.

4. **A.** Malformed bone islands of lateral semicircular canal. Malformed bone islands of lateral semicircular canal are the most common inner ear abnormalities in Down syndrome. This occurs in approximately 50% of affected patients. IAC narrowing occurs in approximately 25% of affected patients, and cochlear aperture stenosis occurs in approximately 20% of patients. Mondini malformation is very uncommon.

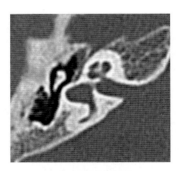

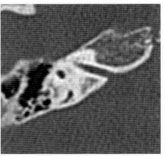

Comment

External and Middle Ear Complications in Down Syndrome

Many patients with Down syndrome suffer from hearing loss from a variety of reasons. The typical pharyngeal and oral cavity anatomy predisposes them to pharyngitis and to obstructive sleep apnea. Because the eustachian tubes are often obstructed when patients with Down syndrome have upper respiratory infections, middle ear effusions and mastoid fluid accumulation are common. "Glue ear" is the condition in which mucoid secretion accumulates in the middle ear and restricts the mobility of ossicles. The mucoid material often becomes infected. The second most common issue concerns the EAC, which is stenosed in approximately 40% to 50% of these patients. Such stenosis often hampers removal and clearance of cerumen and its byproducts, which leads to plug formation. The outer ear and middle ear pathologies invariably lead to conductive hearing loss.

Inner Ear Anomalies and Down Syndrome

Patients with Down syndrome also may have inner ear anomalies (Figures 170-1 and 170-2). Of these, malformation of the bone islands of the lateral semicircular canal is most common. This leads to a strange appearance to the usual symmetric nature of the lateral semicircular canals' interior. In addition to this anomaly, IAC stenosis, dehiscence of the superior semicircular canal, and cochlear aperture stenosis may occur. These findings may result in sensorineural hearing loss in affected patients.

Reference

Intrapiromkul J, Aygun N, Tunkel DE, Carone M, Yousem DM. Inner ear anomalies seen on CT images in people with Down syndrome. *Pediatr Radiol.* 2012;42(12):1449-1455.

Cross-Reference

Neuroradiology: THE REQUISITES, 4th ed, p 400.

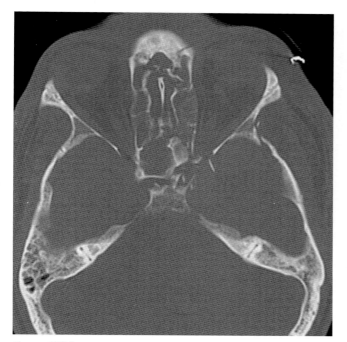

Figure 171-1

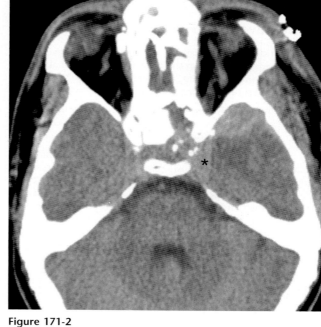

Figure 171-2

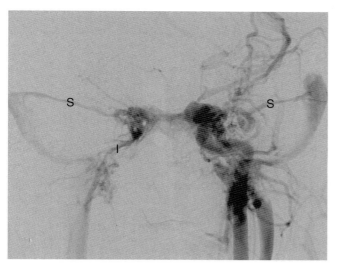

Figure 171-3

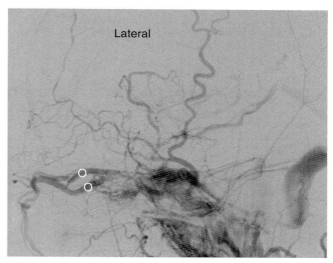

Figure 171-4

HISTORY: Proptosis.

1. What is the best diagnosis?
   A. Vasculitis
   B. Cavernous sinus thrombosis
   C. Carotid-cavernous fistula
   D. Vascular dysplasia

2. What type of carotid-cavernous fistula is this?
   A. A
   B. B
   C. C
   D. D

3. How are direct carotid-cavernous fistulas usually treated?
   A. Surgery
   B. Close follow-up until symptomatic
   C. Radiation
   D. Embolization

4. What is the most common cause of carotid-cavernous fistula?
   A. Congenital
   B. Aneurysm rupture
   C. Trauma
   D. Iatrogenic

CASE 171

Carotid-Cavernous Fistula

1. **C.** Carotid-cavernous fistula. The imaging findings show a communication between the left cavernous internal carotid artery and the cavernous venous sinus, consistent with a carotid-cavernous fistula.

2. **A.** A. This is a type A, which is a direct communication between the intracavernous portion of the internal carotid artery and the cavernous venous sinus.

3. **D.** Embolization. Symptomatic direct carotid-cavernous fistulas (type A) spontaneously resolve only in rare cases. The goal of treatment is to eliminate flow through the fistula and to maintain internal carotid patency when possible. Treatment of direct and indirect fistulas may differ. Direct carotid-cavernous fistulas are usually treated transarterially with detachable coils or balloon embolization tamponading the hole in the internal carotid artery. In the event that a transarterial route is impossible or is ineffective, a transvenous approach using platinum coils may be warranted. This approach can be achieved either via the femoral route or surgically via the superior ophthalmic vein. Complicated carotid-cavernous fistulas, residual carotid-cavernous fistulas after embolization with an arterial approach, and dural arteriovenous fistulas of the cavernous sinus may sometimes need to be treated transvenously. Gamma Knife radiosurgery has also been shown to be effective in treating indirect dural arteriovenous fistulas.

4. **C.** Trauma. Trauma is the most common cause of direct carotid-cavernous fistula formation. The second most common cause is probably aneurysm rupture.

Comment

Classification

There are two basic types of carotid-cavernous vascular malformations, direct (type A) and indirect (dural, types B, C, and D), each of which has a different cause. Carotid-cavernous fistulas represent a direct communication between the intracavernous portion of the internal carotid artery and the cavernous venous sinus. An indirect carotid-cavernous vascular malformation, otherwise known as a dural arteriovenous fistula, is a shunt between meningeal branches of the cavernous internal carotid artery (type B), meningeal branches of the external carotid artery (type C), or meningeal branches of both the intracavernous carotid artery and the external carotid artery (type D) with the cavernous venous sinus.

Clinical

The clinical presentation and imaging findings are normally diagnostic of a direct carotid-cavernous fistula. The typical clinical presentation of a carotid-cavernous fistula is ophthalmologic symptoms, including pulsatile proptosis, pain, chemosis, and orbital bruit. This is because the cavernous sinus directly communicates with the ophthalmic veins, and an abnormal shunt between the sinus and the internal carotid artery can transmit arterial pressure to these veins. In addition, arterial perfusion to the globe is decreased, leading to visual loss. Direct carotid-cavernous fistulas are most commonly the result of head trauma as in this case; however, spontaneous carotid-cavernous fistulas may be seen in a spectrum of disorders, including atherosclerosis in older adults, rupture of a cavernous internal carotid artery aneurysm, or in association with underlying vascular dysplasias. In this case of direct fistula, multiple fractures at the nasal bones, left zygomatic arch, and comminuted fractures involving the lesser wing of the sphenoid, tuberculum sella, and left anterior clinoid process are demonstrated (Figure 171-1).

Imaging

Computed tomography and magnetic resonance (MR) imaging often show enlargement of the superior ophthalmic vein, cavernous sinus, or petrosal venous plexus, as in this case (Figure 171-2). MR angiography and catheter angiography show direct communication between the cavernous internal carotid artery and the cavernous venous sinus as well as early filling of the ipsilateral cavernous sinus, superior or inferior ophthalmic veins, and petrosal venous complex (Figures 171-3 and 171-4). In high-flow lesions, the contralateral venous system may opacify, as in this case, through both intercavernous veins and the petrosal venous complex (see Figures 171-3 and 171-4).

References

Barrow DL, Spector RH, Braun IF, et al. Classification and treatment of spontaneous carotid-cavernous sinus fistulas. *J Neurosurg.* 1985; 62:248-256.

Lewis AI, Tomsick TA, Tew JM. Management of 100 consecutive direct carotid-cavernous fistulas: results of treatment with detachable balloons. *Neurosurgery.* 1995;36:239-244.

Wadlington VR, Terry JB. Endovascular therapy of traumatic carotid-cavernous fistulas. *Crit Care Clin.* 1999;15:831-854.

Cross-Reference

Neuroradiology: THE REQUISITES, 4th ed, pp 332-334.

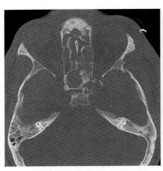
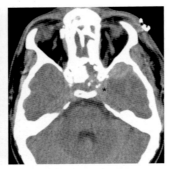
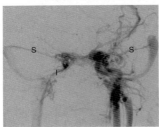
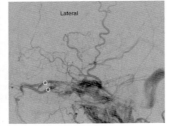

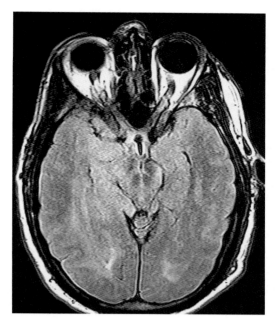

Figure 172-1

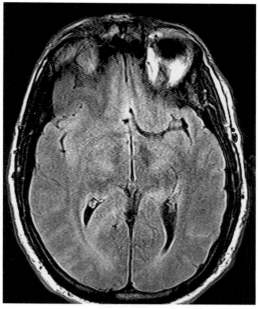

Figure 172-2

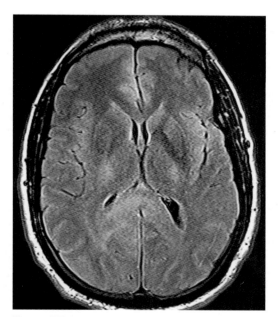

Figure 172-3

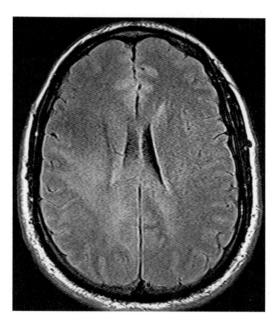

Figure 172-4

HISTORY: Altered personality.

1. Which imaging finding is characteristic of gliomatosis cerebri?
   A. Focal mass spanning the corpus callosum
   B. Extensive white matter signal abnormality in one hemisphere
   C. Gray and white matter signal abnormality involving three or more lobes
   D. Enhancing masses in three or more lobes

2. How often is the corpus callosum involved with gliomatosis cerebri?
   A. 10%
   B. 25%
   C. 50%
   D. 75%

3. What is the survival rate at 1 year in patients diagnosed with this condition?
   A. 25% to 35%
   B. 45% to 55%
   C. 65% to 75%
   D. Greater than 80%

4. Regarding magnetic resonance imaging (MRI) physics, what is the effect of increasing the time to repetition (TR) in spin echo images?
   A. Increased image contrast
   B. Decreased T2 and PD contrast
   C. Decreased scan time
   D. Increased signal

CASE 172

Gliomatosis Cerebri

1. **C.** Gray and white matter signal abnormality involving three or more lobes. This reflects the infiltrative nature of the disease and to be considered must involve three or more lobes. There may or may not be enhancement. No focal mass or involvement of the corpus callosum is necessary.

2. **C.** 50%. The corpus callosum is involved in approximately 50% of the documented cases.

3. **B.** 45% to 55%. The survival rate is reported to be 48% at 1 year.

4. **D.** Increased signal. There is more relaxation/magnetization allowing the next excitation to provide more signal. Increasing the TR results in decreased image contrast, increased T2/PD contrast, and increased scan time.

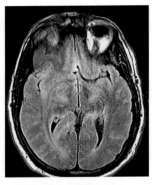

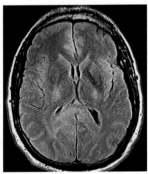

Comment

Case Imaging

This case illustrates the typical radiologic appearance of gliomatosis cerebri. There is extensive abnormality within the brain that affects the white matter (Figures 172-1 through 172-4); however, the gray matter is also involved. This extensively infiltrative process affects large portions of the cerebrum, including the right temporal (see Figures 172-1 and 172-2), occipital (see Figures 172-1 through 172-3), and frontal lobes (see Figures 172-2, 172-3, and 172-4). There is mild gyral swelling and sulcal effacement. There is extension across the splenium of the corpus callosum that is mildly expanded (see Figures 172-2 and 172-3), as well as the anterior commissure (see Figure 172-2), with involvement of the left cerebrum to a lesser extent. There are no regions of necrosis, there is no circumscribed mass, and there is no enhancement (not shown). Also, on Figure 172-1, note the involvement of the optic chiasm and bilateral optic tracts.

Definition

Gliomatosis cerebri is characterized by an extensive infiltrative pattern throughout the involved portions of the brain disproportionate to the remainder of the histologic findings, including a relative paucity of cellularity, anaplasia, and necrosis. In addition to the disproportionate histologic findings relative to the degree of infiltration seen on MRI, clinical symptoms are characteristically mild relative to the degree of brain involvement. Patients often present only with altered mental status or a change in personality. Headaches and seizures may occur. Focal neurologic deficits occur late in the course of disease. Although this tumor may affect patients of any age, it most commonly presents between the third and fifth decades. In addition to the extensive parenchymal involvement and the signal alteration seen on MRI, other findings that may suggest the diagnosis include mild diffuse sulcal and ventricular effacement. Not uncommonly, a large resection or lobectomy is necessary to make the diagnosis pathologically because biopsy may provide insufficient material. Therefore, recognition of the imaging findings, in combination with the patient's history, is important in diagnosing this neoplasm. Radiologists play a critical role by suggesting the diagnosis, mapping the extent of disease, and guiding biopsy.

References

Louis DN, Ohgaki H, Wiestler OD, et al. The 2007 WHO classification of tumours of the central nervous system. *Acta Neuropathol.* 2007;114(2):97-109.

Yip M, Fisch C, Lamarche FB. Gliomatosis cerebri affecting the entire neuraxis. *Radiographics.* 2003;23:247-253.

Cross-Reference

Neuroradiology: THE REQUISITES, 4th ed, pp 61-63.

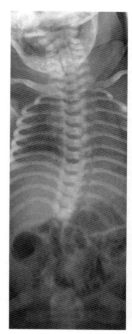
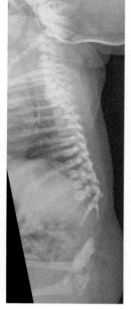
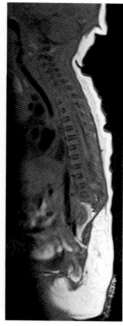
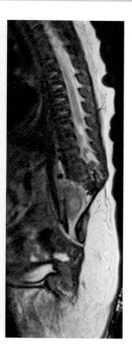

Figure 173-1   Figure 173-2   Figure 173-3   Figure 173-4

HISTORY: A 4-day-old infant has malformed lower extremities.

1. What is the single best diagnosis?
   A. Tethered cord
   B. Myelomeningocele
   C. Sacrococcygeal teratoma
   D. Caudal regression syndrome

2. Which of the following disorders has been linked to this syndrome?
   A. Cretinism
   B. Vitamin K deficiency
   C. Rh incompatibility
   D. Maternal diabetes mellitus

3. Which of the following conditions is associated with this syndrome?
   A. Hemihypertrophy
   B. Lipomeningocele
   C. Capillary hemangioma
   D. Lymphatic malformation of the head and neck

4. Which of the following statements regarding the two types of this syndrome is true?
   A. Caudal agenesis has been categorized into two types depending on the location of the conus medullaris.
   B. Vertebral dysgenesis is less severe in type II caudal agenesis than in type I.
   C. Patients with type I caudal agenesis typically present with tethered cord syndrome.
   D. In patients with type II caudal agenesis, there is abrupt spinal cord terminus that is club-shaped or wedge-shaped.

CASE 173

Caudal Regression Syndrome (Caudal Agenesis)

1. **D.** Caudal regression syndrome. There is absence of the lumbosacral spine and blunting of the conus typical of caudal regression syndrome. There is no evidence of low-lying conus. There is no subcutaneous cystic lesion. There is no sacral mass.

2. **D.** Maternal diabetes mellitus. There is a definite association with maternal diabetes mellitus. Cretinism is related to maternal nutritional deficiency of iodine resulting in congenital hypothyroidism. Neonatal hemorrhagic disease is caused by lack of vitamin K reaching the fetus across the placenta and low levels in breast milk; there is no association with lumbosacral agenesis. Rh incompatibility can result in hydrops fetalis; it is not associated with lumbosacral agenesis seen in this case.

3. **B.** Lipomeningocele. Terminal myelocystocele and lipomeningocele have been associated with this syndrome. Hemihypertrophy is part of Beckwith-Wiedemann syndrome and is not associated with caudal regression syndrome. Capillary hemangioma is not associated with caudal regression syndrome. Capillary malformations of the head and neck are not associated with caudal regression syndrome.

4. **A.** Caudal agenesis has been categorized into two types depending on the location of the conus medullaris. In type I caudal agenesis, vertebral dysgenesis is more severe and ranges from absence of the sacrum and coccyx in most cases to absence of the entire lumbar and lower thoracic vertebrae. Patients with type II caudal agenesis typically present with cord tethering. Patients with type II caudal agenesis typically present with low-lying conus. In type I, there is associated aplasia of the caudal metameres of the spinal cord, resulting in abrupt cord terminus.

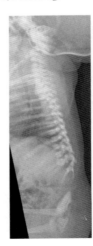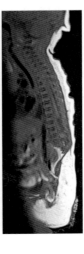

Comment

Background

Caudal agenesis or caudal regression syndrome comprises total or partial agenesis of the spinal column. The congenital spectrum of vertebral abnormalities ranges from agenesis of the coccyx to absence of the sacral, lumbar, and lower thoracic vertebrae. About 16% of infants with caudal regression syndrome have diabetic mothers, and about 1% of diabetic mothers have offspring with the syndrome.

Histopathology

It has been hypothesized that sacral agenesis or dysgenesis may occur as a result of hyperglycemia in a genetically predisposed fetus early in gestation. The insult may prevent canalization and retrogressive differentiation of the caudal cell mass or may promote excessive retrogression resulting in the sacral deformity or anorectal and urogenital malformations.

Imaging

Sacral agenesis or dysgenesis has been categorized into two types on the basis of conus position: type I has a high conus terminating cephalad to the L1 inferior endplate, and type II has a low conus terminating caudal to L1. Patients with type I tend to have a large sacral defect (Figures 173-1 through 173-4), with the sacrum ending above S1. In about 90% of patients with type I, the conus has a blunted wedge-shaped contour (shorter ventrally as a result of a deficiency of anterior horn cells) (see Figures 173-3 and 173-4). The spinal cord terminus is high (T12 level in most cases). The thecal sac tapers below the cord terminus and ends at an unusually high level (see Figures 173-3 and 173-4). Clinically, patients have a stable neurologic deficit. In patients with type II, the conus is often elongated as a result of tethering to a thickened filum, lipoma, or myelocystocele. Sacral dysgenesis is relatively mild; however, the clinical course is more likely to involve neurologic deterioration because of cord tethering. Terminal myelocystoceles and lipomyelomeningoceles are associated with sacral agenesis or dysgenesis in approximately 9% and 6% of cases, respectively. Other anomalies associated with caudal regression include diastematomyelia and anterior sacral meningocele.

Management

Patients may require surgical intervention for decompression and vertebral anomalies. Some authors suggest cutting the filum in cases of cord tethering.

References

Barkovich AJ, Raghavan N, Chuang S, et al. The wedge-shaped cord terminus: a radiographic sign of caudal regression. *AJNR Am J Neuroradiol.* 1989;10(6):1223-1231.

Nievelstein RAJ, Valk J, Smit LME, et al. MR of the caudal regression syndrome: embryologic implications. *AJNR Am J Neuroradiol.* 1994;15(6):1021-1029.

Pang D. Sacral agenesis and caudal spinal cord malformations. *Neurosurgery.* 1993;32(5):755-778, discussion 778-779.

Cross-Reference

Neuroradiology: THE REQUISITES, 4th ed, pp 301, 303.

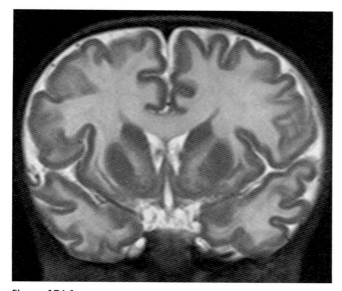

Figure 174-1

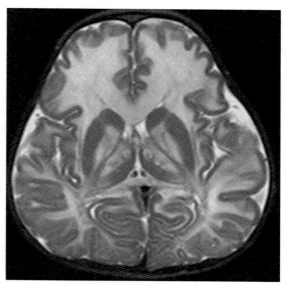

Figure 174-2

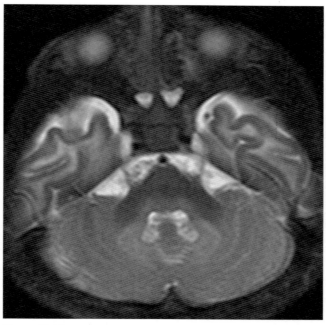

Figure 174-3

HISTORY: An Ashkenazi Jewish patient with hypotonia and macrocephaly.

1. What is the best diagnosis considering both imaging and clinical history?
   A. Canavan disease
   B. Metachromatic leukodystrophy
   C. Alexander disease
   D. Pelizaeus-Merzbacher

2. Which amino acid or derivative is typically elevated in this diagnosis?
   A. Glutamic acid
   B. Aspartic acid
   C. *N*-acetyl aspartic acid
   D. Acetyl-coenzyme A

3. What is the inheritance pattern for this disease?
   A. Autosomal dominant
   B. Autosomal recessive
   C. Sporadic
   D. X-linked

4. Where does Canavan disease begin?
   A. Subcortical white matter
   B. Internal capsule
   C. Basal ganglia
   D. Corpus callosum

CASE 174

Canavan Disease

1. **A.** Canavan disease. Diffuse white matter signal abnormality in a macrocephalic pediatric patient of Ashkenazi Jewish heritage is suggestive of Canavan disease. Metachromatic leukodystrophy presents with symmetric dysmyelination throughout the white matter of both the cerebrum and cerebellum with sparing of the subcortical U-fibers. In this particular case there is involvement of the subcortical U-fibers. Alexander disease does not have a familial pattern. The signal abnormality also tends to be in a more anterior distribution at least initially. Pelizaeus-Merzbacher is not typically associated with macrocephaly. Signal abnormality typically involves the internal capsule, proximal corona radiata, and the optic radiations.

2. **C.** *N*-acetyl aspartic acid. Canavan disease results from a mutation of the gene responsible for *N*-acetylaspartoacylase, resulting in increased *N*-acetyl aspartic acid. The other leukodystrophies result in decreased *N*-acetyl aspartic acid.

3. **B.** Autosomal recessive. The inheritance pattern of Canavan disease is autosomal recessive.

4. **A.** Subcortical white matter. Canavan disease preferentially results in subcortical signal abnormality.

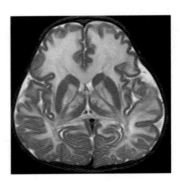

Comment

Leukodystrophies

The leukodystrophies, or dysmyelinating disorders, represent a spectrum of inherited diseases that usually result in both abnormal formation and abnormal maintenance of myelin. Many of the more common of these rare disorders are inherited in an autosomal recessive pattern. In many of the leukodystrophies, specific enzyme deficiencies have been identified as the cause. These diseases cause abnormal growth or development of the myelin sheath. Myelin is made up of at least 10 different chemicals. Each of the leukodystrophies affects one of these substances.

Canavan Disease

Canavan disease is transmitted as an autosomal recessive disorder usually identified in infants of Ashkenazi Jewish descent and in Saudi Arabians. It is the result of a deficiency of *N*-acetylaspartoacylase. Infants may have macrocephaly due to enlargement of the brain. On histologic evaluation, there is diffuse demyelination and the white matter is replaced by microscopic cystic spaces, giving it a "spongy" appearance. In contrast to most of the other dysmyelinating syndromes, Canavan disease preferentially begins in the subcortical white matter and later spreads to diffusely involve the deep white matter (Figures 174-1 and 174-2). There may be sparing of the internal capsules (see Figure 174-2). There may be bilaterally symmetric T2-weighted signal abnormality in the deep gray matter (Figures 174-2 and 174-3), as in this case. The brainstem is involved in late disease (see Figure 174-3). In most cases, the ventricles remain normal or may be slightly small; however, in the late stages of disease, when cerebral atrophy occurs, there may be proportionate enlargement of the ventricles and cerebral sulci. Diffusion-weighted imaging shows diffuse restriction, and spectroscopy shows high levels of *N*-acetyl aspartic acid.

Alexander Disease

Alexander disease is different from many of the leukodystrophies in that no familial pattern has been recognized. Like Canavan disease, it presents with macrocephaly in addition to developmental delay and spasticity. The deep white matter is usually involved early, and the internal capsules are typically involved (in contrast to Canavan disease, in which they are often relatively spared).

Reference

Engelbrecht V, Scherer A, Rassek M, Witsack HJ, Modder U. Diffusion-weighted MR imaging in the brain in children: findings in the normal brain and in the brain with white matter diseases. *Radiology*. 2002;222:410-418.

Cross-Reference

Neuroradiology: THE REQUISITES, 4th ed, p 227.

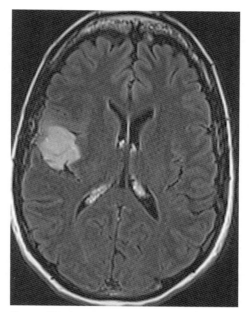

Figure 175-1

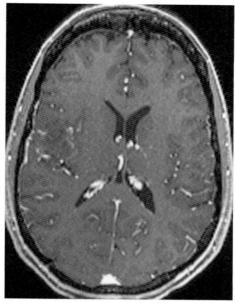

Figure 175-2

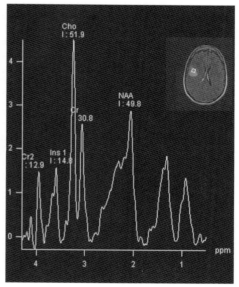

Figure 175-3

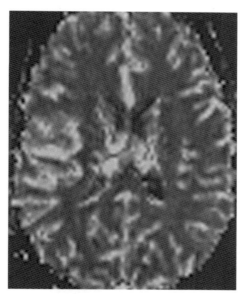

Figure 175-4

HISTORY: A patient presents with seizures.

1. What is the single best diagnosis?
   A. Abscess
   B. Infiltrative glioma
   C. Encephalitis
   D. Tumefactive multiple sclerosis

2. On magnetic resonance spectroscopy (MRS), which markers typically increase in high-grade glioma?
   A. Myoinositol and alanine
   B. Glutamate and glutamine
   C. Creatine and N-acetylaspartate
   D. Choline and lactate

3. Which statement regarding MRS is correct?
   A. Single-voxel MRS takes longer than multivoxel MRS.
   B. Signal-to-noise ratios improve with smaller voxel sizes.
   C. Creatine is often used as a reference value to obtain semi-quantitative ratio measurements.
   D. Longer time to echo (TE) allows for detection of more metabolites than short TE MRS.

4. What histologic feature best allows for characterization of World Health Organization (WHO) grade IV rather than WHO grade III glioma?
   A. Pleomorphism
   B. Cellular density
   C. Number of mitoses
   D. Vascular proliferation

CASE 175

High-Grade Anaplastic Astrocytoma

1. **B.** Infiltrative glioma. The mildly expansile region of signal abnormality on T2-weighted fluid-attenuated inversion recovery (FLAIR) imaging, trace enhancement, elevated choline-to-creatine (Cho/Cr) ratio, and increased perfusion support a diagnosis of neoplasm. Abscess would be a fluid collection with peripheral enhancement. Encephalitis would typically show more enhancement and decreased perfusion centrally, and the MRS spectrum would be variable dependent on the specific cause. Tumefactive multiple sclerosis would show decreased perfusion centrally and peripheral enhancement with an incomplete ring typically.

2. **D.** Choline and lactate. In high-grade gliomas, choline typically increases secondary to high cellularity and lactate increases secondary to necrosis.

3. **C.** Creatine is often used as a reference value to obtain semi-quantitative ratio measurements. The concentration of creatine remains relatively stable in multiple pathologies and therefore is a useful reference for semi-quantitative assessment.

4. **D.** Vascular proliferation. According to the WHO grading of gliomas, grade III tumors demonstrate pleomorphism, high cellularity, and a high number of mitoses. Vascular proliferation and necrosis are characteristic of WHO grade IV tumor.

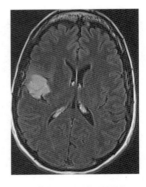

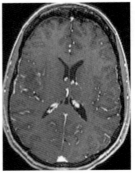

Comment

Imaging

This case shows abnormal signal intensity in the superficial cortex and subcortical white matter of the inferior right frontal lobe and superior right temporal lobe (Figure 175-1). There is mild local mass effect manifested by gyral expansion and sulcal effacement. No avid contrast enhancement is identified (Figure 175-2). These features on conventional FLAIR and gadolinium-enhanced images suggest a low-grade astrocytoma (see Figures 175-1 and 175-2). On proton MRS, an increased choline peak is highly suggestive of a malignant neoplasm (Figure 175-3). Perfusion imaging shows markedly elevated regional cerebral blood volume, also highly suggestive of a high-grade astrocytoma (Figure 175-4).

Classification/Grading

There are two classes of astrocytic tumors: tumors with narrow zones of infiltration (pilocytic astrocytoma, subependymal giant cell astrocytoma, pleomorphic xanthoastrocytoma) and tumors with diffuse zones of infiltration. According to the WHO classification, infiltrating astrocytic tumors may be divided into three subtypes: low-grade astrocytoma, anaplastic astrocytoma, and glioblastoma (GBM). The histologic criteria for these subdivisions depend on the cellular density, number of mitoses, presence of necrosis, nuclear and cytoplasmic pleomorphism, and vascular endothelial proliferation. GBM typically has all of these histologic features, whereas low-grade astrocytomas may show only minimal increased cellularity and cellular pleomorphism. The presence of necrosis and vascular endothelial proliferation, in particular, favors GBM. Histologically, anaplastic astrocytomas have features that are between those of a low-grade astrocytoma and those of a GBM. Necrosis is much less common than seen in the more malignant GBM. Anaplastic astrocytomas are highly malignant, with an average survival time of 2.5 years after diagnosis.

Reference

Lupo JM, Cha S, Chang SM, Nelson SJ. Analysis of metabolic indices in regions of abnormal perfusion in patients with high grade glioma. *AJNR Am J Neuroradiol.* 2007;28:1455-1461.

Cross-Reference

Neuroradiology: THE REQUISITES, 4th ed, p 59.

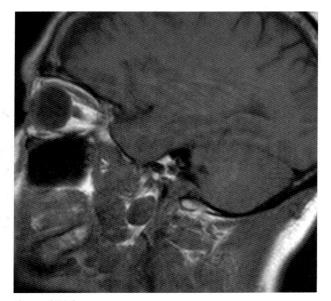

Figure 176-1

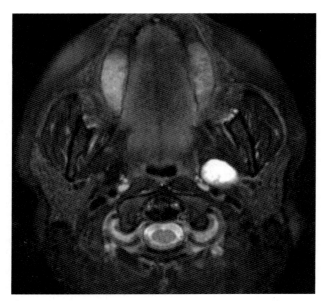

Figure 176-2

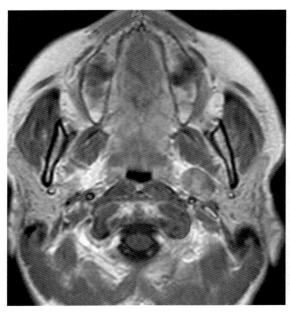

Figure 176-3

HISTORY: A 44-year-old woman has a 6-month history of depression and progressive weakness in the lower extremities. As part of her work-up, she underwent brain and cervical spine magnetic resonance imaging (MRI).

1. What should be *excluded* from the differential diagnosis of a lesion in this location?
   A. Rhabdomyosarcoma
   B. Pleomorphic adenoma
   C. Schwannoma
   D. Node

2. What is the most common lesion to populate the prestyloid parapharyngeal space (PPS)?
   A. Pleomorphic adenoma
   B. Schwannoma
   C. Paraganglioma
   D. Direct spread from primary site of mucosal carcinoma

3. Which of the following is the most common primary site of carcinoma whose metastases invade the PPS?
   A. Parotid gland
   B. Nasopharynx
   C. Oropharynx
   D. Paranasal sinuses

4. What percentage of benign prestyloid PPS lesions are pleomorphic adenomas?
   A. 0% to 20%
   B. 21% to 40%
   C. 41% to 60%
   D. 61% to 80%

CASE 176

Parapharyngeal Pleomorphic Adenoma

1. **A.** Rhabdomyosarcoma. Pleomorphic adenoma arises in this location from minor salivary gland rests, not parotid tissue. Schwannoma arises from the branches of cranial nerve V. Nodes can occur in the PPS. Rhabdomyosarcoma does not occur in this location. Abscesses are extremely rare in this location without oropharyngeal infection.

2. **D.** Direct spread from primary site of mucosal carcinoma. Direct spread from primary site of mucosal carcinoma is the most common lesion to populate the prestyloid PPS. This is the most common malignant tumor of the PPS. Schwannoma is the second most common benign tumor after pleomorphic adenoma, and paraganglioma is the third. Nodal metastasis from primary site of squamous cell carcinoma is the second most common malignant spread after direct spread.

3. **B.** Nasopharynx. The most common primary site of carcinoma to invade the PPS is the nasopharynx. The oropharynx is the second most common primary site; the parotid gland is the third. Lymphoma and cancers of the paranasal sinuses are rare.

4. **D.** 61% to 80%. Of benign prestyloid PPS lesions, 61% to 80% are pleomorphic adenomas.

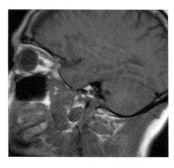

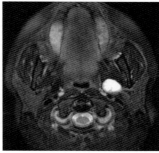

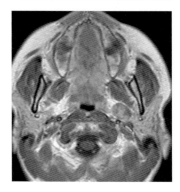

Comment

Identifying Parapharyngeal Space Lesions

Most PPS lesions are discovered incidentally, as in this case. The mass had nothing to do with the patient's lower extremity weakness, but it was discovered on the brain MRI study (Figures 176-1 through 176-3). When patients do have complaints, there may be parotid or neck swelling or pain.

Types of Lesions

Although pleomorphic adenomas, derived from minor salivary gland rests in the prestyloid PPS, are the most common primary lesion in the prestyloid PPS, the most common lesion to invade the space is carcinoma from the nasopharynx. When nasopharyngeal carcinoma invades the PPS, the cancer grade is advanced from T1 to T2.

Mucosal carcinomas, including oropharyngeal squamous cell carcinomas, invade the PPS from the anteromedial border of the PPS more commonly than do parotid masses spreading posterolaterally.

Incidence of Pleomorphic Adenomas

In older patients, the pleomorphic adenomas of the PPS can be monitored expectantly because the rate of malignant degeneration is sufficiently low (approximately 5% to 10% in 10 years) that the surgery to remove the adenoma may not be indicated, according to life expectancy statistics. In a younger patient such as this one, however, surgical removal to prevent carcinoma ex pleomorphic adenoma would be advised. Carcinoma ex pleomorphic adenoma represents fewer than 5% of all salivary gland tumors and approximately 10% of malignant parotid masses.

Imaging Findings

Pleomorphic adenomas are characterized by their bright signal intensity on T2-weighted scans and their avid enhancement. The enhancement pattern shows progressive gradual enhancement for up to 10 minutes after injection. The enhancement persists with delayed washout for as long as 20 to 25 minutes. Apparent diffusion coefficient (ADC) values may increase diagnostic specificity and sensitivity. Higher ADC values are suggestive of pleomorphic adenoma rather than malignancy and Warthin tumor.

References

AJCC. Pharynx. In: Edge SB, Byrd DR, Compton CC, et al., eds. *AJCC Cancer Staging Manual.* 7th ed. New York: Springer; 2010: 41-56.

Gangopadhyay M, Bandopadhyay A, Sinha S, Chakroborty S. Clinicopathologic study of parapharyngeal tumors. *J Cytol.* 2012;29(1): 26-29.

Hisatomi M, Asaumi J, Yanagi Y, et al. Assessment of pleomorphic adenomas using MRI and dynamic contrast enhanced MRI. *Oral Oncol.* 2003;39(6):574-579.

Cross-Reference

Neuroradiology: THE REQUISITES, 4th ed, pp 457-458.

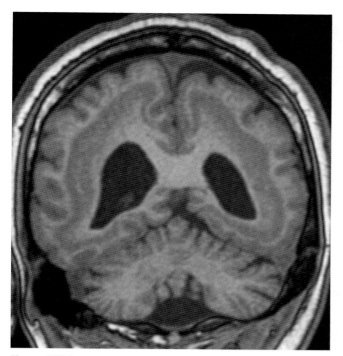

Figure 177-1

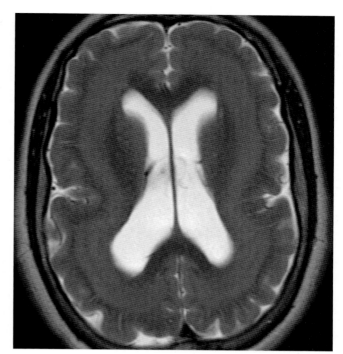

Figure 177-2

HISTORY: A patient presents with seizures and developmental delay.

1. What is the diagnosis?
   A. Congenital toxoplasmosis infection
   B. Tuberous sclerosis
   C. Schizencephaly
   D. Band heterotopia

2. Which of the following infections is most highly associated with pachygyria?
   A. Toxoplasmosis
   B. Cytomegalovirus
   C. Rubella
   D. Herpes simplex virus

3. Which of the following statements is correct with regard to cortical dysplasias and heterotopias?
   A. Cortical dysplasias are due to failure in normal migration.
   B. Heterotopia is associated with an increased risk for brain malignancy.
   C. Subependymal nodules in tuberous sclerosis are heterotopias.
   D. Cortical dysplasia and heterotopias are frequently seen in the same patient.

4. What tumor is associated with cortical dysplasia?
   A. Dysembryoplastic neuroepithelial tumor
   B. Desmoplastic infantile ganglioglioma
   C. Oligodendroglioma
   D. Pleomorphic xanthoastrocytoma

CASE 177

Band Heterotopia and Pachygyria

1. **D.** Band heterotopia. This is the classical appearance for band heterotopia. There are confluent areas of signal abnormality in the periventricular regions that follow the signal of cortex. There are also cortical abnormalities compatible with pachygyria. Toxoplasmosis usually manifests with scattered parenchymal and periventricular calcifications. Tuberous sclerosis manifests with subependymal nodules that may or may not bulge into the ventricular lumen. Schizencephaly is a cleft typically lined with gray matter seen within the parenchyma.

2. **B.** Cytomegalovirus. Cytomegalovirus has a high association with pachygyria.

3. **D.** Cortical dysplasia and heterotopias are frequently seen in the same patient. Cortical dysplasias result from abnormal maturation of cortical tissue, not failure to migrate. Heterotopias are not at risk for malignancy. Subependymal nodules in tuberous sclerosis are neoplastic, not heterotopic.

4. **A.** Dysembryoplastic neuroepithelial tumor. Dysembryoplastic neuroepithelial tumors are associated with cortical dysplasia in approximately 80% of cases.

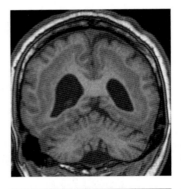

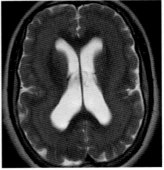

Comment

Heterotopias

Heterotopias are abnormalities of migration in which normal neurons occur in abnormal locations as a result of failure of migration along the radial glial fibers from the germinal region to the cortex. Three well-recognized types of heterotopia are focal, subependymal, and diffuse (laminar, band). *Subcortical heterotopia* is a newer term that refers to a specific entity in which neurons are abnormally located, predominantly in the subcortical white matter.

Diffuse or Band Heterotopia

Diffuse or band heterotopia refers to a layer of gray matter, the migration of which has arrested such that it is localized between the subcortical white matter laterally and the deep white matter medially (Figures 177-1 and 177-2). The inner and outer margins of the heterotopic neurons are well demarcated. The band of gray matter is separated from the overlying cortex by a mantle of subcortical white matter. Band heterotopias are frequently associated with overlying cortical dysplasias (pachygyria, polymicrogyria), as in this case (see Figures 177-1 and 177-2). The severity of the cortical dysplasia is directly related to the severity of the band heterotopia: the thicker the band is, the more severe the overlying dysplasia will be. Similarly, patients with band heterotopia tend to have more pronounced clinical symptoms. In addition to seizures, which may have an age of onset ranging from infancy to young adulthood, many children with band heterotopia have moderate to severe developmental delay.

Cortical Dysplasia

Cortical dysplasias differ from heterotopias in that they do not represent a failure of normal migration but rather a failure in the development of a normal six-layered cortex after migration from the germinal matrix to the cortical region.

References

Barkovich AJ. Morphologic characteristics of subcortical heterotopia: MR imaging study. *AJNR Am J Neuroradiol*. 2000;21:290-295.

Blümcke I, Thom M, Aronica E, et al. The clinicopathologic spectrum of focal cortical dysplasias: a consensus classification proposed by an ad hoc task force of the ILAE Diagnostic Methods Commission. *Epilepsia*. 2011;52(1):158-174.

Cross-Reference

Neuroradiology: THE REQUISITES, 4th ed, pp 274-275.

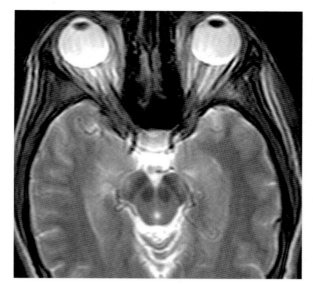

Figure 178-1

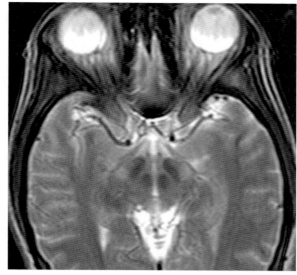

Figure 178-2

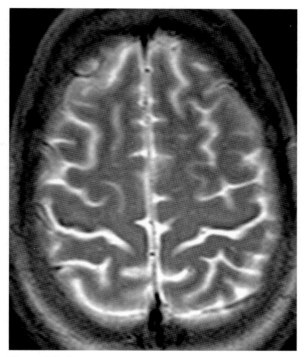

Figure 178-3

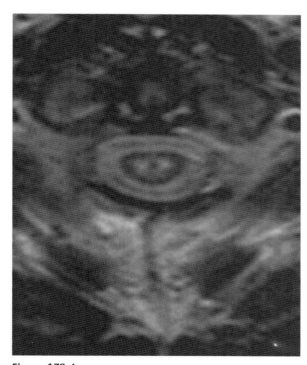

Figure 178-4

HISTORY: A patient presents with loss of motor strength in limbs.

1. What is the single best diagnosis?
   A. Poliovirus
   B. Multiple sclerosis
   C. Amyotrophic lateral sclerosis
   D. Lupus

2. What is the usual cause of death in patients with this disease?
   A. Pulmonary infections
   B. Cardiac arrest
   C. Stroke
   D. Sepsis

3. Which cranial nerve (CN) is most commonly affected in this disease?
   A. CN IX
   B. CN X
   C. CN XI
   D. CN XII

4. What causes T2 hypointensity in the precentral gyrus in this disease?
   A. Calcium in microglia
   B. Iron in microglia
   C. Hemosiderin
   D. Demyelination

CASE 178

Amyotrophic Lateral Sclerosis

1. **C.** Amyotrophic lateral sclerosis (ALS). ALS is the best answer considering the brain and spinal cord findings and the history of loss of motor strength. The brain and spinal cord findings exclusive of the clinical history are less specific. The symmetry of signal abnormality in the lateral columns is less common for multiple sclerosis. Polio usually affects the dorsal spinal cord. Magnetic resonance imaging findings in lupus are most often associated with ischemic changes.

2. **A.** Pulmonary infections. Although the cited cause of death is usually respiratory failure, this is usually hastened by infection, as proven in postmortem series.

3. **D.** CN XII. The hypoglossal nerve, CN XII, is the most commonly affected cranial nerve in ALS.

4. **B.** Iron in microglia. Although usually a late finding, iron accumulation in microglia may result in hypointense T2 signal in the precentral gyrus.

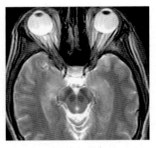

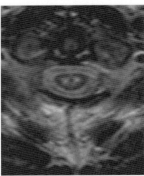

Comment

Background

ALS (Lou Gehrig disease) is the most common neurodegenerative disorder involving the motor neurons. It occurs in approximately 1 in 100,000 people annually. Most cases are sporadic, although autosomal dominant transmission may occur. It is a syndrome of upper and lower motor neuron dysfunction of the arms, legs, and bulbar or respiratory motor systems that slowly progresses over months to years in adults without primary involvement of any other part of the nervous system or the presence of any specific cause. Patients typically present in the sixth decade; clinical manifestations include hyperreflexia, weakness of the hands and forearms, spasticity, and cranial neuropathies. The hypoglossal nerve is most commonly affected, and its involvement may be detected on imaging as denervation atrophy with fatty replacement of the tongue.

Histopathology

Histopathologic examination shows selective degeneration of the somatic motor neurons of the brainstem nuclei and spinal cord (anterior horn cells) as well as the large pyramidal neurons of the motor cortex. Associated degeneration of the corticospinal tracts has been tracked in postmortem specimens from the cerebral cortex to the conus medullaris.

Imaging

In extreme cases, abnormal T2-weighted signal intensity may extend from the cortex, along the precentral gyrus of the motor strip (pyramidal Betz cells or upper motor neurons) (Figure 178-3); through the corona radiata, the posterior part of the posterior limb of the internal capsule, the cerebral peduncles, and brainstem (Figures 178-1 and 178-2); and down to the ventral and lateral portions of the spinal cord (Figure 178-4). Abnormal T2-weighted hypointensity, believed to be related to the deposition of iron or other minerals, may be present along the cerebral cortex in the motor strip, as in this case. High signal intensity on T1-weighted images in the anterolateral columns of the spinal cord has also been reported in patients with ALS.

Single-Photon Emission Computed Tomography

Single-photon emission computed tomography (SPECT) with N-isopropyl-p-I-123 iodoamphetamine may show decreased uptake in the cerebral cortex, including the motor cortex.

Magnetic Resonance Spectroscopy

Spectroscopy of the precentral gyrus region has shown a strong correlation between reduced N-acetylaspartate and glutamate levels and elevated choline and myo-inositol levels and severity of disease.

Management

ALS is a fatal disease and is incurable. Glutamate pathway antagonists are the only medications that have shown efficacy in extending life in patients with ALS.

References

Bowen BC, Pattany PM, Bradley WG, et al. MR imaging and localized proton spectroscopy of the precentral gyrus in amyotrophic lateral sclerosis. *AJNR Am J Neuroradiol.* 2000;21:647-658.

Sperfeld AD, Bretschneider V, Flaith L, et al. MR-pathologic comparison of the upper spinal cord in different motor neuron diseases. *Eur Neurol.* 2005;53(2):74-77.

Waragai M, Shinotoh H, Hayashi M, et al. High signal intensity on T1-weighted MRI of the anterolateral column of the spinal cord in amyotrophic lateral sclerosis. *J Neurol Neurosurg Psychiatry.* 1997;62(1):88-91.

Cross-Reference

Neuroradiology: THE REQUISITES, 4th ed, pp 247-248.

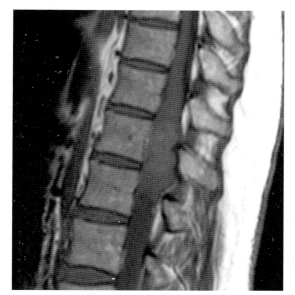

Figure 179-1

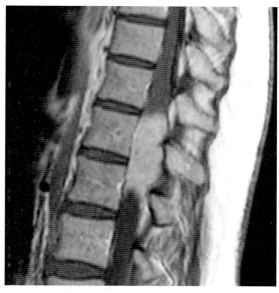

Figure 179-2

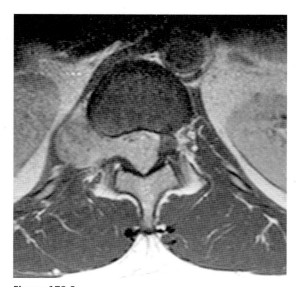

Figure 179-3

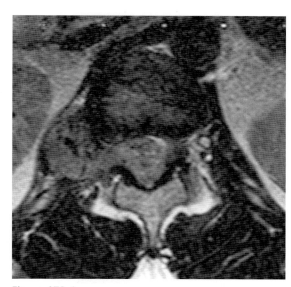

Figure 179-4

HISTORY: A 33-year-old man presents with back pain and leg numbness.

1. Which is the correct statement regarding central nervous system hemangiopericytomas?
   A. These tumors are meningioma variants.
   B. These tumors are most often intra-axial when intracranial.
   C. Radiation therapy, often without surgery, is the treatment of choice for hemangiopericytoma of the spine.
   D. Hemangiopericytomas are usually World Health Organization (WHO) grade II tumors.

2. When these masses occur in the spine, where are most of them located?
   A. Intramedullary
   B. Intradural extramedullary
   C. Interdural
   D. Extradural

3. In what age group do these tumors most often present?
   A. 0 to 20 years
   B. 30 to 50 years
   C. 51 to 70 years
   D. Older than 70 years

4. Which feature on magnetic resonance imaging (MRI) is the most helpful in differentiating hemangiopericytoma from meningioma?
   A. Hypointense T1 signal relative to cord
   B. Intense enhancement
   C. Intratumoral and peritumoral flow voids
   D. Dural-based lesion

CASE 179

Hemangiopericytoma of the Lumbar Spine

1. **D.** Hemangiopericytomas are usually WHO grade II tumors. Hemangiopericytomas are most often WHO grade II tumors in contrast to the etiopathologic different meningioma. When intracranial, these are often extra-axial arising from meningeal pericytes. Surgical resection (often with preoperative embolization) and postoperative radiation therapy is the preferred treatment plan for these lesions.

2. **D.** Extradural. Although rare, when these occur in the spine, the most common location is extradural.

3. **B.** 30 to 50 years. Patients with hemangiopericytomas most often present between 30 and 50 years of age. There is a smaller peak in childhood.

4. **C.** Intratumoral and peritumoral flow voids. Intratumoral and peritumoral flow voids are a hallmark of hemangiopericytoma. Most of both of these tumors are iso-hypointense on T1-weighted imaging and they tend to avidly enhance. Both are often dural based.

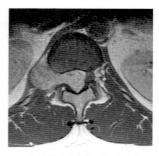

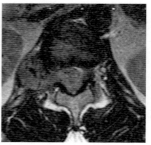

Comment

Background

Hemangiopericytomas are hypervascular tumors that most commonly occur between the ages of 30 and 50 and equally affect men and women. Hemangiopericytomas mostly involve the musculoskeletal system and are rarely found in the central nervous system, arising primarily within the epidural space. Within the spinal column, they are usually extradural in location, although intradural lesions have been described.

Histopathology

Hemangiopericytomas are thought to arise from the pericytes of Zimmerman, which are modified smooth muscle cells surrounding capillaries and postcapillary venules.

Imaging

Hemangiopericytomas are predominantly iso-intense to spinal cord parenchyma on T1-weighted (Figure 179-1) and T2-weighted MRI images (Figure 179-2). They may be distinguished by prominent intratumoral flow voids (see Figure 179-2) and intense enhancement (Figures 179-3 and 179-4), consistent with the known hypervascularity of these neoplasms. Preoperative identification of these tumors is important because of their aggressive nature, high rate of local recurrence, and propensity for late distant metastases. On angiography, hemangiopericytoma is a highly vascular lesion demonstrating corkscrew vessels and long-lasting dense tumor stain.

Management

Surgical excision is the mainstay of therapy. Adjuvant postoperative radiotherapy has been recommended because of the high incidence of local recurrence. Preoperative embolization may prevent excessive intraoperative blood loss.

Reference

Santillan A, Zink W, Lavi E, et al. Endovascular embolization of cervical hemangiopericytoma with Onyx-18: case report and review of the literature. *J Neurointerv Surg*. 2011;3(3):304-307.

Cross-Reference

Neuroradiology: THE REQUISITES, 4th ed, p 44.

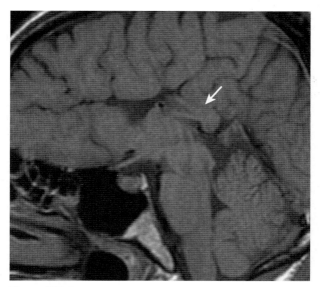

Figure 180-1

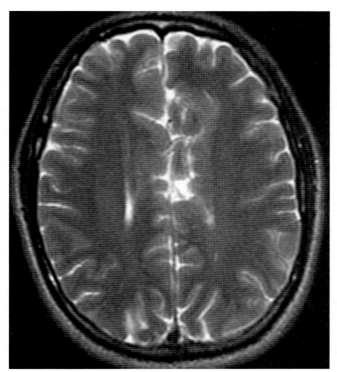

Figure 180-2

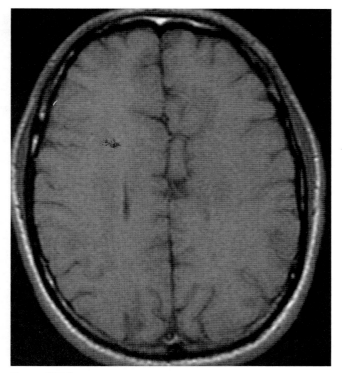

Figure 180-3

HISTORY: A patient presents with seizures.

1. What causes the imaging findings presented in this case?
   A. Failure of prosencephalon cleavage
   B. Intrauterine infarct or hemorrhage
   C. Perinatal infection
   D. Cortical migrational anomaly

2. What structure is missing in alobar, semilobar, and lobar holoprosencephaly (HPE)?
   A. Corpus callosum
   B. Septum pellucidum
   C. Interhemispheric fissure
   D. Frontal horns

3. What form of HPE is present in this patient?
   A. Alobar
   B. Semilobar
   C. Lobar
   D. Middle interhemispheric variant

4. What part of the corpus callosum is most often affected in syntelencephaly?
   A. Rostrum
   B. Genu
   C. Body
   D. Splenium

CASE 180

Lobar Holoprosencephaly

1. **A.** Failure of prosencephalon cleavage. This is a case of semilobar HPE caused by partial failure of the prosencephalon to segment or cleave into the distinct cerebral hemispheres.

2. **B.** Septum pellucidum. The absence of the septum pellucidum is the common missing structure. The corpus callosum, interhemispheric fissure, and the frontal horns may be abnormal or partially absent.

3. **B.** Semilobar. There is partial fusion of the bilateral cerebral hemispheres with dysgenesis of the corpus callosum. The third ventricle is present, and there are separate occipital horns and bodies of the lateral ventricles.

4. **C.** Body. The middle interhemispheric variant of HPE, also called syntelencephaly, is characterized by fusion of the posterior frontal and parietal lobes across the midline, involving the posterior body of the corpus callosum.

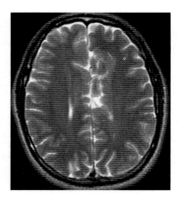

Comment

Background

HPE comprises a spectrum of disorders characterized by hypoplasia of the rostral end of the neural tube and the premaxillary segment of the face (lack of forebrain induction). HPE is characterized by failure of cleavage of the embryonic prosencephalon, which is normally complete by embryonic day 35. With this failure of cleavage comes partial to complete failure of separation of the telencephalon and diencephalon into the right and left cerebral hemispheres and basal ganglia or thalami. Because the optic vesicles and olfactory bulbs evaginate from the prosencephalon, visual disturbances and incomplete formation of the olfactory system are frequently present. Hypoplasia of the premaxillary segment results in facial anomalies, including cleft lip and palate; abnormalities of the orbit such as cyclopia and hypotelorism; and forehead proboscis.

Classification

HPE may be divided into subtypes: alobar (the most severe form), semilobar, lobar (the mildest form of the major subtypes), and middle interhemispheric variant. There is no clear distinction between subtypes; rather, they are on a continuum. In alobar HPE, the falx, interhemispheric fissure, and septum pellucidum are absent. There is failure of separation of the cerebrum and the ventricular system, resulting in a monoventricle contiguous with a dorsal cyst. In semilobar HPE, the interhemispheric fissure and falx cerebri are usually formed posteriorly and are absent anteriorly. In lobar HPE, the interhemispheric fissure and falx anteriorly are hypoplastic (Figures 180-2 and 180-3). Often the posterior corpus callosum or splenium is formed, as in this case (*arrow* in Figure 180-1). The third ventricle is usually well formed. In the semilobar and lobar forms of HPE, the ventricular system shows variable degrees of development. The middle interhemispheric variant differs from classic HPE in that the posterior frontal and parietal lobes are most significantly affected rather than the basal forebrain. The anterior frontal lobes and occipital lobes are separated, and the genu and splenium of the corpus callosum are formed, but the callosal body is absent. The hypothalamus and lentiform nuclei appear separated, but the caudate nuclei and thalami are incompletely separated in many cases.

Associations

Heterotopias and cortical dysplasia are common associated anomalies of HPE, as seen in this case, in the left more than right medial frontal lobes.

Reference

Simon EM, Hevner RF, Pinter JD, et al. The middle interhemispheric variant of holoprosencephaly. *AJNR Am J Neuroradiol.* 2002; 23:151-155.

Cross-Reference

Neuroradiology: THE REQUISITES, 4th ed, pp 265-267.

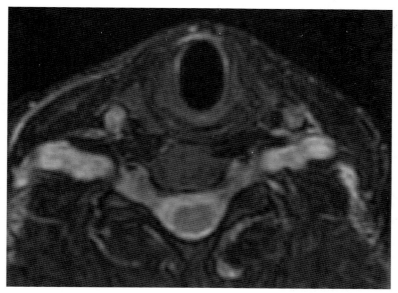

Figure 181-1

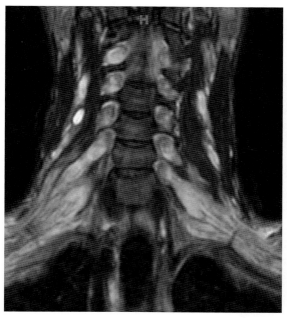

Figure 181-2

HISTORY: A young adult has bilateral neck swelling and discomfort.

1. This patient also has an optic pathway glioma. What is the most likely diagnosis?
   A. Neurofibromatosis type 1
   B. Chronic inflammatory demyelinating polyneuropathy (CIDP)
   C. Dejerine-Sottas disease
   D. Charcot-Marie-Tooth disease

2. Which of the following is a feature of neurofibromatosis type 1?
   A. Vestibular schwannoma
   B. Sphenoid wing dysplasia
   C. Meningiomas
   D. Ependymomas

3. How are Dejerine-Sottas and Charcot-Marie-Tooth diseases classified?
   A. Demyelinating disorders
   B. Hereditary motor and sensory neuropathies
   C. Glycogen storage diseases
   D. Mitochondrial disorders

4. Which of the following groups correctly lists the parts of the brachial plexus from central to peripheral?
   A. Roots, trunks, cords, divisions, branches
   B. Roots, divisions, trunks, cords, branches
   C. Roots, trunks, branches, cords, divisions
   D. Roots, trunks, divisions, cords, branches

CASE 181

Neurofibromatosis Type 1

1. **A.** Neurofibromatosis type 1 (NF1). NF1, CIDP, Dejerine-Sottas disease, and Charcot-Marie-Tooth disease can all account for the bilateral enlargement of the cervical nerves, but when a patient also has an optic pathway glioma, the diagnosis is NF1.

2. **B.** Sphenoid wing dysplasia. Sphenoid wing dysplasia is a characteristic of NF1, not NF2, as are optic pathway gliomas and plexiform neurofibromas. Vestibular schwannoma and meningiomas are common tumors in patients with NF2 (vestibular schwannoma is most common). Ependymomas may occur in the spinal cords of patients with NF2, whereas astrocytomas of the spinal cord are more common in NF1.

3. **B.** Hereditary motor and sensory neuropathies (HMSNs). Dejerine-Sottas and Charcot-Marie-Tooth diseases are HMSNs, types III and I, respectively. HMSN types II, V, and VI are also variants of Charcot-Marie-Tooth disease, and HMSN type IV is also called *Refsum disease*.

4. **D.** Roots, trunks, divisions, cords, branches. From central to peripheral, the parts of the brachial plexus are as follows: roots, trunks, divisions, cords, branches. One mnemonic for remembering this order is "Radiology Techs Drink Cold Beverages."

Comment

Features of Neurofibromatosis

In the brachial plexus, neurofibromas are more common than schwannomas. Plexiform neurofibromas are more common in patients with NF1 and increase the potential for malignant tumors of the peripheral nerve sheath. Causes of symmetric bilateral nerve enlargement besides neurofibromatosis include CIDP, HMSN syndromes, multifocal motor neuropathy syndromes, amyloidosis, and lymphomatous infiltration (Figures 181-1 and 181-2).

Relevant Anatomy

The brachial plexus includes the roots of the cervical spinal segments C5 to T1. From the roots, the neuronal structures evolve into the trunks, divisions, cords, and branches. The brachial plexus passes between the anterior and middle scalene muscles and is intimately associated with the subclavian and axillary arteries.

Reference

Reilly MM. Classification and diagnosis of the inherited neuropathies. *Ann Indian Acad Neurol.* 2009;12(2):80-88.

Cross-Reference

Neuroradiology: THE REQUISITES, 4th ed, pp 291-293.

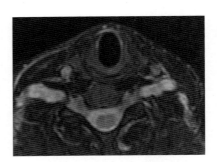

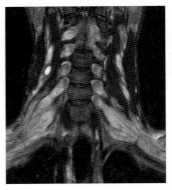

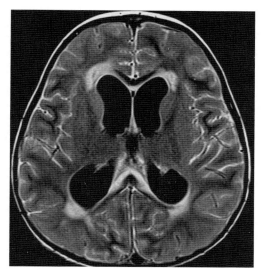

Figure 182-1

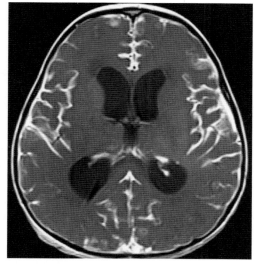

Figure 182-2

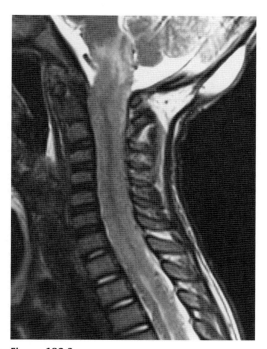

Figure 182-3

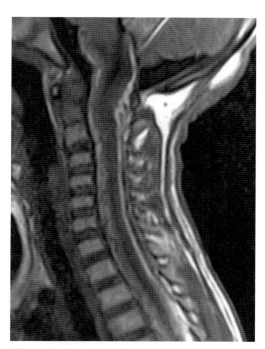

Figure 182-4

HISTORY: A 3-year-old with altered mental status and multiple odd birthmarks, according to her mother.

1. What is the best diagnosis?
   A. Infectious meningitis
   B. Neurocutaneous melanosis
   C. Intracranial hypotension
   D. Nonaccidental trauma with subarachnoid hemorrhage

2. Regarding inversion recovery techniques, which statement is correct?
   A. The time to inversion (TI) in fluid-attenuated inversion recovery (FLAIR) is shorter than it is in short-tau inversion recovery (STIR).
   B. At 1.5 tesla (T), the TI to null cerebrospinal fluid is at approximately 2000 to 2500 msec.
   C. At 1.5 T, the TI to null fat is at approximately 800 to 900 msec.
   D. FLAIR is only applied to T2-weighted images.

3. How does gadolinium result in increased signal intensity on a T1-weighted image?
   A. Gadolinium is directly visualized as iodinated contrast is in computed tomography (CT).
   B. Gadolinium is ferromagnetic, altering local magnetic fields.
   C. Unpaired electrons in the element result in paramagnetic effects.
   D. Gadolinium results in local susceptibility, prolonging T1 relaxation.

4. What is included in the diagnostic criteria for primary leptomeningeal melanosis?
   A. Focal dural based masses are present.
   B. Elevated protein in cerebrospinal fluid is identified.
   C. There is invasion of adjacent brain or spinal cord.
   D. There is absence of cutaneous or ocular melanoma.

CASE 182

Neurocutaneous Melanosis

1. **B.** Neurocutaneous melanosis. There is diffuse leptomeningeal thickening and enhancement and nonsuppression on T2-weighted FLAIR imaging. This appears to coat the brainstem and the spinal cord. The odd birthmarks, mentioned in the history obtained from the patient's mother, are likely cutaneous nevi and point toward a diagnosis of neurocutaneous melanosis.

2. **B.** At 1.5 T, the TI to null cerebrospinal fluid is at approximately 2000 to 2500 msec. This is the inversion time used in FLAIR imaging. The TI in FLAIR is longer than the TI in STIR imaging. In STIR, the inversion time at 1.5 T is typically 175 msec to null fat. FLAIR can be used with T1-weighted images.

3. **C.** Unpaired electrons in the element result in paramagnetic effects. This results in T1 relaxation time shortening and therefore increased T1 signal. Gadolinium is not directly visualized. It alters the local magnetic field. It is not ferromagnetic.

4. **D.** There is absence of cutaneous or ocular melanoma. The diagnostic criteria are demonstration of proliferation of melanocytes in the meninges, absence of cutaneous or ocular melanoma, and absence of metastasis.

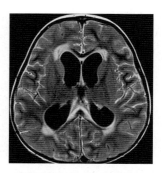

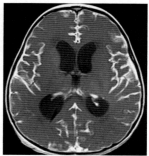

Comment

Background

Leptomeningeal melanosis refers to an increase in the number of melanocytes in the leptomeninges. Melanoblasts (precursors to melanocytes) are derived from the neural crest. Proliferation of melanocytes along the leptomeninges may be seen in various forms, including primary leptomeningeal melanosis, primary leptomeningeal melanoma, and metastatic melanoma. Metastatic melanoma is the most common cause of such proliferation.

Neurocutaneous Melanosis

Leptomeningeal melanosis associated with cutaneous nevi is referred to as neurocutaneous melanosis and is classified as a phakomatosis. These patients typically have multiple congenital hyperpigmented or giant hairy pigmented cutaneous nevi as this patient did. Malignant transformation of meningeal melanosis may occur in 50% of patients and often manifests with seizures when the intracranial compartment is involved because of invasion. Leptomeningeal melanosis responds poorly to radiation and chemotherapy. Reported cases suggest that intrathecal recombinant interleukin-2 may provide a more promising response.

Primary Leptomeningeal Melanosis

The diagnosis of primary leptomeningeal melanosis can be made when the following criteria are met: (1) There is a proliferation of melanocytes within the meninges or melanocytosis (high melanocyte count in the cerebrospinal fluid); (2) there is no cutaneous or ocular melanoma; and (3) an extensive work-up (including a bone scan and CT of the chest, abdomen, and pelvis) shows no metastatic lesions. Primary central nervous system melanocytic proliferation carries a poor prognosis. Patients may present with signs of increased intracranial pressure, seizures, and cranial neuropathies. Leptomeningeal melanosis may be benign or malignant. When malignant, there is characteristically invasion of the adjacent brain or the spinal cord.

Because melanocytosis in the cerebrospinal fluid may be associated with a high protein content, non–contrast-enhanced CT may show a hyperdense exudate in the subarachnoid spaces that may be mistaken for acute hemorrhage. On magnetic resonance imaging, T2-FLAIR (Figure 182-1) shows hyperintensity along the leptomeninges and within the subarachnoid spaces. There is diffuse enhancement throughout the same areas on postcontrast T1-weighted images (Figure 182-2). Note hydrocephalus secondary to impaired cerebrospinal fluid resorption (see Figures 182-1 and 182-2). Involved leptomeninges may show regions of T2-weighted hypointensity (Figure 182-3) because of the paramagnetic effects of melanin. Hyperintense signal is present in the leptomeninges of the posterior fossa and spine on precontrast T1-weighted images (Figure 182-4).

References

Byrd SE, Reyes-Mugica M, Darling CF, Chou P, Tomita T. MR of leptomeningeal melanosis in children. *Eur J Radiol*. 1995;20:93-99.

Di Rocco F, Sabatino G, Koutzoglou M, et al. Neurocutaneous melanosis. *Childs Nerv Syst*. 2004;20(1):23-28.

Hayashi M, Maeda M, Majji T, et al. Diffuse leptomeningeal hyperintensity on fluid attenuated inversion recovery MR images in neurocutaneous melanosis. *AJNR Am J Neuroradiol*. 2004;25:138-141.

Cross-Reference

Neuroradiology: THE REQUISITES, 4th ed, p 298.

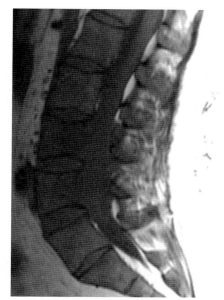

Figure 183-1

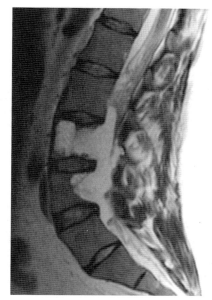

Figure 183-2

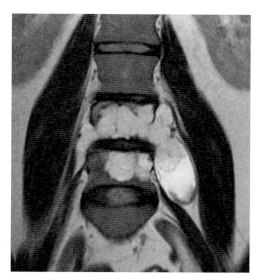

Figure 183-3

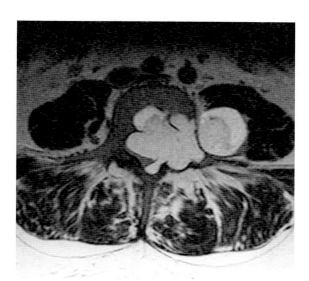

Figure 183-4

HISTORY: A 28-year-old woman presents with back pain and lower extremity pain.

1. What is the most likely diagnosis of those listed?
   A. Nerve sheath tumor
   B. Hemangioma
   C. Chordoma
   D. Discitis osteomyelitis

2. What percentage of these lesions originate in the lumbar vertebrae?
   A. 1% to 10%
   B. 11% to 20%
   C. 21% to 30%
   D. Greater than 50%

3. What finding on magnetic resonance imaging suggests the diagnosis?
   A. Hypointense signal on T1-weighted images
   B. Hyperintense signal with multiple hypointense septa on T2-weighted images
   C. Sparing of the disc spaces
   D. Heterogeneous signal on T2-weighted images

4. Which of the following statements regarding chordoma is true?
   A. Lumbar chordomas are often diagnosed early because of symptoms arising from compression of the anterior column and roots.
   B. The most common presenting symptom of lumbar chordomas is paraplegia.
   C. The most likely cause of death in cases of lumbar chordoma is distant metastasis.
   D. Forty percent of chordomas develop late metastasis after treatment.

CASE 183

Chordoma of the Lumbar Spine

1. **C.** Chordoma. The imaging findings of hyperintense cystic and mucinous features on T2-weighted images are typical of chordomas. The mass does not follow the course of the spinal nerves on axial images, and the sagittal image shows evidence of L3 and L4 vertebral body involvement. Hemangiomas usually do not extend beyond the cortex and are usually not as hyperintense on T2-weighted imaging. Discitis osteomyelitis is less likely because the disc spaces and endplates are relatively spared.

2. **A.** 1% to 10%. The lumbar spine is an uncommon location for chordomas, accounting for only 6% of spinal chordomas. Approximately 15% of chordomas occur in the vertebral column, mostly in the cervical region. The remainder occur in either the sacrum (≈50%) or the clivus (≈35%).

3. **B.** Hyperintense signal with multiple hypointense septa on T2-weighted images. The pattern of hyperintense lobules separated by hypointense septations is shown on the axial image. Most tumors are hypointense on T1-weighted images. Tumors tend to spare the disc space. Chordoma is typically inhomogeneous on both T1- and T2-weighted images; however, this finding is nonspecific and may be seen in other tumors.

4. **D.** Forty percent of chordomas develop late metastasis after treatment. Because symptoms are often confused with discogenic or nonspecific pathology, diagnosis is often delayed. The most frequent symptoms are pain and paresthesia. Paraplegia is rare. Local aggressiveness rather than metastases is more likely to cause death and disability.

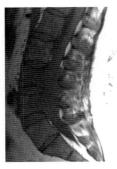

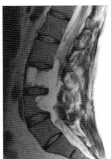

Comment

Background

Chordomas are rare, slow-growing, locally invasive malignant tumors. The age range is 27 to 80 years with a mean age at diagnosis of 56. Symptoms most commonly arise from compression of the anterior column and roots. The most frequent complaint in patients with lumbar chordomas is pain and paresthesia. Symptoms often appear to be a result of discogenic or nonspecific pathology, resulting in delayed diagnosis.

Histopathology

Chordomas are thought to arise from notochord remnants (mesodermal precursor of the vertebral column). They appear as lobules of cells arranged in long strands, or "cords," with a mucinous background separated by fibrous bands.

Imaging

Chordomas appear hypointense or isointense on T1-weighted images (Figure 183-1). Lesions demonstrating high signal intensity on T1-weighted images have been reported. Signal intensity is usually inhomogeneous because a combination of cystic and solid components frequently exists. On T2-weighted images (Figures 183-2 through 183-4), inhomogeneous signal intensity is also observed, with some regions of the tumor equaling or exceeding the intensity of cerebrospinal fluid. Septa of low signal intensity radiating throughout the predominantly high signal intensity mass on T2-weighted images (see Figure 183-4) may help in differentiating chordomas from more common paraspinal or spinal masses.

Management

Chordomas are well known for their high local recurrence rates, and distant metastases following treatment are reported in greater than 40% of patients. Complete surgical en bloc resection with wide, histologically proven tumor-free margins is the treatment of choice for patients with chordomas.

Reference

Sivabalan P, Li J, Mobbs RJ. Extensive lumbar chordoma and unique reconstructive approach. *Eur Spine J.* 2011;20(suppl 2): S336-S342.

Cross-Reference

Neuroradiology: THE REQUISITES, 4th ed, p 583.

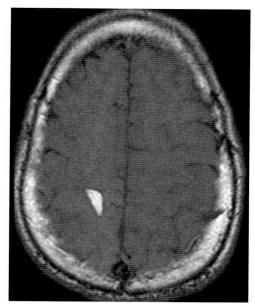

Figure 184-1

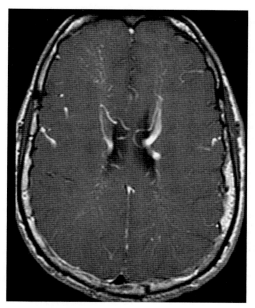

Figure 184-2

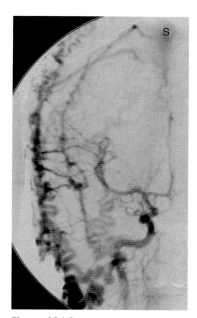

Figure 184-3

HISTORY: A patient presents with headache.

1. What is the single best diagnosis considering the image findings presented in this case?
   A. Amyloid angiopathy
   B. Cavernoma and developmental venous anomalies
   C. Dural arteriovenous fistula
   D. Cerebral arteriovenous malformation

2. What is the most widely accepted proposed mechanism for development of this lesion?
   A. Trauma
   B. Venous thrombosis
   C. Surgery
   D. Venous hypertension

3. What is the best predictor of intracranial hemorrhage in patients with these lesions?
   A. Drainage to the cavernous sinus
   B. Retrograde flow in the dural venous sinuses
   C. Multiple channels or holes at the fistula
   D. Cortical venous drainage

4. What is the whole body annual dose limit to radiation workers?
   A. 5 millisievert (mSv)
   B. 20 mSv
   C. 50 mSv
   D. 150 mSv

CASE 184

Dural Arteriovenous Fistula

1. **C.** Dural arteriovenous fistula (DAVF). In Figure 184-1 (T1-weighted image), there is a focal hematoma in the right frontal/parietal region. In Figure 184-2 (contrast-enhanced T1-weighted image), there are dilated cortical and periventricular veins. In Figure 184-3, the right common carotid artery injection demonstrates enlarged external carotid artery branches feeding the superior sagittal sinus that fills during the arterial phase, consistent with DAVF.

2. **B.** Venous thrombosis. Dural venous thrombosis is the common mechanism in theories regarding the mechanism of DAVF formation. Trauma has been implicated, and post-surgical fistulas are found. Venous hypertension is likely a result of thrombosis or fistula formation rather than the cause of it.

3. **D.** Cortical venous drainage. In both Cognard and Borden classification systems, the presence of cortical venous drainage is the greatest risk factor for intracranial hemorrhage.

4. **C.** 50 mSv. The occupational dose limits for radiation workers in SI (International System) units is 50/150/500 mSv for the whole body/lens of eye/extremities.

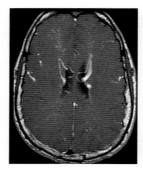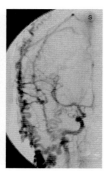

Comment

Background

Intracranial DAVFs account for approximately 10% to 15% of all intracranial vascular malformations. More than half occur in the posterior fossa, and they may be categorized based on the dural venous sinus involved by the vascular abnormality. These vascular malformations most commonly involve the sigmoid or transverse sinuses, accounting for 70% of all of these lesions. DAVFs are distinguished from parenchymal or pial arteriovenous malformations (AVMs) by the absence of a parenchymal nidus and presence of dural arterial feeders.

Clinical

Most dural vascular malformations manifest clinically in older adults. They are believed to be acquired lesions that typically arise as a consequence of dural venous sinus thrombosis. A collateral network of vessels develops, including enlargement of normally present microscopic arteriovenous shunts within the dura (Figure 184-3). In addition, as arteriovenous shunting increases, venous hypertension develops. In certain DAVFs, venous hypertension may result in retrograde filling of leptomeningeal or cortical veins that communicate with the involved sinus, as in this case (Figure 184-2). Pulsatile tinnitus is a common symptom. Lesions involving the cavernous sinus may result in ophthalmoplegia, chemosis, and proptosis. Severe cases can be associated with impaired cognition, dementia, seizures, and other neurologic symptoms. In such cases, rupture of the enlarged venous collaterals may occur. Approximately 10% to 15% of DAVMs are associated with intracranial hemorrhage (Figure 184-1), which is usually intraparenchymal or subarachnoid. Hemorrhage is associated with lesions in which there is development of dilated leptomeningeal veins. DAVFs that drain strictly to the dural venous sinuses are not usually associated with hemorrhage.

Imaging

DAVFs are difficult to diagnose on traditional computed tomography (CT) and magnetic resonance (MR) imaging. Imaging findings may include venous thrombosis, dilated cortical veins, or intracranial hemorrhage (see Figure 184-1). Imaging findings may be normal, however, and a high index of suspicion is required. Time-resolved four-dimensional CT angiography performed on 320-slice scanners and time-resolved MR angiography techniques have increased sensitivity and specificity of cross-sectional imaging techniques for the identification and characterization of fistulas. Digital subtraction angiography remains the mainstay for diagnosis. Flat detector CT is an adjunct to angiography.

Classification

The two accepted classification systems in the literature were proposed by Borden and colleagues (1995) and Cognard and coworkers (1995). These systems account for characteristics of the lesions and allow for prognostication. In both systems, the presence of cortical venous drainage (CVD) is associated with increased risk of intracranial hemorrhage and nonhemorrhagic deficits. The Borden system characterizes lesions based on the drainage site, presence of CVD, and whether the lesions have one hole or multiple holes. Cognard classification relies on more details, incorporating drainage location, flow direction in the sinus, and presence of CVD.

Treatment

Endovascular approaches have become the mainstay of treatment with transarterial, transvenous, and combined techniques dependent on fistula and other patient factors. Surgery has become a second-line treatment for those cases in which endovascular treatment fails or is not possible to perform. Stereotactic radiosurgery may have a role in treatment as well.

References

Borden JA, Wu JK, Shucart WA. A proposed classification for spinal and cranial dural arteriovenous fistulous malformations and implications for treatment. *J Neurosurg.* 1995;82:166-179.

Cognard C, Gobin YP, Pierot L, et al. Cerebral dural arteriovenous fistulas: clinical and angiographic correlation with a revised classification of venous drainage. *Radiology.* 1995;194:671-680.

Gandhi D, Chen J, Pearl M, et al. Intracranial dural arteriovenous fistulas: classification, imaging findings, and treatment. *AJNR Am J Neuroradiol.* 2012;33(6):1007-1013.

Cross-Reference

Neuroradiology: THE REQUISITES, 4th ed, pp 147-149.

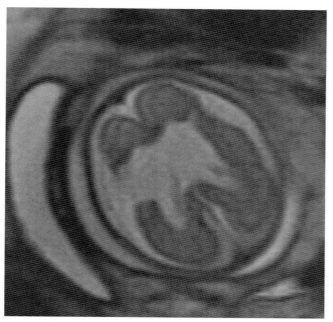

Figure 185-1

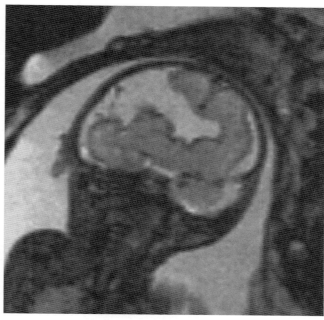

Figure 185-2

HISTORY: A patient presents with seizures.

1. What is the best diagnosis given the imaging findings?
   A. Hydrocephalus
   B. Schizencephaly
   C. Porencephaly
   D. Semilobar holoprosencephaly

2. What frequency is septo-optic dysplasia associated with this entity?
   A. 0% to 24%
   B. 25% to 50%
   C. 51% to 74%
   D. 75% to 100%

3. What is the greatest technical limitation for fetal magnetic resonance imaging (MRI)?
   A. Inability to use contrast agents
   B. Maternal discomfort and size
   C. Fetal motion
   D. Fetal size

4. What can be done to reduce the specific absorption rate (SAR) in MRI?
   A. Increase the field strength of the magnet
   B. Use multiple echo pulse sequences
   C. Increase flip angles
   D. Increase repetition times

CASE 185

Schizencephaly

1. **B.** Schizencephaly. There is a cleft in the brain parenchyma extending from the ventricle to the extra-axial space which appears to be lined by gray matter compatible with an open lip schizencephaly.

2. **B.** 25% to 50%. Septo-optic dysplasia is present in 25% to 50% of patients with schizencephaly.

3. **C.** Fetal motion. There are techniques utilized in fetal MRI that allow for rapid acquisition of images, although this remains the greatest technical limitation.

4. **D.** Increase repetition times. Lower field strength magnets produce less SAR; techniques using multiple echos and increased flip angles increase the SAR. Increasing the repetition rate and using lower flip angles can reduce SAR, although this results in potential loss of image contrast.

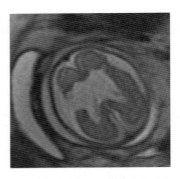

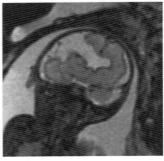

Comment

Fetal MRI

Fetal MRI is an increasingly available technique used to evaluate the fetal neural axis. Ultrafast T2-weighted sequences, parallel imaging, and new coil designs have allowed fetal MRI to be used to evaluate processes that cannot be evaluated by other imaging techniques. Fetal MRI allows assessment of in vivo brain development and early diagnosis of congenital abnormalities potentially inadequately evaluated by prenatal sonography. It has been especially useful in the evaluation of sonographically diagnosed ventriculomegaly, suspected abnormalities of the corpus callosum, and posterior fossa lesions.

Schizencephaly

Schizencephaly is a migrational abnormality that results from an injury to the germinal matrix and causes failure of normal migration and neuronal differentiation. This anomaly is thought to be the result of an in utero watershed ischemic event leading to damage not only to the germinal matrix but also to the radial glial fibers along which the neurons normally migrate from the germinal region to their final destination in the cortex. Recent research reveals a potential association with the *COL4A1* gene.

Imaging

Schizencephaly extends from the ventricular surface to the subarachnoid surface of the brain and is lined by dysplastic gray matter (Figures 185-1 and 185-2). Usually, there is a cerebrospinal fluid (CSF) cleft between the layers of gray matter. When the CSF cleft is large and gaping, it is referred to as "open-lip" schizencephaly. When the layers of gray matter are in apposition or when there is only a thin layer of CSF between them, the condition is referred to as "closed-lip" schizencephaly. MRI is the imaging modality of choice to assess these abnormalities. Closed-lip schizencephaly, when the gray matter layers are apposed, may be difficult to detect. A small ventricular "dimple" or diverticulum may be a clue to the diagnosis and should prompt a close search for closed-lip schizencephaly. Other conditions that may cause dimpling of the ventricle are previous injuries, such as periventricular ischemia or infection.

Associations

Septo-optic dysplasia is present in 25% to 50% of patients with schizencephaly. Patients with migrational anomalies usually present with a seizure disorder. Depending on the size of the migrational abnormality, there may also be focal neurologic deficits, such as hemiparesis.

References

Ceccherini AF, Twining P, Varied S. Schizencephaly: antenatal detection using ultrasound. *Clin Radiol*. 1999;54:620-622.

Glenn OA, Barkovich J. Magnetic resonance imaging of the fetal brain and spine: an increasingly important tool in prenatal diagnosis: part 2. *AJNR Am J Neuroradiol*. 2006;27:1807-1814.

Yoneda Y, Haginoya K, Kato M, et al. Phenotypic spectrum of COL4A1 mutations: porencephaly to schizencephaly. *Ann Neurol*. 2013;73: 48-57.

Cross-Reference

Neuroradiology: THE REQUISITES, 4th ed, pp 278-280.

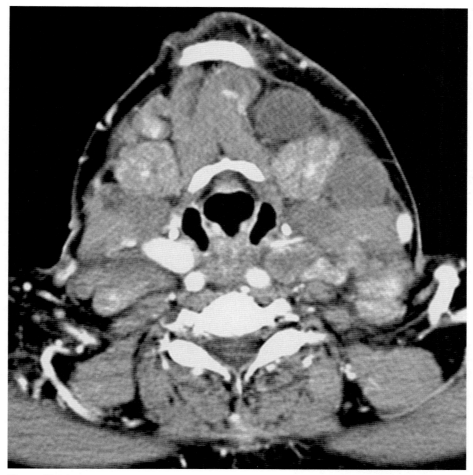

Figure 186-1

HISTORY: A middle-aged adult presents with multiple neck masses.

1. For bilateral nonnecrotic massive lymphadenopathy, which of the following is the most likely diagnosis?
   A. Human immunodeficiency virus (HIV) disease
   B. Squamous cell carcinoma
   C. Mycobacterial infection
   D. Sinus histiocytosis

2. Which of the following is true of Rosai-Dorfman disease?
   A. It is more common in adults than in children.
   B. It is characterized by massive lymphadenopathy.
   C. It is rarely accompanied by extranodal disease.
   D. It is related to Epstein-Barr virus exposure.

3. The incidence of posttransplantation lymphoproliferative disease (PTLD) is highest after which tissue transplant?
   A. Bone marrow
   B. Liver
   C. Lung
   D. Kidney

4. What is the most common site of extranodal Rosai-Dorfman disease in the head and neck?
   A. Brain
   B. Sinonasal cavity
   C. Masticator space
   D. Orbit

CASE 186

Rosai-Dorfman

1. **D.** Sinus histiocytosis. Bilateral nonnecrotic massive lymphadenopathy is common in lymphoma and sinus histiocytosis. Necrosis is a feature of squamous cell carcinoma and tuberculous adenitis. HIV nodes are usually not massive.

2. **B.** It is characterized by massive lymphadenopathy. Rosai-Dorfman disease is characterized by massive lymphadenopathy and is more common in children and adolescents than in adults. More than 40% of affected patients have extranodal manifestations.

3. **C.** Lung. PTLD has the highest incidence among lung transplant recipients. PTLD after renal transplantation is not as common. The incidence of PTLD after liver transplantation is quoted as 2%.

4. **B.** Sinonasal cavity. The most common site of extranodal Rosai-Dorfman disease in the head and neck is the sinonasal cavity. The salivary glands are the second most common site. The masticator space and orbit are not as commonly affected.

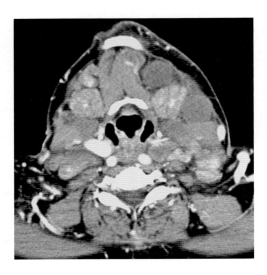

Comment

Differential Diagnosis

Rosai-Dorfman disease is also called *sinus histiocytosis with massive lymphadenopathy.* It is a disease of childhood (80% of affected patients are younger than 20 years, and 67% are younger than 10 years) and causes bilateral massive cervical lymphadenopathy (Figure 186-1). Therefore, it is included in the differential diagnosis with mononucleosis, cat scratch disease, lymphoma, and mastocytosis, which also affect younger patients. Affected patients may have fever, elevated erythrocyte sedimentation rates, and polyclonal hypergammaglobulinemia.

Imaging Findings

Imaging features are that of large, nonnecrotic lymphadenopathy. The nodes are usually hot on gallium scanning and positron emission tomography (PET). Extranodal deposits occur in approximately half of affected patients and may be in the skin, the sinonasal cavity, the salivary glands, the orbits, and the bones. Hypointensity of sinonasal sinus histiocytosis on T2-weighted scans implies a differential diagnosis of lymphoma, sarcoidosis, fungal disease, pseudotumor, and granulomatous infections. The most common manifestation in the orbit is an extraconal mass that causes proptosis.

Relevant Anatomy

Intracranially, Rosai-Dorfman disease may infiltrate the dura of the sella, cavernous sinus, periclival regions, and foramen magnum. The dura around venous sinuses may also be affected.

Treatment of Rosai-Dorfman Disease

Treatment is watchful waiting at first. The disease is often self-limited. However, interferon, steroids, chemotherapy, radiation therapy, or a combination of these may be administered to patients with advanced disease. Surgery is confined to cases of progressive, obstructive disease.

Reference

La Barge DV 3rd, Salzman KL, Harnsberger HR, et al. Sinus histiocytosis with massive lymphadenopathy (Rosai-Dorfman disease): imaging manifestations in the head and neck. *AJR Am J Roentgenol.* 2008;191(6):W299-W306.

Cross-Reference

Neuroradiology: THE REQUISITES, 4th ed, p 448.

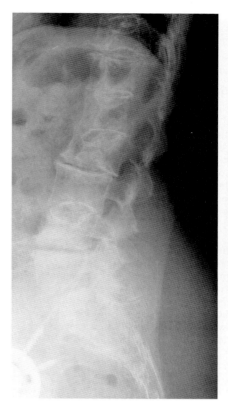

Figure 187-1

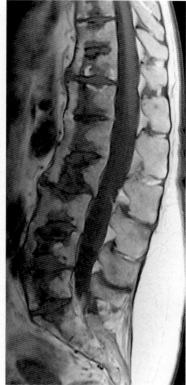

Figure 187-2

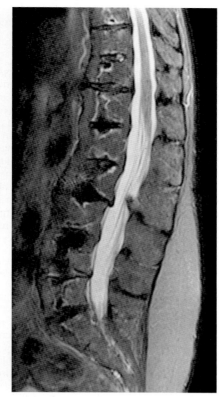

Figure 187-3

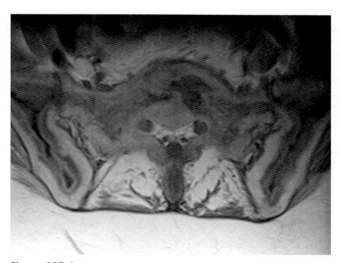

Figure 187-4

HISTORY: A 56-year-old man presents with back pain.

1. Which of the following is the most likely diagnosis?
   A. Metastasis
   B. Multiple myeloma
   C. Lymphoma
   D. Gaucher disease

2. H-shaped vertebrae are classically seen in which of the following conditions?
   A. Hurler syndrome
   B. Scheuermann disease
   C. Renal osteodystrophy
   D. Sickle cell disease

3. All of the following are skeletal manifestations of Gaucher disease *except:*
   A. Osteopoikilosis
   B. Osteonecrosis
   C. Osteosclerosis
   D. Osteopenia

4. Which of the following magnetic resonance imaging (MRI) marrow signal changes are seen in Gaucher disease?
   A. Hyperintense T1 and T2 signal
   B. Hypointense T1 and T2 signal
   C. Hyperintense T1 and hypointense T2 signal
   D. Hypointense T1 and hyperintense T2 signal

CASE 187

Gaucher Disease

1. **D.** Gaucher disease. The findings of osteopenia and osteonecrosis with development of vertebral body compression sparing the anterior and posterior margins are skeletal manifestations of Gaucher disease. The differential diagnosis would include sickle cell disease, in which central endplate depressions with sparing of the anterior and posterior margins of the endplate are typical findings. There are no discrete vertebral body lesions and no epidural or paravertebral soft tissue abnormalities to suggest metastatic disease. The marrow abnormality in this case involves the central aspect of the vertebral body. Involvement of the spine by multiple myeloma is typically focal or diffuse with heterogeneous marrow signal. Although bone marrow necrosis can be seen in lymphoma before and after chemotherapy, H-shaped vertebrae are not typically seen.

2. **D.** Sickle cell disease. H-shaped vertebrae are a characteristic finding classically seen in approximately 10% of patients with sickle cell anemia and are secondary to infarction causing growth retardation of the central aspect of the vertebral body. Hurler syndrome results in bullet-shaped vertebrae, not H-shaped vertebrae. Scheuermann disease is associated with multilevel vertebral body Schmorl nodes and wedge-shaped vertebral body deformities resulting in kyphosis. Renal osteodystrophy can result in sclerosis of the vertebral body endplates known as rugger jersey spine.

3. **A.** Osteopoikilosis. Osteopoikilosis is a benign, autosomal dominant, sclerosing dysplasia of bone characterized by the presence of numerous bone islands in the skeleton. Skeletal complications of Gaucher disease include osteonecrosis. Osteonecrosis is bone death, believed to be secondary to ischemia from chronic infarction caused by Gaucher cells. Osteosclerosis can occur as aberrant remodeling after bone infarction with deposition of calcium into the bone. Generalized osteopenia is believed to result from abnormally high rates of bone resorption and reduced rates of bone formation.

4. **B.** Hypointense T1 and T2 signal. MRI typically shows reduced T1 and T2 signal secondary to bone marrow infiltration and features of osteonecrosis.

Comment

Background

Gaucher disease is the most prevalent inherited, lysosomal storage disease and occurs most commonly in Ashkenazi Jews.

Pathophysiology

Gaucher disease is a rare autosomal recessive lysosomal storage disorder caused by β-glucocerebrosidase deficiency, which leads to accumulation of the lipid glucocerebroside in the reticuloendothelial system. The symptoms and pathology of Gaucher disease result from the accumulation of Gaucher cells in various organ systems. Musculoskeletal complications include osteopenia, abnormal bone remodeling, delayed bone healing, pathologic fracture, increased propensity for infection, and bleeding from involvement of the bone marrow.

Imaging

Radiologic findings include Erlenmeyer flask deformity, osteopenia, osteosclerosis, osteonecrosis, pathologic fractures, and bone marrow infiltration (Figure 187-1). H-shaped vertebrae may be seen in Gaucher disease and are secondary to infarction of the end vessels supplying the vertebral body, causing growth retardation of the central aspect of the vertebral body (Figure 187-2). MRI shows reduced T1 and T2 signal secondary to bone marrow infiltration and features of osteonecrosis (Figures 187-3 and 187-4).

Management

Depending on the status of the patient, the mainstay of treatment is enzyme replacement and substrate reduction.

References

Ozcan HN, Kara M, Kara O, et al. Severe skeletal involvement in a patient with Gaucher's disease. *J Orthop Sci.* 2009;14(4):465-468.
Wenstrup RJ, Roca-Espiau M, Weinreb NJ, et al. Skeletal aspects of Gaucher disease: a review. *Br J Radiol.* 2002;75(suppl 1):A2-A12.

Cross-Reference

Neuroradiology: THE REQUISITES, 4th ed, pp 258-259.

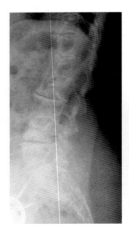

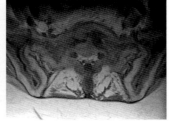

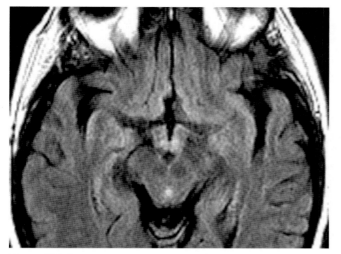

Figure 188-1

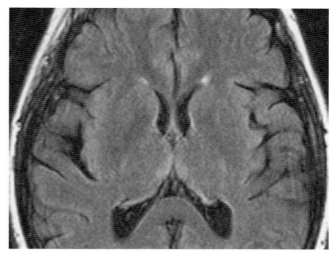

Figure 188-2

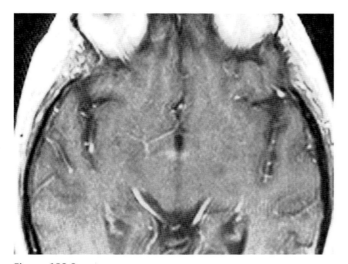

Figure 188-3

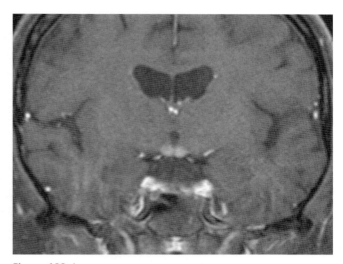

Figure 188-4

HISTORY: Confusion, nystagmus, and ataxia.

1. What is the best diagnosis?
   A. Friedreich ataxia
   B. Wernicke encephalopathy
   C. Deep venous ischemia
   D. Wilson disease

2. What causes this entity?
   A. Vitamin B_{12} deficiency
   B. Folate deficiency
   C. Vitamin C deficiency
   D. Vitamin B_1 deficiency

3. Which of the following conditions is associated with thiamine deficiency?
   A. Hyperemesis gravidarum
   B. Trauma
   C. Enzyme deficiency
   D. Mercury poisoning

4. What type of amnesia is seen in Korsakoff psychosis?
   A. Transient global
   B. Antegrade
   C. Retrograde
   D. Dissociative

CASE 188

Wernicke Encephalopathy

1. **B.** Wernicke encephalopathy. Signal alteration in the periaqueductal region, the mammillary bodies, and the paramedian thalami in a patient with ataxia and confusion are consistent with Wernicke encephalopathy and must be recognized because duration of illness before treatment is directly related to worsening long-term prognosis. Friedreich ataxia is an autosomal disorder associated with cerebellar atrophy and with cardiac anomalies, particularly affecting the conduction pathway. There is no abnormal signal in the thalami. Deep venous infarct may result in bilateral and symmetric basal ganglia and thalamic signal alteration but would tend to be more diffuse. Wilson disease, which often presents with parkinsonism and upper extremity weakness, results from abnormal copper metabolism.

2. **D.** Vitamin B_1 deficiency. Vitamin B_1 (thiamine) is depleted in patients with Wernicke encephalopathy. Vitamin B_{12} deficiency causes megaloblastic anemia and subacute combined degeneration of the spinal cord. Women with folate deficiency who become pregnant are more likely to give birth to low-birth-weight infants and infants with neural tube defects. A deficiency of vitamin C results in scurvy, characterized by soft gums, skin hemorrhages, capillary weakness, anemia, and slow wound healing.

3. **A.** Hyperemesis gravidarum. Thiamine deficiency has been associated with hyperemesis gravidarum, chronic alcoholism, bariatric surgery, prolonged infectious conditions, carcinoma, and anorexia nervosa.

4. **C.** Retrograde. Korsakoff psychosis is manifested by a retrograde amnesia, which is an inability to recall events that happened before the onset of the amnesia.

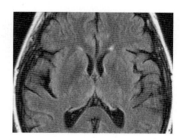

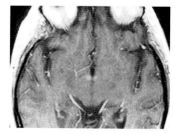

Comment

Background

Wernicke encephalopathy is a neurologic disorder of acute onset. Wernicke encephalopathy is related to thiamine deficiency and is found most commonly in the setting of chronic alcoholism; however, this vitamin deficiency may also be present in other conditions that result in chronic malnutrition, such as anorexia nervosa, prolonged infectious or febrile conditions, and hyperemesis gravidarum. Wernicke syndrome has also been reported in association with long-term parenteral therapy. Thiamine reserves are depleted in 4 to 6 weeks if dietary intake is absent.

Presentation

The classical presentation (16% to 38%) is ocular signs (nystagmus, oculomotor, and abducens palsy), altered consciousness, and ataxia. Tremors, confusion, and delusions are often observed. Korsakoff manifests with retrograde amnesia and difficulty acquiring new information. The two not uncommonly occur together.

Imaging

This case shows many of the radiologic findings seen in Wernicke encephalopathy. There is high T2-weighted and fluid-attenuated inversion recovery (FLAIR) signal intensity (Figure 188-1) and enhancement in the mammillary bodies (Figures 188-3 and 188-4) and high signal intensity in the medial thalami (Figure 188-2). Wernicke encephalopathy is typically associated with generalized cerebral cortical and cerebellar vermian atrophy. In addition, specific deep structures are involved and are best assessed with magnetic resonance imaging, which is more sensitive than computed tomography in evaluating the small structures involved in this entity. Abnormal T2-weighted and FLAIR hyperintensity is seen in the mammillary bodies (in essentially all patients) (see Figure 188-1) and may be seen in the hypothalamus, periaqueductal gray matter, and medial thalami (see Figure 188-2). Imaging findings are often bilaterally symmetric. In the acute setting, mild swelling may be associated with the signal alteration, and enhancement (Figures 188-3 and 188-4) has been reported. Resolution of the signal alterations after treatment with thiamine has been reported. In the late stages, atrophy (particularly of the mammillary bodies) may be the main finding.

References

Mascalchi M, Belli G, Guerrini L, Nistri M, Del Seppia I, Villari N. Proton MR spectroscopy of Wernicke encephalopathy. *AJNR Am J Neuroradiol*. 2002;23:1803-1806.

Weidauer S, Nichtweiss M, Lanfermann H, Zanella FE. Wernicke encephalopathy: MR findings and clinical presentation. *Eur Radiol*. 2003;13:1001-1009.

Zuccoli G, Pipitone N. Neuroimaging findings in acute Wernicke's encephalopathy: review of the literature. *AJR Am J Roentgenol*. 2009;192:501-508.

Cross-Reference

Neuroradiology: THE REQUISITES, 4th ed, p 223.

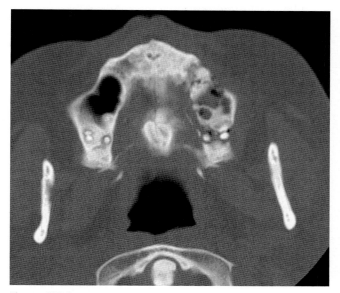

Figure 189-1

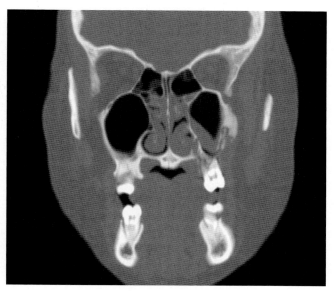

Figure 189-2

HISTORY: A female patient being treated for metastatic breast cancer experiences jaw pain.

1. Which of the following is a known risk factor for osteonecrosis related to bisphosphonate therapy?
   A. Male sex
   B. Age older than 60
   C. Intact dentition
   D. Oral administration of the medication

2. What is the mechanism of action of simple bisphosphonates?
   A. Induction of osteoclast apoptosis
   B. Osteoblast proliferation and differentiation
   C. Increased calcium absorption in the gut
   D. Inhibition of parathyroid glands

3. What is the incidence of jaw necrosis in patients with bone metastases who are being treated with bisphosphonates?
   A. Less than 25%
   B. 26% to 50%
   C. 51% to 75%
   D. Greater than 75%

4. What is the approximate ratio of involvement of the mandible versus the maxilla in bisphosphonate-induced osteonecrosis?
   A. 10 : 1 in favor of the mandible
   B. 10 : 1 in favor of the maxilla
   C. 3 : 1 in favor of the maxilla
   D. 3 : 1 in favor of the mandible

CASE 189

Bisphosphonate Osteonecrosis

1. **B.** Age older than 60. The risk factors for development of osteonecrosis include female sex, recent dental extractions, intravenous administration of bisphosphonates, high dose of bisphosphonates, and age older than 60 years.

2. **A.** Induction of osteoclast apoptosis. Bisphosphonates are metabolized by osteoclasts to metabolites that exchange with the terminal pyrophosphate moiety of adenosine triphosphate (ATP), resulting in an ATP that is nonfunctional and ultimately in apoptosis.

3. **A.** Less than 25%. Jaw necrosis occurs in less than 25% of patients with bone metastases who are being treated with bisphosphonates.

4. **D.** 3:1 in favor of the mandible. The approximate ratio of involvement in bisphosphonate-induced osteonecrosis is 3:1 in favor of the mandible over the maxilla.

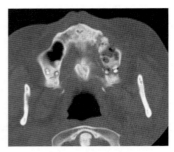

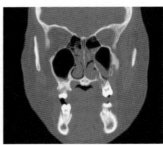

Comment

Complications of Bisphosphonate Therapy

Osteonecrosis of the maxilla is one potential complication of the use of bisphosphonates to treat the bone metastases of breast cancer, lung cancer, prostate cancer, and myeloma. These agents are also used to treat hypercalcemia, Paget disease, and generalized osteoporosis. The onset of osteonecrosis occurs sooner (2 to 3 years) after use for cancer treatment than for treatment of osteoporosis (6 years). The risk factors for development of osteonecrosis include female sex, recent dental extractions, intravenous administration of bisphosphonates, high dose of bisphosphonates, and age older than 60 years. This complication of therapy is very difficult to treat, and withdrawal of the agent does not necessarily lead to reversal of the process. Recommendations from the Canadian Association of Oral and Maxillofacial Surgeons are as follows:

- Dental examination and radiographs before the initiation of intravenous bisphosphonate therapy
- Completion of urgent surgical dental procedures before the initiation of high-dose bisphosphonate therapy and completion of nonurgent procedures 3 to 6 months after cessation of bisphosphonate therapy
- Cessation of smoking, limiting of alcohol intake, and maintenance of good oral hygiene
- If osteonecrosis occurs, initiate supportive care, management of pain, treatment of secondary infection, and removal of necrotic debris and sequestrum

Imaging Findings

Imaging features reveal a mixed pattern of both osteolytic lesions and sclerotic regions in the mandible or maxilla, but lucent lesions predominate on computed tomographic images (Figures 189-1 and 189-2). Periosteal reaction is variable but more commonly seen than not. On T1-weighted magnetic resonance images, the normal marrow signal is replaced with hypointense signal. Enhancement in the cortex and subcortical bone is present, and the enhancement may involve the adjacent muscles of mastication.

Reference

Thumbigere-Math V, Sabino MC, Gopalakrishnan R, et al. Bisphosphonate-related osteonecrosis of the jaw: clinical features, risk factors, management, and treatment outcomes of 26 patients. *J Oral Maxillofac Surg.* 2009;67(9):1904-1913.

Cross-Reference

Neuroradiology: THE REQUISITES, 4th ed, pp 462, 480.

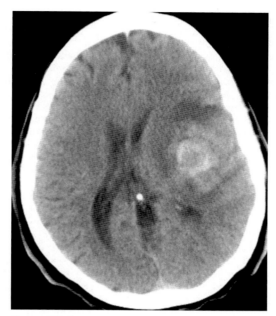

Figure 190-1

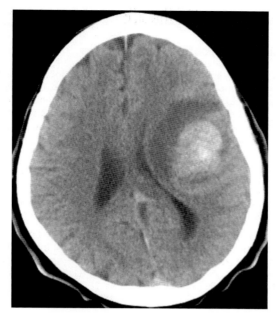

Figure 190-2

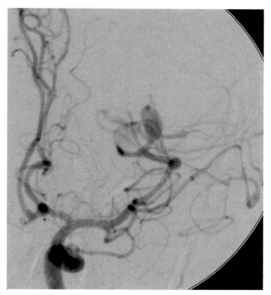

Figure 190-3

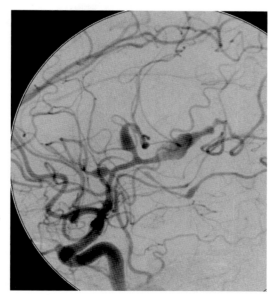

Figure 190-4

HISTORY: Human immunodeficiency virus (HIV) positive with fever and mental status change.

1. What is the best diagnosis?
   A. Hematoma following thrombolysis
   B. Hemorrhagic neoplasm
   C. Trauma
   D. Mycotic aneurysm rupture

2. Where is the most common site for this entity?
   A. Anterior cerebral artery
   B. Posterior cerebral artery
   C. Middle cerebral artery
   D. Vertebral and basilar arteries

3. What percentage of patients affected have multiple aneurysms?
   A. 10%
   B. 20%
   C. 30%
   D. 40%

4. Modern contrast agents used in angiography are characterized as which of the following?
   A. High-osmolar ionic
   B. High-osmolar non-ionic
   C. Low-osmolar ionic
   D. Low-osmolar non-ionic

CASE 190

Ruptured Mycotic Aneurysm

1. **D.** Mycotic aneurysm rupture. There is a lobar hematoma and the digital subtraction angiographic (DSA) images show multiple fusiform aneurysms with irregular morphology. In the absence of the DSA images, the differential would include hematoma following thrombolysis, a hemorrhagic mass, trauma, and vasculitis.

2. **C.** Middle cerebral artery. Overall, 75% to 80% of intracranial mycotic aneurysms are found in the distal branches of the middle cerebral artery.

3. **B.** 20%. Approximately 20% of patients will present with multiple mycotic aneurysms.

4. **D.** Low-osmolar, non-ionic. Currently used iodinated contrast has low osmolarity, nearly iso-osmolar to human blood. Non-ionic contrast is used. High-osmolar agents result in deleterious effects such as endothelial damage, thrombosis, and pulmonary hypertension.

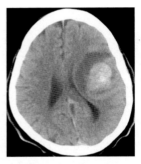

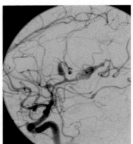

Comment

Background

Fifteen percent of patients with acute subarachnoid hemorrhage die before reaching the hospital. The incidence of aneurysmal rebleeding is approximately 2% per day in the first 2 weeks after the initial hemorrhage. The angiographer must address several issues, including identifying the vessel from which the aneurysm arises, the size of the aneurysm, the presence or absence of an aneurysm neck, the orientation of the aneurysm, and the anatomy of the circle of Willis. A search for multiple aneurysms is necessary. If there is more than one aneurysm, it is necessary to try to determine which aneurysm bled.

Mycotic Aneurysms

A mycotic aneurysm results from an infectious process that involves the arterial wall. Viridans streptococci and *Streptococcus aureus* are the most common pathogens. These aneurysms may be caused by a septic embolus that causes inflammatory destruction of the arterial wall, beginning with the endothelial surface. Infected embolic material also reaches the adventitia through the vasa vasorum. Inflammation disrupts the adventitia and muscularis, resulting in aneurysmal dilation. Mycotic aneurysms are estimated to account for 2% to 3% of all intracranial aneurysms. They have an increased incidence in the setting of drug abuse and in a spectrum of immunocompromised states. The thoracic aorta is reported to be the most common site of mycotic aneurysms. Intracranial mycotic aneurysms are less common. They occur with greater frequency in children and are often found on vessels distal to the circle of Willis. They frequently manifest with a cerebral hematoma (Figures 190-1 and 190-2), as in this case of middle cerebral artery mycotic aneurysm (Figures 190-3 and 190-4). Mycotic aneurysms generally have a fusiform morphologic appearance and are usually very friable (see Figures 190-3 and 190-4).

Management

Treatment is difficult and risky. Most cases are treated emergently with antibiotics, which are continued for 4 to 6 weeks. Serial angiography helps to document the effectiveness of medical therapy. Even if aneurysms seem to be shrinking, they may subsequently grow, and new aneurysms may form. Delayed clipping or coiling may be more feasible. Indications for this treatment approach include subarachnoid hemorrhage, increasing size of the aneurysm during treatment with antibiotics (this is controversial), and failure of the aneurysm to shrink after 4 to 6 weeks of antibiotic treatment. Patients with subacute bacterial endocarditis who require valve replacement should have bioprosthetic (i.e., tissue) valves instead of mechanical valves to eliminate the need for risky anticoagulation therapy.

References

Cloft HJ, Kallmes DF, Jensen ME, Lanzino G, Dion JE. Endovascular treatment of ruptured, peripheral cerebral aneurysms: parent artery occlusion with short Guglielmi detachable coils. *AJNR Am J Neuroradiol*. 1999;20:308-310.

Loevner LA, Ting TY, Hurst RW, Goldberg H, Schut L. Spontaneous thrombosis of a basilar artery traumatic aneurysm in a child. *AJNR Am J Neuroradiol*. 1998;19:386-388.

Cross-Reference

Neuroradiology: THE REQUISITES, 4th ed, pp 179, 183.

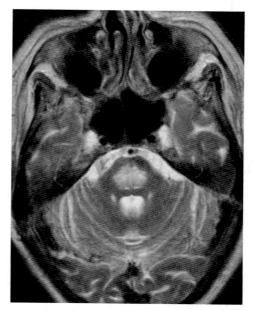

Figure 191-1   Patient A.

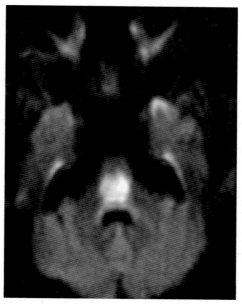

Figure 191-2   Patient A.

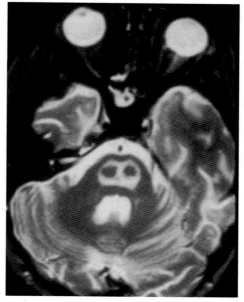

Figure 191-3   Patient B.

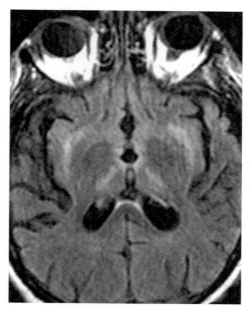

Figure 191-4   Patient C.

HISTORY: Patient A (Figures 191-1 and 191-2) developed a rapid decline in mental status and soon died. Patients B (Figure 191-3) and C (Figure 191-4) presented with coma.

1. What is the single best diagnosis common to each patient?
   A. Brainstem glioma
   B. Wallerian degeneration
   C. Vertebrobasilar ischemia
   D. Osmotic demyelination

2. This condition is frequently associated with overzealous correction of what abnormality?
   A. Hyponatremia
   B. Hypernatremia
   C. Hypokalemia
   D. Hyperkalemia

3. Which patients typically present with this condition?
   A. Cancer patients
   B. Alcoholic patients
   C. Postoperative patients
   D. Septic patients

4. What are the chances of full recovery after having this condition?
   A. 10%
   B. 30%
   C. 50%
   D. 70%

CASE 191

Osmotic Demyelination

1. **D.** Osmotic demyelination. There is abnormal signal in the pons of Patients A and B (Figures 191-1 through 191-3) with sparing of the corticospinal tracts (Patient B); a neoplasm would manifest as an expansile mass involving almost the entirety of the pons. Wallerian degeneration typically manifests with abnormal signal along a white matter tract, with associated atrophy. There is no atrophy of the pons in these cases and no evidence of encephalomalacia in the cortex. The signal abnormality in the thalamus and eternal capsule of Patient C (Figure 191-4) would not be seen in vertebrobasilar ischemia.

2. **A.** Hyponatremia. When hyponatremia is rigorously corrected, osmotic demyelination can result.

3. **B.** Alcoholic patients. This condition is most frequently seen in alcoholics and malnourished patients.

4. **B.** 30%. It's a rule of thirds: approximately one third of patients fully recover, one third survive with neurologic deficits, and one third die or have serious neurologic deficits.

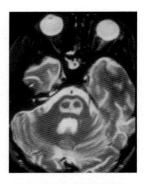

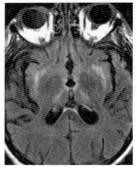

Comment

Background

Osmotic demyelination may be seen with underlying systemic processes that have a predilection for electrolyte abnormalities. It is most commonly seen in alcoholics and in chronically debilitated and malnourished patients after rapid correction of hyponatremia. It is not the low serum level but rather the rapidity with which it is corrected that is believed to be responsible for this disorder. Overzealous correction of serum sodium levels may be followed by acute or subacute clinical deterioration, including change in mental status, coma, quadriparesis, extrapyramidal signs, and, if the condition is unrecognized, death. This process commonly involves extrapontine structures, as in Patient C (Figure 191-4). Pathologically, demyelination is noted without a significant inflammatory response, with relative sparing of axons. There is an associated reactive astrocytosis.

Imaging

It is characterized by hyperintensity on T2-weighted images in the central pons, with relative sparing of the peripheral pons. The corticospinal tracts are usually spared (Figure 191-3). The T2 image (Figure 191-1) and the diffusion trace (Figure 191-2) show acute demyelination in the central pons. The T2 fluid-attenuated inversion recovery (FLAIR) image of Patient C (Figure 191-4) shows abnormal signal in the thalami and external capsules. Usually, osmotic demyelination is not associated with enhancement or significant mass effect.

Differential Diagnosis

When osmotic demyelination is localized only to the pons, the radiologic diagnosis is usually easy. If there is pontine and extrapontine involvement or involvement only in extrapontine structures, the differential diagnosis is broad, including other demyelinating disorders, encephalitis, and ischemia.

Reference

Sterns RH, Riggs JE, Schochette SS. Osmotic demyelination syndrome following correction of hyponatremia. *N Engl J Med.* 1986;314: 1535-1542.

Cross-Reference

Neuroradiology: THE REQUISITES, 4th ed, p 222.

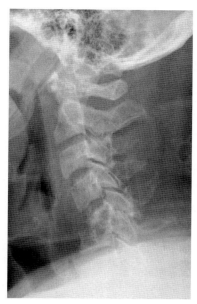

Figure 192-1

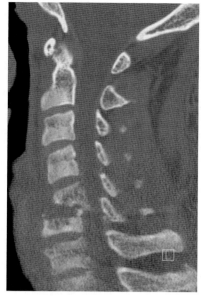

Figure 192-2

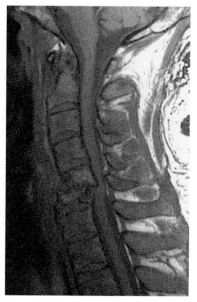

Figure 192-3

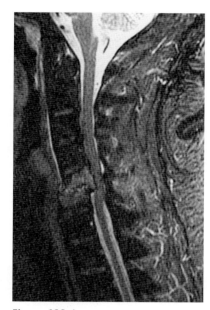

Figure 192-4

HISTORY: A 55-year-old man with end-stage renal disease who is on long-term hemodialysis presents with recent severe neck pain, upper extremity numbness, and weakness.

1. Considering the patient history and imaging, what is the single best diagnosis?
   A. Discitis osteomyelitis
   B. Neuropathic spondyloarthropathy (Charcot spine)
   C. Dialysis-induced spondyloarthropathy
   D. Degenerative spondylarthritis

2. All of the following are underlying mechanisms of dialysis-induced spondyloarthropathy *except:*
   A. β_2-Microglobulin amyloidosis
   B. Crystal-induced arthropathy
   C. Aluminum-induced spondyloarthropathy
   D. Calcium toxicity

3. Which finding on magnetic resonance imaging (MRI) is characteristic in dialysis-induced spondyloarthropathy?
   A. Erosive endplate changes
   B. High T2 endplate signal
   C. High T2 signal in the disc
   D. High T1 endplate signal

4. What is the most reliable way to differentiate between an infectious versus a noninfectious cause in patients with chronic renal disease and rapidly progressive spondyloarthropathy?
   A. Computed tomography (CT)
   B. MRI
   C. Laboratory data (sedimentation rate and white blood cell count)
   D. Biopsy

CASE 192

Dialysis-Induced Spondyloarthropathy

1. **C.** Dialysis-induced spondyloarthropathy. The findings presented fit the characteristic features of dialysis-induced spondyloarthropathy. This entity typically manifests with significant vertebral endplate erosions, subluxation, reactive endplate changes of sclerosis on CT scan, and occasionally areas of abnormal increased T2 signal of the discovertebral junctions, owing to the associated inflammatory process.

2. **D.** Calcium toxicity. Calcium per se is unlikely to cause discovertebral erosions and destruction of the intervertebral discs; rather, secondary hyperparathyroidism in patients with renal osteodystrophy with elevated serum levels of parathormone leads to subchondral bone reabsorption and erosive arthropathy related to abnormal osteoclastic activity. β_2-Microglobulin amyloidosis is a condition that affects patients undergoing long-term hemodialysis or continuous ambulatory peritoneal dialysis. The association of crystal deposits and chronic renal disease in patients undergoing dialysis is well recognized. Calcium hydroxyapatite and calcium pyrophosphate have been recovered from specimens of affected areas. Patients with toxic accumulation of aluminum may develop erosive spondyloarthropathy.

3. **A.** Erosive endplate changes. Erosive endplate changes are characteristic findings in the segment of the spine affected by dialysis-induced spondyloarthropathy. High T2 signal of the endplates is not a characteristic finding of dialysis-induced spondyloarthropathy. Typically, there is no increase or minimal increased T2 signal in the intervertebral disc, as opposed to infection, in which the affected disc is characteristically bright on T2-weighted images. Low T1 endplate signal is characteristic of dialysis-induced spondyloarthropathy.

4. **D.** Biopsy. Biopsy and culture of the segment of the spine affected provides information about the causative organism in cases of infection. In dialysis-induced spondyloarthropathy, the presence of crystals and β-amyloid particles is diagnostic.

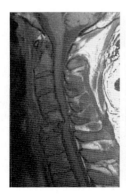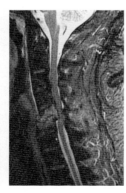

Comment

Background

In patients undergoing long-term dialysis for chronic renal disease, a destructive spondyloarthropathy that resembles infection may develop. The process tends to affect primarily the cervical spine followed by the thoracic spine and thoracolumbar junction. Clinically, patients present with pain, radiculopathy, and signs of compressive myelopathy in the absence of symptoms of obvious infection.

Histopathology

Dialysis-induced spondyloarthropathy may be related to the deposition of crystals in the intervertebral discs and adjacent endplates as demonstrated by transmission electron microscopy. Aluminum toxicity and accumulation in the disc space may produce similar destructive changes as well as secondary hyperparathyroidism in patients with renal osteodystrophy. This can lead to subperiosteal and subchondral reabsorption of bone and erosive arthropathy. Dialysis-related amyloidosis is caused by the deposition of β_2-microglobulin as amyloid fibrils that are known to accumulate in synovial membranes and osteoarticular sites, particularly in the spine, evoking an inflammatory reaction, which leads to destructive osteoarthropathy.

Imaging

Characteristic imaging features include marked disc space narrowing, vertebral body erosions, and sclerosis on CT or plain films; cartilaginous node formation in the absence of significant osteophyte formation; and epidural spinal masses (Figures 192-1 and 192-2). On MRI, the disc typically appears low or minimally bright in signal on T2-weighted images. There is also evidence of abnormal low T1 signal and low T2 signal in the eroded subchondral endplates, although occasionally, because of the presence of inflammatory cells, the subchondral endplates may show bright T2 signal, making differentiation from infection very difficult (Figures 192-3 and 192-4).

Management

Treatment includes medical care and, in more severe cases, decompression and surgical stabilization.

References

Danish FR, Klinkmann J, Yokoo H, et al. Fatal cervical spondyloarthropathy in a hemodialysis patient with systemic deposition of beta2-microglobulin amyloid. *Am J Kidney Dis*. 1999;33(3): 563-566.

Kaplan P, Resnick D, Murphey M, et al. Destructive noninfectious spondyloarthropathy in hemodialysis patients: a report of four cases. *Radiology*. 1987;162(1 Pt 1):241-244.

Kiss E, Keusch G, Zenetti M, et al. Dialysis-related amyloidosis revisited. *AJR Am J Roentgenol*. 2005;185(6):1460-1467.

Cross-Reference

Neuroradiology: THE REQUISITES, 4th ed, p 562.

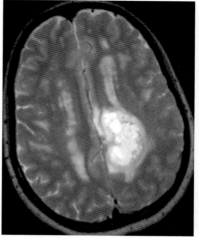

Figure 193-1

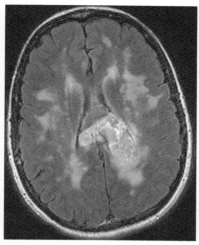

Figure 193-2

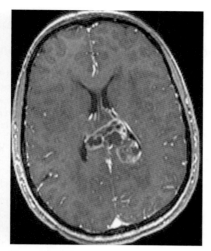

Figure 193-3

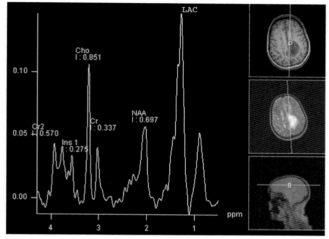

Figure 193-4

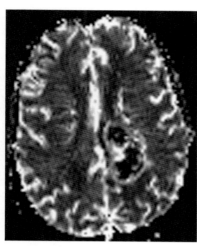

Figure 193-5

HISTORY: History of multiple sclerosis with weakness and headache.

1. What is the most likely diagnosis in light of all of the imaging and magnetic resonance spectroscopy (MRS) findings?
   A. Glioblastoma
   B. Abscess
   C. Central neurocytoma
   D. Tumefactive demyelination

2. If the glutamate or glutamine peaks were elevated and instead of increased perfusion there was decreased perfusion, what would the best diagnosis be?
   A. Glioblastoma
   B. Abscess
   C. Central neurocytoma
   D. Tumefactive demyelination

3. Concerning MRS techniques (point-resolved spectroscopy [PRESS] and stimulated echo acquisition mode [STEAM]), which statement is correct?
   A. Signal-to-noise ratio (SNR) is greater in PRESS than in STEAM.
   B. PRESS is better for metabolites with short T2.
   C. Specific absorption ratio (SAR) is higher in STEAM.
   D. Localization is better in PRESS.

4. What is the resonance frequency of water on MRS?
   A. 1.3 parts per million (ppm)
   B. 3.0 ppm
   C. 4.7 ppm
   D. 5.9 ppm

CASE 193

Multiple Sclerosis and Glioblastoma

1. **A.** Glioblastoma. Tumefactive demyelination as implied by its name may appear as a mass. The rim of increased perfusion on the cerebral blood volume map (Figure 193-5) is more suggestive of glioma than tumefactive multiple sclerosis. This patient had biopsy-proven glioblastoma.

2. **D.** Tumefactive demyelination. In the absence of increased perfusion at the periphery of the mass lesion and if there were elevated glutamate or glutamine levels, tumefactive multiple sclerosis would be the more likely diagnosis.

3. **A.** SNR is greater in PRESS than in STEAM. PRESS and STEAM are the two most common acquisition techniques in MRS. PRESS utilizes a single 90-degree and two 180-degree slice selective pulses in orthogonal planes. STEAM utilizes three 90-degree slice selection pulses. PRESS has twice as much SNR as STEAM. STEAM is better for metabolites with short T2. SAR is lower in STEAM. Localization is better in STEAM.

4. **C.** 4.7 ppm. The resonance frequency of water on MRS is 4.7 ppm.

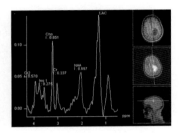

Comment

Background

Tumefactive multiple sclerosis, high-grade glioma (glioblastoma), and occasionally an abscess can appear similar on imaging, particularly in the absence of a clinical history (Figures 193-1 through 193-3). Multiple sclerosis typically occurs in younger patients, and there are often additional clinical or imaging findings to suggest this diagnosis. On close questioning, patients often have neurologic symptoms that are spaced both in time and location. Furthermore, magnetic resonance imaging may demonstrate white matter lesions separate from the mass that are suggestive of multiple sclerosis (see Figures 193-1 and 193-2).

Value of Advanced Techniques

Perfusion imaging in this case shows markedly elevated regional cerebral blood volume (Figure 193-5) in the enhancing rim of the necrotic mass, suggesting a high-grade glioma or glioblastoma rather than demyelination. Glioblastoma was confirmed at surgical biopsy. Nonspecific spectroscopic findings in tumefactive multiple sclerosis include an increase in choline, lactate, and lipid peaks and a decrease in the *N*-acetylaspartate peak (Figure 193-4). These spectroscopic characteristics reflect the histologic correlate of marked demyelination in the absence of significant inflammation. Gliomas also consistently show reductions in *N*-acetylaspartate and increases in phospholipids, reflecting the replacement of normal neuronal tissue with a proliferating cellular process. Increases in lactate are not uncommon as a result of tissue ischemia and necrosis, as in this case. Variable increases in lipid levels may be seen.

Increase in glutamate or glutamine peaks favors tumefactive demyelination and is typically not seen in aggressive neoplasms (not present in this case). Serial proton MRS can be a useful, noninvasive method of overcoming the diagnostic dilemma of differentiating glioma from acute tumefactive demyelination. Persistent elevation of choline and lactate levels favors a glioma. Normalization of the initial increases in phospholipids, lipid, and lactate peaks within 3 to 4 weeks, followed by persistent, marked reductions of the neuronal marker *N*-acetylaspartate, has been described over time in tumefactive demyelination.

References

Cianfoni A, Niku S, Imbesi SG. Metabolite findings in tumefactive demyelinating lesions utilizing short echo time proton magnetic resonance spectroscopy. *AJNR Am J Neuroradiol.* 2007;28:272-277.

Jamroz-Wiśniewska A, Janczarek M, Belniak E, et al. Tumour-like lesions in multiple sclerosis. *Neurol Neurochir Pol.* 2008;42: 161-167.

Cross-Reference

Neuroradiology: THE REQUISITES, 4th ed, pp 59-62, 206-212.

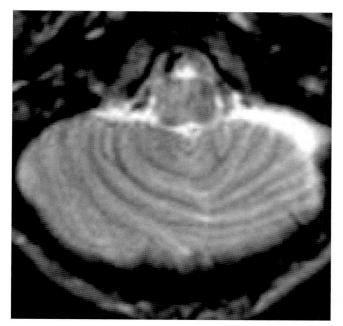

Figure 194-1

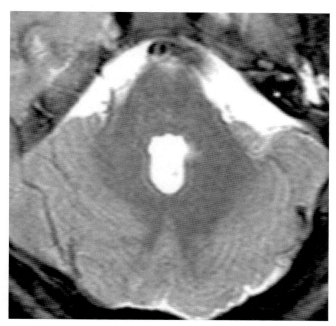

Figure 194-2

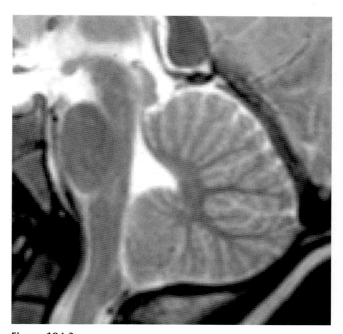

Figure 194-3

HISTORY: A patient with developmental delay presents with ataxia.

1. What is the diagnosis?
   A. Lhermitte-Duclos
   B. Dyke-Davidoff-Masson
   C. Joubert
   D. Rhombencephalosynapsis

2. What structure is absent?
   A. Vermis
   B. Pons
   C. Cerebellar peduncle
   D. Dentate nuclei

3. What disease is characterized by elongation of the superior cerebellar peduncles and vermian hypoplasia?
   A. Rhombencephalosynapsis
   B. Aqueductal stenosis
   C. Joubert syndrome
   D. Dandy-Walker malformation

4. By what age would you expect to see myelination of the cerebellar white matter on a T1-weighted image in a patient born at term?
   A. Birth
   B. 3 months
   C. 6 months
   D. 9 months

CASE 194

Rhombencephalosynapsis

1. **D.** Rhombencephalosynapsis. There is fusion of the cerebellar hemispheres across midline with absence of the cerebellar vermis. Lhermitte-Duclos is a probably hamartomatous tumor of the cerebellum associated with Cowden syndrome. Dyke-Davidoff-Masson is ex vacuo enlargement of the calvarium, paranasal sinuses, and mastoids in response to volume loss in the ipsilateral cerebral hemisphere. Joubert is described in the answer for question 3.

2. **A.** Vermis. The vermis is absent. The pons, cerebellar peduncles, and dentate nuclei are present, although the later two pairs are fused at the midline.

3. **C.** Joubert syndrome. This disease is typically autosomal recessive, characterized by the molar tooth deformity that results when the superior cerebellar peduncles are thin and elongated in the anteroposterior direction and the vermis is hypoplastic without cerebellar hemispheric fusion.

4. **B.** 3 months. At 3 months, a T1-weighted image should show myelination of the cerebellar white matter.

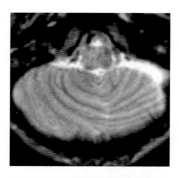

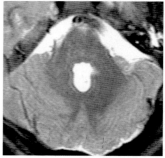

Comment

Rhombencephalosynapsis

Rhombencephalosynapsis is an anomaly resulting from agenesis or hypoplasia of the cerebellar vermis. There is fusion of the cerebellar hemispheres (Figures 194-1 and 194-2), with variable fusion of other posterior fossa structures, including the middle cerebellar peduncles, cerebellar dentate nuclei, and superior and inferior colliculi. In the cerebellar hemispheres, the orientation of the folia is disorganized. They are usually transverse in configuration, extending across the midline without intervening vermis. Magnetic resonance imaging typically shows an absent or severely hypoplastic vermis, with fusion of the cerebellar hemispheres (see Figures 194-1 through 194-3). There is usually posterior pointing of the fourth ventricle. Associated supratentorial anomalies include partial or complete absence of the septum pellucidum, a hypoplastic anterior commissure, ex vacuo enlargement of the ventricular system related to surrounding volume loss of the brain parenchyma, and fusion of the thalami. Hypertelorism and migrational anomalies have also been reported with this condition. The clinical presentation is more commonly related to the associated supratentorial anomalies.

Joubert Syndrome

Joubert syndrome, another dysplasia of the posterior fossa contents, is characterized by severe hypoplasia or aplasia of the cerebellar vermis. It has a characteristic imaging appearance, including a "bat-wing" configuration of the fourth ventricle and a horizontal orientation of the superior cerebellar peduncles. In contrast to rhombencephalosynapsis, the cerebellar hemispheres are apposed in the midline but are not fused. Associated supratentorial anomalies are uncommon.

References

Montull C, Mercader JM, Peri J, Martinez FM, Bonaventura I. Neuroradiological and clinical findings in rhombencephalosynapsis. *Neuroradiology*. 2000;42:272-274.

Utsunomiya H, Takano K, Ogasawara T, et al. Rhombencephalosynapsis: cerebellar embryogenesis. *AJNR Am J Neuroradiol*. 1998;19: 547-549.

Cross-Reference

Neuroradiology: THE REQUISITES, 4th ed, pp 281-282.

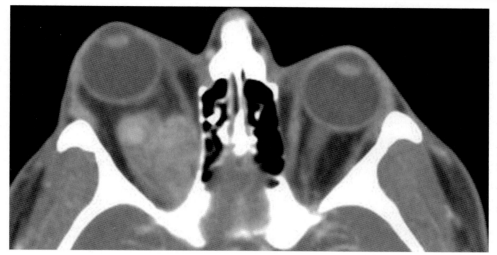

Figure 195-1

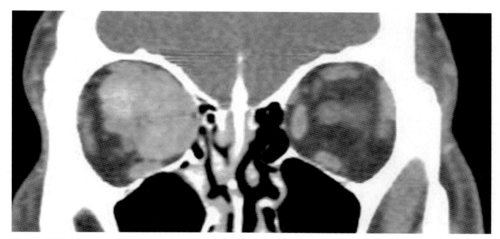

Figure 195-2

HISTORY: A patient presents with right-sided proptosis.

1. Which of the following is the most common primary mesenchymal tumor of the orbit in adults?
   A. Fibrous histiocytoma
   B. Schwannoma
   C. Hemangioma
   D. Rhabdomyosarcoma

2. What is the most common primary mesenchymal tumor of the orbit in children?
   A. Fibrous histiocytoma
   B. Schwannoma
   C. Hemangioma
   D. Rhabdomyosarcoma

3. Which of the following is true with regard to orbital fibrous histiocytomas (OFHs)?
   A. They have benign and malignant forms.
   B. They are benign lesions.
   C. They are malignant lesions.
   D. They are non-neoplastic.

4. What cranial nerve is the source of most schwannomas of the orbit?
   A. II
   B. III
   C. IV
   D. V

CASE 195

Orbital Fibrous Histiocytoma

1. **A.** Fibrous histiocytoma. The most common primary mesenchymal tumor of the orbit in adults is fibrous histiocytoma. Schwannoma and rhabdomyosarcoma are less common. Hemangioma is not considered mesenchymal.

2. **D.** Rhabdomyosarcoma. The most common primary mesenchymal tumor of the orbit in children is rhabdomyosarcoma.

3. **A.** They have benign and malignant forms. OFH is a neoplasm with benign (85%) and malignant (15%) forms. One fourth of malignant OFHs are locally aggressive.

4. **D.** V. Cranial nerve V (the trigeminal nerve) is the source of most schwannomas of the orbit. Optic nerve tumors are not schwannomas; rather, they are gliomas.

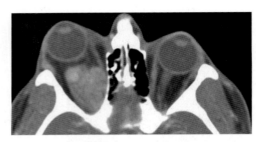

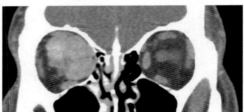

Comment

Features of Orbital Fibrous Histiocytoma

The fibrous lesions of the orbit include OFH, fibroma, solitary fibrous tumor, fibrosarcoma, fibromatosis, and nodular fasciitis. Fibrous histiocytoma usually occurs in adults and commonly manifests as a mass with proptosis and visual disturbance. The aggressiveness of the tumor varies from completely benign (60%) to locally aggressive (25%) to malignant (15%). It may invade the intracranial space from its origin in the orbit, and metastases have also been described. Recurrence rates also vary, depending on the aggressiveness of the tumor, from 25% (benign) to 64% (malignant). Treatment is surgical. Solitary fibrous tumors of the orbit have a more benign course but can look similar to OFHs. They are in the same category of disease.

Imaging Findings

The OFH mass is usually a well-defined process with a predilection for the upper, nasal portion of the orbit (Figures 195-1 and 195-2). Remodeling of the bone in the benign form, as in this case, is common. When benign, the lesion enhances homogeneously. More aggressive features on imaging include bone destruction, inhomogeneous enhancement, spiculated margins, low T2 signal, and perineural spread. Many of these tumors are periocular.

Reference

Font RL, Hidayat AA. Fibrous histiocytoma of the orbit. A clinicopathologic study of 150 cases. *Hum Pathol.* 1982;13(3):199-209.

Cross-Reference

Neuroradiology: THE REQUISITES, 4th ed, p 340.

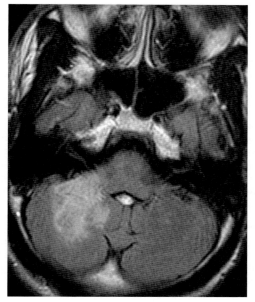

Figure 196-1

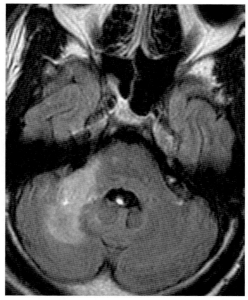

Figure 196-2

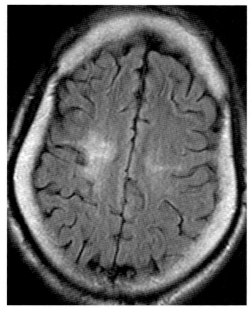

Figure 196-3

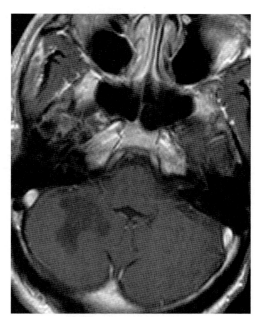

Figure 196-4

HISTORY: An immunocompromised patient presents with hemiparesis.

1. What is the diagnosis?
   A. Metastasis
   B. Toxoplasmosis
   C. Progressive multifocal leukoencephalopathy (PML)
   D. Immune reconstitution inflammatory syndrome (IRIS)

2. What is the infectious agent responsible for this entity?
   A. Human immunodeficiency virus (HIV)
   B. Cytomegalovirus (CMV)
   C. John Cunningham (JC) virus
   D. Herpes simplex virus (HSV)

3. What structure is *least* likely affected by this entity?
   A. Frontal white matter
   B. Cerebellum
   C. Thalamus
   D. Spinal cord

4. Which cell does the JC virus infect?
   A. Astrocytes
   B. Endothelial cells
   C. Ependymocytes
   D. Oligodendrocytes

CASE 196

Progressive Multifocal Leukoencephalopathy

1. **C.** Progressive multifocal leukoencephalopathy (PML). Most metastatic lesions enhance, and the lesions in this case do not enhance on the postcontrast scan. There is also lack of significant mass effect. Toxoplasmosis is seen in immunosuppressed patients but typically manifests with ring-enhancing lesions. The differential diagnosis could include demyelination from HIV. Immune reconstitution inflammatory syndrome can be associated with PML, although there also tends to be enhancement.

2. **C.** John Cunningham virus. The JC virus is a papovavirus responsible for PML. HIV does not cause PML, nor does CMV or HSV.

3. **D.** Spinal cord. The spinal cord and optic nerves are typically (but not always) spared.

4. **D.** Oligodendrocytes. The JC virus preferentially affects oligodendrocytes.

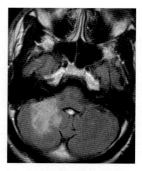

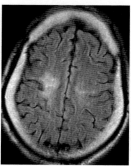

Comment

Background

Before the acquired immunodeficiency syndrome (AIDS) epidemic, PML was largely seen in a spectrum of immunocompromised patients, including patients with hematologic malignancies (leukemia and lymphoma), patients who had undergone organ transplantation, patients taking immunosuppressive drugs, and patients with autoimmune disorders. In recent decades, however, most cases of PML have been noted in patients with HIV infection. More recently, medications utilized for the treatment of multiple sclerosis have been implicated in PML occurrence, namely, natalizumab. PML is caused by infection of the oligodendrocytes with a papovavirus (JC virus). Histologically, multifocal regions of demyelination involve the subcortical U-fibers.

Clinical

The clinical presentation of PML includes focal neurologic deficits (hemiparesis), visual symptoms, and especially progressive cognitive decline. The infection is rapidly progressive, with continued neurologic decline, central nervous system demyelination, and death usually occurring within 6 months to 1 year from the onset of symptoms.

Imaging

Magnetic resonance imaging (MRI) is far more sensitive than computed tomography (CT) in defining the number and extent of lesions in PML. On CT, PML usually appears as focal regions of hypodensity within the white matter, usually without mass effect or enhancement. On MRI, increased T2-weighted signal intensity with associated T1-weighted hypointensity is noted in the involved white matter (Figures 196-1 through 196-4). PML has a predilection to involve the subcortical white matter, although the deep white matter is also commonly involved. There is a slight preference for involvement of the parietal and occipital white matter, but any area of the brain may be affected, including the cerebellum (see Figures 196-1 through 196-4), as in this case. Although single focal lesions may be seen, multifocal lesions typically occur and may or may not be bilaterally symmetric in distribution. Unilateral multifocal distribution may also occur. Mass effect or enhancement is less common in PML, occurring in 5% to 10% of cases.

PML-IRIS

IRIS is a T-cell–mediated encephalitis commonly associated with the initiation of highly active antiretroviral therapy (HAART) or after completion of treatment in patients with autoimmune disease such as multiple sclerosis. Imaging can be variable but is usually characterized by patchy enhancement and white matter signal abnormality.

References

Kleinschmidt-DeMasters BK, Miravalle A, Schowinsky J, et al. Update on PML and PML-IRIS occurring in multiple sclerosis patients treated with natalizumab. *J Neuropathol Exp Neurol.* 2012; 71(7):604-617.

Mader I, Herrlinger U, Klose U, Schmidt F, Kuker W. Progressive multifocal leukoencephalopathy: analysis of lesion development with diffusion-weighted MRI. *Neuroradiology.* 2003;45:717-721.

Selewski DT, Shah GV, Segal BM, et al. Natalizumab (Tysabri). *AJNR Am J Neuroradiol.* 2010;31(9):1588-1590.

Thurnher MM, Post MJ, Rieger A, Kleibl-Popov C, Loewe C, Schindler E. Initial and follow-up MR imaging findings in AIDS-related progressive multifocal leukoencephalopathy treated with highly active antiretroviral therapy. *AJNR Am J Neuroradiol.* 2001;22:977-984.

Cross-Reference

Neuroradiology: THE REQUISITES, 4th ed, pp 217-218.

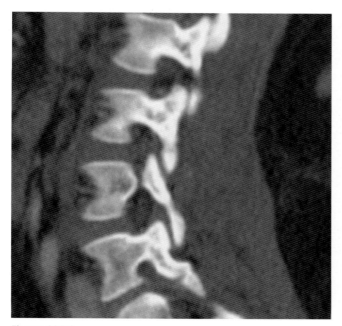

Figure 197-1

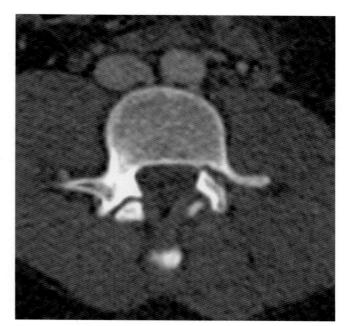

Figure 197-2

HISTORY: A 25-year-old woman was involved in a motor vehicle collision.

1. What is the diagnosis?
   A. Fracture of the pedicle
   B. Retrosomatic cleft
   C. Pars interarticularis defect
   D. Congenital absence of the pedicle

2. Where along the spinal axis is this most common?
   A. Cervical spine
   B. Thoracic spine
   C. Lumbar spine
   D. Sacrum

3. Osseous abnormalities frequently reported in association with this entity include all of the following *except:*
   A. Spina bifida occulta
   B. Vertebral body fusion
   C. Additional hypoplastic pedicles
   D. Limbus vertebra

4. What other finding or disease is this entity associated with?
   A. Neurofibromatosis type 1
   B. Chiari type I malformation
   C. Mega cisterna magna
   D. Von Hippel–Lindau

CASE 197

Congenital Absence of Pedicle

1. **D.** Congenital absence of the pedicle. The findings of absence of the pedicle with deformed articular facet and hypoplastic transverse process make this diagnosis the most likely. There is a linear defect in the pedicle in cases of retrosomatic cleft. The affected pedicle is either normal in size or may be elongated, shortened, or thickened but is not hypoplastic as seen in this case. There is no defect noted in the pars interarticularis.

2. **C.** Lumbar spine. The lumbar spine is the most common location for this to occur.

3. **D.** Limbus vertebra. There is no association with limbus vertebra. Spina bifida occulta, vertebral body fusion anomalies, and additional hypoplastic pedicles have been reported.

4. **A.** Neurofibromatosis type 1. There is an association with NF1 and not with the other options presented. There is an association with genitourinary and other congenital abnormalities.

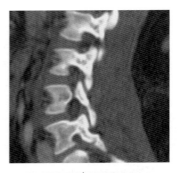

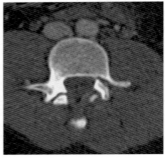

Comment

Background

Congenital absence of the pedicle or hypoplasia of a lumbar pedicle is an uncommon anomaly. Most cases are asymptomatic and discovered incidentally or are found in patients who present with low back pain. The anomaly occurs most frequently in the lumbar spine followed by the cervical spine. It has been observed in association with genitourinary and other congenital abnormalities and in patients with neurofibromatosis.

Pathophysiology

In a patient with congenital absence of the pedicle, the biomechanical dysfunction from concomitant deformity or abnormal function of the facet joint is a cause of lumbar spine instability in axial rotation and flexion. In addition, because the facet shares the axial load at a specific level, the contralateral joint in patients with congenital absence of the pedicle must bear a greater load, resulting in the development of severe degenerative changes.

Imaging

A computed tomography (CT) scan is performed to detect bony anomalies (Figures 197-1 and 197-2). Three-dimensional CT is effective in determining the relationships between the deformed bones. Magnetic resonance imaging helps to distinguish this condition from pedicle destruction by tumor or infection by the presence of fat, nerves, and vessels rather than a soft tissue mass in the intervertebral foramen and by the dorsally positioned abnormal articular processes.

Management

Most patients are asymptomatic or complain of low back pain that can be managed by conservative therapy. In rare cases with neurologic impairment, surgical intervention may be required.

Reference

Kaito T, Kato Y, Sakaura H, et al. Congenital absence of a lumbar pedicle presenting with contralateral lumbar radiculopathy. *J Spinal Disord Tech.* 2005;18(2):203-205.

Cross-Reference

Neuroradiology: THE REQUISITES, 4th ed, p 550.

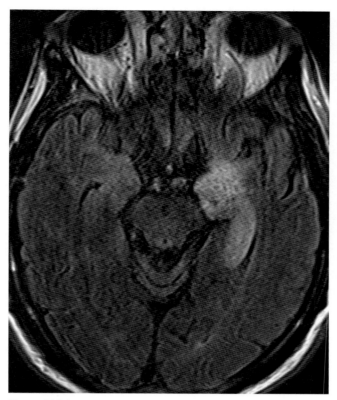

Figure 198-1

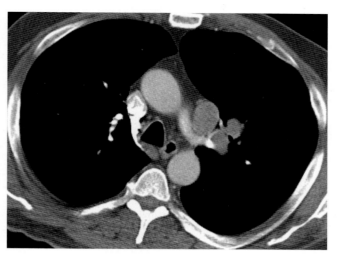

Figure 198-2

HISTORY: Cognitive dysfunction in a patient with lung carcinoma.

1. What is the best diagnosis?
   A. Seizures
   B. Gliomatosis cerebri
   C. Limbic encephalitis
   D. Low-grade diffuse astrocytoma

2. What is the most likely disease present in this patient's chest?
   A. Hodgkin lymphoma
   B. Small cell lung cancer
   C. Mucinous adenocarcinoma
   D. Non–small cell lung cancer

3. Which circulating autoantibody is most likely present in this patient?
   A. Anti-Hu
   B. Anti-Ri
   C. Anti-Yo
   D. Anti-Tr

4. What percentage of cancer patients develop a paraneoplastic syndrome?
   A. Less than 2%
   B. 2% to 5%
   C. 6% to 10%
   D. 11% to 15%

CASE 198

Limbic Encephalitis—Paraneoplastic Syndrome

1. **C.** Limbic encephalitis. Although seizures and low-grade neoplasms may appear as signal abnormality in the medial temporal lobe, the best answer from among these options is limbic encephalitis, which is a paraneoplastic syndrome often associated with small cell lung carcinoma.

2. **B.** Small cell lung cancer. Lung cancer, particularly small cell carcinoma, is the most common malignancy associated with neurologic paraneoplastic syndromes. However, these syndromes may be seen in ovarian carcinoma, testicular germ cell tumors, gastrointestinal cancer, Hodgkin disease, breast cancer, and neuroblastoma in children.

3. **A.** Anti-Hu. Anti-Hu antibodies have been associated more specifically with limbic encephalitis than have other antibodies.

4. **A.** Less than 2%. In fact, less than 1% of patients with cancer develop a paraneoplastic syndrome.

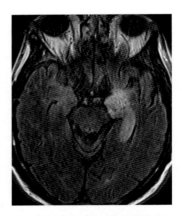

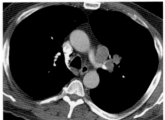

Comment

Background

Paraneoplastic syndromes affecting the central nervous system represent a spectrum of neurologic manifestations that are associated with extracranial cancers but are not the result of direct invasion of the central nervous system by tumor. They occur in less than 1% of patients with cancer; however, in 33% to 50% of patients with a paraneoplastic syndrome, the syndrome develops before the diagnosis of systemic neoplasm is made. Such syndromes include limbic encephalopathy, cerebellar degeneration, opsoclonus or myoclonus, retinal degeneration, Lambert-Eaton myasthenic syndrome, and myelopathy. Lung cancer, particularly small cell carcinoma, is the most common malignancy associated with neurologic paraneoplastic syndromes (Figure 198-2). However, these syndromes may be seen in ovarian carcinoma, testicular germ cell tumors, gastrointestinal cancer, Hodgkin disease, breast cancer, and neuroblastoma in children.

Etiology

The cause of paraneoplastic syndromes is unknown; however, the most widely accepted theory is that they occur as a result of an autoimmune disorder. Circulating autoantibodies have been identified in several paraneoplastic syndromes. Anti-Yo is specific to paraneoplastic cerebellar degeneration associated with breast and ovarian cancer, and anti-Hu is most often associated with paraneoplastic limbic encephalitis.

Clinical

Paraneoplastic limbic encephalitis may present with a change in mental status, personality changes, and memory impairment.

Imaging and Pathology

Computed tomography may be unremarkable. On magnetic resonance imaging, high signal intensity may be identified in the medial temporal lobes on T2-weighted images such as the T2 fluid-attenuated inversion recovery (FLAIR) image shown in this case (Figure 198-1). Mild enhancement may occur. Involvement of the hypothalamus may also be noted. On pathologic evaluation, nonspecific inflammatory changes and cellular infiltrates are identified without the presence of tumor or viral inclusions.

Management

Treatment of the primary malignancy may result in improvement of the neurologic symptoms.

References

Aguirre-Cruz L, Charuel JL, Carpentier AF, et al. Clinical relevance of non-neuronal auto-antibodies in patients with anti-Hu or anti-Yo paraneoplastic diseases. *J Neurooncol*. 2005;71:39-41.

Ances BM, Vitaliani R, Taylor RA, et al. Treatment-responsive limbic encephalitis identified by neuropil antibodies: MRI and PET correlates. *Brain*. 2005;128:1764-1777.

Cross-Reference

Neuroradiology: THE REQUISITES, 4th ed, pp 81-83.

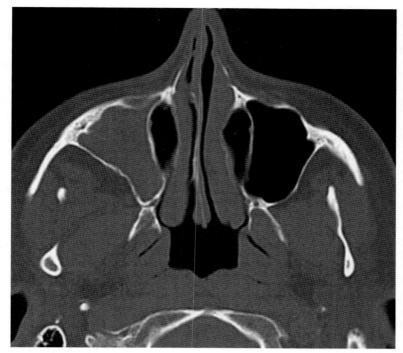

Figure 199-1

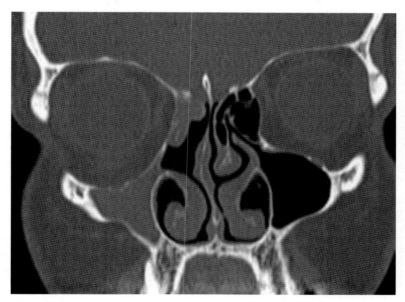

Figure 199-2

HISTORY: A 35-year-old patient presents with enophthalmos.

1. Which of the following is the best diagnosis?
   A. Maxillary sinus hypoplasia
   B. Polyps
   C. Silent sinus syndrome
   D. Fungus ball

2. What is the presumed cause of this entity?
   A. Decreased pressure, which leads to sinus "atelectasis," pulling the walls of the sinus inward
   B. Increased pressure, which causes bone remodeling
   C. Chronic sinusitis
   D. Obstruction of ostia, which leads to opacification

3. Which of the following is the correct definition of *hypoglobus?*
   A. Low pressure in orbit
   B. Enophthalmos
   C. Downward displacement of the globe in the orbit
   D. Small globe

4. Which is *not* a feature of this entity and is often seen in maxillary sinus hypoplasia?
   A. Increased fat outside the walls of the sinus
   B. Downward displacement of the orbital floor
   C. Hypoplasia of the uncinate process
   D. Small sinus volume

CASE 199

Silent Sinus Syndrome

1. **C.** Silent sinus syndrome (SSS). SSS accounts for this "atel-ectatic" sinus. Polyps and fungus ball would not be seen as a cause of a small maxillary sinus. This specific case, showing enophthalmos, does not indicate maxillary sinus hypoplasia. Hypoglobus and increased retromaxillary fat are unusual with sinus hypoplasia but are seen in SSS.

2. **A.** Decreased pressure, which leads to sinus "atelectasis" pulling the walls of the sinus inward. Negative pressure retraction in SSS causes the walls of the maxillary sinus to be pulled inward. This also leads to the orbital floor depression and hypoglobus.

3. **C.** Downward displacement of the globe in the orbit. Hypoglobus is the downward displacement of the globe in the orbit. Low pressure in the orbit is called *hypotony*. Inward displacement is *enophthalmos*, and a small globe is *microglobia* or *microphthalmos*. Hypoglobus is a feature of SSS.

4. **C.** Hypoplasia of the uncinate process. This is not characteristic of SSS, although it is often seen in maxillary sinus hypoplasia. Some features of SSS include increased fat outside the walls of the sinus, downward displacement of the orbital floor, and small sinus volume.

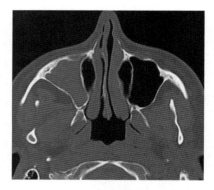

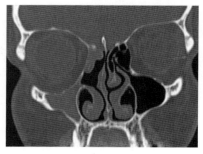

Comment

Symptoms and Complications of Silent Sinus Syndrome

As the volume of the affected sinus decreases, the orbital volume has a commensurate increase. This leads to enophthalmos, which is the most common complaint associated with SSS, not the chronic sinusitis, which is the etiologic feature. Because of the depression of the orbital floor into the collapsing maxillary antrum, the globe may also show inferior depression *(hypoglobus)*. Most affected patients have complete opacification of the "atelectatic" sinus and obstruction at the ostium (Figures 199-1 and 199-2). The entity affects the maxillary sinus exclusively, and documented negative pressure within the sinus accounts for the retraction.

Classification of Silent Sinus Syndrome

Why is this not simply maxillary sinus hypoplasia, which is many times more common than SSS? Criteria for diagnosing maxillary sinus hypoplasia include a small maxillary sinus, often with thickened walls; vertical enlargement of the orbit; elevated canine fossa; enlarged superior orbital and pterygopalatine fossa; and lateral position of the infraorbital nerve canal. The uncinate process is usually hypoplastic as well. A classification of maxillary sinus hypoplasia has been developed:

- Type I: normal uncinate process, a well-defined infundibular passage, and mild sinus hypoplasia
- Type II: absent or hypoplastic uncinate process, ill-defined infundibular passage, and soft tissue–density opacification of a significantly hypoplastic sinus
- Type III: absent uncinate process and profoundly hypoplastic, cleftlike sinus

Reference

Hourany R, Aygun N, Della Santina CC, Zinreich SJ. Silent sinus syndrome: an acquired condition. *AJNR Am J Neuroradiol*. 2005; 26(9):2390-2392.

Cross-Reference

Neuroradiology: THE REQUISITES, 4th ed, p 417.

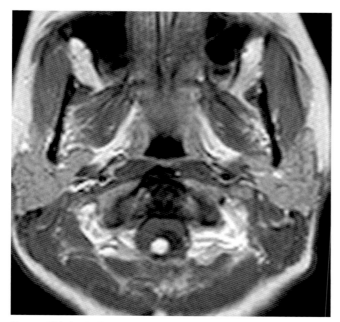

Figure 200-1 Patient A.

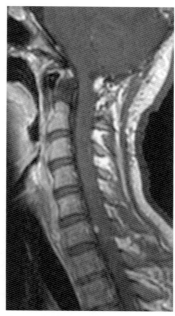

Figure 200-2 Patient A.

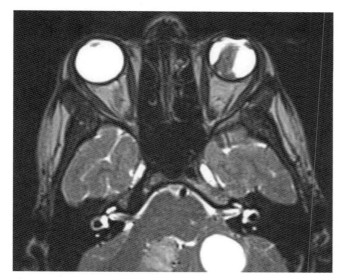

Figure 200-3 Patient B.

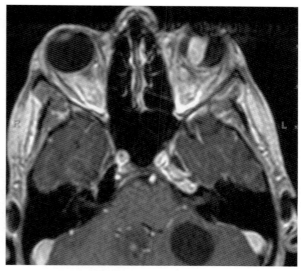

Figure 200-4 Patient B.

HISTORY: Patient A (Figures 200-1 and 200-2) presents with seizure, and Patient B (Figures 200-3 and 200-4) presents with left visual blurring.

1. What is the common diagnosis for both patients?
   A. Tuberous sclerosis
   B. Neurofibromatosis type 2
   C. Sturge-Weber
   D. Von Hippel–Lindau

2. In an adult, what is the most common enhancing posterior fossa mass?
   A. Multiple arteriovenous malformations
   B. Hemangioblastomas
   C. Metastasis
   D. Cysticercosis

3. In what percentage of patients with this disease are the ocular manifestations the presenting symptoms?
   A. 0% to 20%
   B. 21% to 40%
   C. 41% to 60%
   D. Greater than 60%

4. What percentage of patients with a cerebellar hemangioblastoma also have this disease?
   A. 0% to 15%
   B. 16% to 25%
   C. 26% to 35%
   D. Greater than 35%

CASE 200

Von Hippel–Lindau Disease

1. **D.** Von Hippel–Lindau (VHL). Multiple enhancing cerebellar lesions, spinal ependymal lesions, and retinal lesions consistent with hemangioblastomas in an adult are diagnostic of VHL disease. Metastases could be included in the differential diagnosis. Subependymal nodules and subependymal giant cell tumors are seen in tuberous sclerosis. Meningiomas, schwannomas, and ependymoma are seen in neurofibromatosis type 2. Sturge-Weber syndrome manifests with cortical calcifications, brain atrophy, and pial angiomatosis; in this case, there are focal enhancing lesions along the spinal cord and in the cerebellum with no cortical calcifications or atrophy.

2. **C.** Metastasis. Metastasis is the most common cause of multiple enhancing cerebellar lesions.

3. **C.** 41% to 60%. The ocular manifestations are the presenting symptoms in 50% of patients with VHL disease.

4. **B.** 16% to 25%. Of patients with cerebellar hemangioblastomas, 20% also have VHL disease.

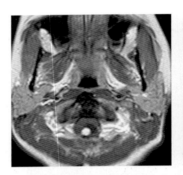
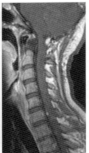
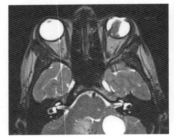
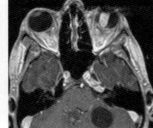

Comment

Patient A

These images show a cystic mass with a solid enhancing mural nodule in the region of the area postrema of the medulla (Figures 200-1 and 200-2) and multiple small enhancing cerebellar lesions. One of many superficial enhancing nodules along the pial surface of the spinal cord is visible at the level of C6 (see Figure 200-2). Because this patient is an adult and the lesions are multiple, juvenile pilocytic astrocytoma is not a consideration. The differential diagnosis includes multiple hemangioblastomas seen in VHL disease and, less likely, metastatic disease.

Patient B

These images show a unilateral ocular/retinal hemangioblastoma; at the edges of the images, cystic and solid masses in the posterior fossa represent cerebellar hemangioblastomas (Figures 200-3 and 200-4). The lesions typically appear in patients in their 20s and cause visual abnormalities. They may be multiple at initial presentation or may multiply in the follow-up period.

Diagnosing von Hippel–Lindau Disease

For formal diagnosis of VHL disease, the following must be manifest:

- In an individual with no known family history of VHL disease, there must be two or more characteristic lesions:
  - Two or more hemangioblastomas of the retina, spine, or brain or a single hemangioblastoma in association with a visceral manifestation (e.g., multiple kidney or pancreatic cysts)
  - Renal cell carcinoma
  - Adrenal or extra-adrenal pheochromocytomas
  - Endolymphatic sac tumors, papillary cystadenomas of the epididymis or broad ligament, or neuroendocrine tumors of the pancreas
- In an individual with a family history of VHL disease, there must be one or more of the following disease manifestations:
  - Retinal hemangioblastoma
  - Spinal or cerebellar hemangioblastoma
  - Adrenal or extra-adrenal pheochromocytoma
  - Renal cell carcinoma
  - Multiple renal and pancreatic cysts

Approximately 20% of patients with hemangioblastomas have VHL disease. Conversely, 45% of patients with VHL disease may have central nervous system (CNS) hemangioblastomas. In VHL disease, these neoplasms are multiple in at least 40% of cases. Hemangioblastomas occur most commonly in the cerebellum and retina, although they may also arise in the brainstem (especially the medulla), the spinal cord, and (rarely) the cerebrum and viscera outside of the CNS. There is an approximately 10-fold increase in the incidence of pheochromocytomas in these patients. Polycythemia related to the production of erythropoietin by hemangioblastomas is common.

Reference

Slater A, Moore NR, Huson SM. The natural history of cerebellar hemangioblastomas in von Hippel-Lindau disease. *AJNR Am J Neuroradiol.* 2003;24:1570-1574.

Cross-Reference

Neuroradiology: THE REQUISITES, 4th ed, pp 297-298.

Page numbers followed by *f* indicate figures.